Ultimate Health

Ultimate Health

Twelve Keys to Abundant
Health and Happiness

DR JOHN BRIFFA

MICHAEL JOSEPH
an imprint of
PENGUIN BOOKS

MICHAEL JOSEPH

Published by the Penguin Group

Penguin Books Ltd, 80 Strand, London WC2R 0RL, England
Penguin Putnam Inc., 375 Hudson Street, New York, New York 10014, USA
Penguin Books Australia Ltd, 250 Camberwell Road, Camberwell, Victoria 3124, Australia
Penguin Books Canada Ltd, 10 Alcorn Avenue, Toronto, Ontario, Canada M4V 3B2
Penguin Books India (P) Ltd, 11 Community Centre, Panchsheel Park, New Delhi – 110 017, India
Penguin Books (NZ) Ltd, Cnr Rosedale and Airborne Roads, Albany, Auckland, New Zealand
Penguin Books (South Africa) (Pty) Ltd, 24 Sturdee Avenue, Rosebank 2196, South Africa

Penguin Books Ltd, Registered Offices: 80 Strand, London WC2R 0RL, England

www.penguin.com

First published 2002

3

Set in 12/14.75 pt Monotype Bembo
Typeset by Rowland Phototypesetting Ltd,
Bury St Edmunds, Suffolk
Printed in Great Britain by Clays Ltd, St Ives plc

A CIP catalogue record for this book is available from the British Library

ISBN 0-7181-4498-8

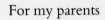

For my parents

Contents

Acknowledgements

First and foremost, I would like to thank my patients, past and present. The knowledge contained in this book is essentially a distillation of the experiences I have had in clinical practice over the years. It is only through working with real people with real problems that the writing of *Ultimate Health* has been possible. I acknowledge and am grateful for the contribution my patients have made to this book.

In addition, I would also like to acknowledge some special people in my life. To Eileen Campbell at Penguin for putting her immediate faith in the project and supporting me throughout. To Debby Vandepeer, my fantastic assistant, for her organizational skills and sense of humour, and for ensuring that I keep my feet firmly on the ground! To my brother Joe for reading through some early drafts of the emotional section of the book and giving valuable feedback. To Leo Wheeler for being a dear friend and for introducing me to many concepts that have been instrumental in my personal development over the last few years. To Gillian Hamer, my 'surrogate aunt', for her continuous love and support. To Michael (OS!) and Jennifer Grice for their friendship, and for their support during the last few weeks of the writing of this book. To Hazel Courteney, for being such a wonderful selfless friend and for inspiring so much of my work. To Lianne Campbell and Jyotish Patel, for so many wonderful insights, lots of laughs and simple truth. To Marlene and Peter Richardson, for their tireless help in so many ways. To Stewart Andersen for giving me the nudge which was so instrumental in my spiritual development. To Ron and Helen Clarke, for putting their faith in me all those years ago. To Roger Dwek, whose wonderful massage during the writing of this book was a real godsend. And to Sara Pankhurst, for giving me space when I needed it but was there when I needed that too.

Introduction

Our health and happiness are subject to an enormous array of factors and influences. Some of these elements are what might be regarded as physical in nature. For instance, exercise, diet, and medicinal herbs have been proven to affect the well-being of both body and mind. There is also a wealth of evidence which shows that our emotions can influence health. Stress, for instance, has been shown to suppress the function of the immune system, and in the long term can lead to a slew of imbalances in the body's physiology and biochemistry.

It is clear that, as human beings, we have two fundamental aspects: *physical* and *emotional*. This means that we can use either physiological or emotionally oriented approaches to overcome illness and enhance well-being. For example, while meditation may help an individual break through a problem with depression, the herb St John's Wort may also be effective here. Vitamin C and zinc may help to boost the immune system, but so may t'ai chi. Yet, while either a physical or mind-body approach may heal a health issue, it has been my experience that they are most powerful and effective when applied *together*. To this end, *Ultimate Health* is designed to provide you with a synergistic blend of body and mind approaches to achieving true health and happiness.

Ultimate Health is divided into three main parts. The first section sets out what I believe to be the most important physiological components of health. During my time in practice, I have come to realize that the causes of ill-health and disease issues are often highly individual in nature. My belief is that the most effective approach to any health issue is to identify the specific imbalances that are relevant to the individual, and to correct these. However, while what underlies a health issue is very much an individual affair, my experience is that certain factors tend to be common to many. The first six chapters of the book explore these themes. Briefly, these are breathing, water consumption, detoxification of the body, blood sugar balance and adrenal gland health, thyroid function and exercise. Where appropriate, I have included questionnaires and other information to help you identify your individual imbalances. Each chapter also gives specific and practical guidelines on how to restore health using these key physiological approaches.

The second section of *Ultimate Health* is concerned with the emotional aspects of health and happiness. Our beliefs, and our feelings towards ourselves, other people and the world around us are clearly important for our sense of contentment and fulfilment. What is also apparent is that our emotions can have a very important bearing on our physical health. Very often in practice I have seen people whose health issues are related, at least in part, to emotionally based concerns. I have also witnessed people transform their physical health by addressing and resolving their emotional issues. But don't take my word for it: science has done much in recent years to unravel the link between our emotions and physical health. So great has the interest been in this area that it has spawned a whole new brand of medicine called 'psychoneuroimmunology'.

As with the physical factors, the emotional issues which may underlie illness can be very individual in nature. However, here again, I have found that certain things are common to many. The second half of the book deals with what I regard as the most important emotional tools for transforming the health of both body and mind. These core principles explore the concepts of honouring our true selves, trusting our intuition, living in the moment, seeing life as a mirror of ourselves, seeing the positive in all experiences and using love as a tool to better relationships with ourselves and others. In each chapter I have set out the common emotional 'glitches' which can erode our health and happiness, and offer ways to dissolve them through changing our approach to life.

Throughout the twelve chapters, I use case studies for illustration. To protect anonymity, I have changed the names and other details which are not relevant to the central theme. In the section on emotional health, I have included details and experiences from my own life. This may seem a little self-indulgent, but the truth is, I wanted to put some of myself into this book. While I hope this book offers a lot of positive advice, I simply do not want to give the impression that I never have issues of my own. I am not impervious to the challenges we all face from time to time. Sharing some of my own issues with you serves to illustrate the point that I am human too, and in that sense am no different from you.

The twelve chapters of *Ultimate Health* are intended to form important foundational tools for creating powerful shifts in physical health, as well as catalysing positive change in how we experience our lives. It is my belief that putting into practice the advice contained in these chapters can be effective in healing many, many health issues. While this may be the case, it doesn't do any harm (and in fact may do a lot of good) to provide a little extra help wherever possible. With this in mind, the last section of the book is an A–Z of health. In it, I explore specific natural health approaches to over 150 medical conditions and symptoms. Dietary and lifestyle approaches, often coupled with recommendations of specific natural supplements, form the basis of the advice here. The information in this A–Z of health is based on what has been found to work in practice, and much of it is scientifically validated. I have designed the information presented in this A–Z so that it may be used as an adjunct to the twelve fundamental principles.

While I have intended *Ultimate Health* to be a complete guide to achieving physical and emotional well-being, it is no last word. However useful the information in this book turns out to be for you, there is no reason why you should not find other worthwhile information elsewhere. Some of this may conflict with concepts and themes explored here. It is my belief that no information, whatever the source, is inherently 'right' or 'wrong'. The only person who can really determine what is right for you, is *you*. That said, I do sincerely hope that *Ultimate Health* proves an invaluable aid in your quest for abundant health and happiness.

For more information about all aspects of health and to email Dr Briffa visit his website at www.drbriffa.com

1. Give Your Body Oxygen

While the human body can survive a few weeks without food, and perhaps a few days without water, it can't do without oxygen for more than a few minutes. Oxygen is an essential ingredient in the reactions which burn food to make energy, and any shortfall in the supply of this gas can therefore impair our sense of vitality and well-being. Not only that, but *all* the body's cells require oxygen to function normally. From the cells in the liver which neutralize toxins from the gut, to the cells in the glands which secrete essential hormones into the bloodstream, one thing they all have in common is their need for oxygen.

Oxygen is supplied to the body through the act of breathing. Breathing is something we generally don't have to think about, so there's a tendency for us to feel it's something we do perfectly well. However, experience shows that many of us don't breathe nearly as well as we might, and this can have a significant impact on both our physical and emotional health. Learning and practising proper breathing is, quite simply, fundamental to abundant health and vitality.

The essential role that oxygen plays in the function of the body's organs is most evident in conditions such as heart attack and stroke. Here, parts of the body become starved of oxygen due to an interruption in blood supply, leading to death in the body's tissues. Also, in conditions where the lungs fail to absorb adequate amounts of oxygen from the atmosphere, such as chronic bronchitis and emphysema, breathlessness, fatigue and a reduced capacity for exercise and activity are the result. Let's make no mistake about it, oxygen is of prime importance to life and health.

Breathing fulfils two main functions in the body. As we know, all the cells in the body require oxygen to function, and the act of breathing allows this gas to be absorbed from the air into the bloodstream. While the cells use oxygen, they also generate a waste product – carbon dioxide. The other main function of breathing is to allow the body to rid itself of this unwanted gas. The process of oxygen absorption and carbon dioxide elimination by the body is sometimes referred to as 'gas exchange'.

Beyond the physiological roles that breathing appears to fulfil, lie other benefits. In Eastern medicine, breathing exercises are often used as an integral part of many different therapies which link mind and body. In many traditional forms of therapy, including yoga, t'ai chi and ki gong, proper breathing is believed to help harmonize the whole self and is thought to offer diverse healing effects. Breathing exercises are often used in treating conditions and symptoms as diverse as high blood pressure, menopausal hot flushes, migraine, panic attacks and depression. Many individuals find that practising efficient breathing has a calming, balancing effect on their mood and sense of well-being, but also leaves them feeling energized and focused.

Are you breathing right?

While many of us assume breathing is something we do well enough, this may not be the case. We know that the efficiency of basic systems in the body can vary enormously between individuals. For instance, while some people have cast-iron digestions, and are able to break down and absorb any food without ill-effect, others may not be so lucky and therefore run into problems with nutrient deficiency and food sensitivity as a result. While certain people may have strong immune systems and get through the year without so much as a sniffle, others may be susceptible to just about any bug that happens to be lurking in their immediate environment. The same is true of breathing. Some people get all the oxygen they need for optimum health through their complete and efficient breathing habits, though many others don't. To understand what efficient breathing is all about, and what can go wrong, it helps to know a little about the structure and function of the lungs.

The structure and function of the lungs

Oxygen is taken into the body from the air via the lungs. Air which is inhaled through the nose and/or mouth first travels down the windpipe (trachea) to enter two tubes called the 'bronchi', each of which takes the air into the lung itself. The bronchi divide again and again, forming a branching network of tubes which get ever smaller in size as they approach the outer reaches of the lung tissue. Finally, these tubes end in the form of tiny sacs called 'alveoli'. It is in the alveoli that gas exchange takes place. Surrounding the alveoli is an intimate network of tiny blood vessels known as capillaries. Oxygen and carbon dioxide can pass back and forth between the alveoli and the blood in the capillaries, and this allows the lungs to perform their function of gas exchange.

When oxygen is taken into the lungs, some of it will transfer across the wall of the alveoli into the blood contained in the capillaries. This blood (known as 'oxygenated blood') eventually travels to the heart in a vessel called the pulmonary vein. The heart then pumps this blood to the body's tissues, where the oxygen is used, and swapped for carbon dioxide. This blood (known as 'deoxygenated blood') travels back to the heart, so that it can pump it once again to the lungs. In the lungs, the carbon dioxide leaves the bloodstream and enters the alveoli, after which it can be removed from the body as the lungs breathe out. On the in-breath, more oxygen is absorbed into the bloodstream from the air, and this then travels to the heart to be pumped to the rest of the body. And so this cycle repeats.

The act of breathing and the process of gas exchange depend on the mechanics which get air in and out of the lungs. Inspiration (breathing in) and expiration (breathing out) is controlled by muscular contractions in and around the chest.

The chest cavity is essentially made up of the spine at the back, the sternum or breastbone at the front, and ribs on either side which connect the two. After breathing out, the curved ribs hang down somewhat, rather like bucket handles. Between the ribs there are muscles (called the 'intercostal muscles') which contract during inspir-ation. The effect of the intercostal muscle contraction is to draw the

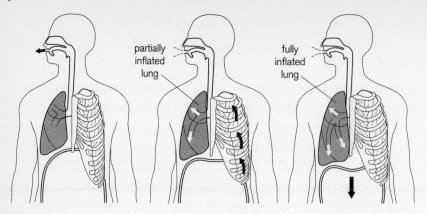

1. Exhalation   **2. Chest inhalation**   **3. Belly inhalation**

ribs up, increasing the size of the chest which in turn causes air to be drawn into the lungs (inspiration).

Apart from the intercostal muscles, there are other muscles involved in the act of breathing, the most important of which is the 'diaphragm'. The diaphragm is a dome-shaped thin muscular sheet which lines the base of the chest and separates it from the abdomen. During inspiration, the diaphragm contracts and flattens, and this causes air to be drawn into the lungs.

Broadly speaking, individuals can be classified as chest breathers or diaphragmatic (belly) breathers. Chest breathers tend to breathe in and out using mainly their intercostal muscles. The breaths tend to be shallow and often relatively short. In chest breathing, air is drawn into the smaller upper parts of the lungs, but may never make it into the lower reaches of the lung where much of gas exchange takes place. In Eastern medicine, this type of breathing is viewed as inefficient and incomplete.

Belly breathing on the other hand is viewed as both healthy and important to well-being. Here, instead of the intercostal muscles doing the bulk of the work, it is the diaphragm which contracts to draw air into the lungs. In diaphragmatic breathing, inspired air can make its way into the expansive lung tissue at the base of the chest. Belly breathing goes a long way to optimizing the process of oxygen absorption and carbon dioxide removal.

Assessing your breathing

This simple exercise will enable you to get a good idea about whether you are predominantly a chest breather or belly breather:

> Put your left hand in the middle of your chest with your right hand over your navel. Breathe normally. Look at your hands and take a note of which hand moves more when you breathe. If your left hand is moving more than your right, it is a sign that you are a chest breather. If your right is moving more than your left, however, it is likely that your breathing is essentially diaphragmatic in nature.

Is inefficient breathing your problem?

The questions in the following questionnaire are designed to help you assess the efficiency of your breathing. Score each question as indicated, and then add up your total score.

1. Having done the exercise above, do you rate yourself as a:

chest breather?	8 points
belly breather?	0 points
somewhere in between?	4 points

2. Can walking up just one or two flights of stairs make you very breathless?

never	0 points
sometimes	2 points
often or always	4 points

3. You are sometimes aware of the need to take a big breath of air at rest?

never	0 points
sometimes	2 points
often	4 points

4. Do you consider yourself as a:
generally relaxed individual who is not prone to bouts of
anxiety or stress?   0 points
highly strung and anxious individual who quite often feels
anxious or stressed out?   4 points
somewhere in between?   2 points

**5. Count the number of breaths you take in a minute at rest (no
sooner than an hour after any form of exercise). Do this three
times during the day and average the result. Is the number
of breaths you take in a minute:**
between 5 and 9?   0 points
between 10 and 15?   3 points
16 or more?   6 points

Interpreting your score
0–9: your answers to the questionnaire suggest that you have good breathing habits, and that poor breathing is unlikely to be an issue in your weight
or health issues
10–16: your answers to the questionnaire suggest that your breathing
habits may benefit from the breathing exercises outlined in this chapter
more than 16: your answers to the questionnaire suggest that your breathing pattern is not healthy and that you would almost certainly benefit from
practising the breathing techniques outlined in this chapter on a regular
basis

Hyperventilation and health

As we discussed earlier in this chapter, many of us can take rapid,
shallow breaths that simply do not allow enough oxygen to be
absorbed into the system. Another effect of hyperventilation is that
we can end up with lower than normal levels of carbon dioxide in
the body. Now, while carbon dioxide is essentially a waste product,
we do need some of it. Why? Well, one thing about carbon dioxide
is that it is acidic. The more carbon dioxide we have in the blood, the
more acidic the blood is. If through hyperventilation carbon dioxide

levels drop, then the blood becomes more alkaline. Now for a bit of physiology: due to something called the Bohr effect, as the blood becomes more alkaline, less oxygen is released from haemoglobin in the red blood cells into the tissue. Basically, when we over-breathe, our tissues become starved of oxygen.

Over forty years ago, a Russian scientist by the name of Professor Buteyko developed a breathing system designed to reduce over-breathing and reduce the effects of chronic illnesses including asthma and emphysema. The Buteyko method is becoming increasingly recognized as a useful tool in the treatment of ill-health.

Do you need the Buteyko method?

Professor Buteyko developed a test designed to measure depth of breathing and the consequent levels of carbon dioxide and oxygen in the body. It is called the 'control pause breathing test':

1. Breathe in gently for two seconds
2. Exhale gently for three seconds
3. Close your mouth, pinch your nose and hold your breath
4. Start timing
5. Stop timing when it becomes difficult to continue to hold your breath.

According to Professor Buteyko, less than 10 seconds suggests a very significant problem with hyperventilation. Between 10 and 25 is also significant, though less severe. Around 25 to 40 seconds generally means some attention is needed. More than 45 seconds is good and more than 60 is excellent.

The Buteyko method is taught by specially trained practitioners. It normally involves a series of five or more hourly tuition sessions. More details about the Buteyko method can be obtained via the website www.buteyko.com.

Belly breathing

If you have identified yourself as a chest breather, it will almost certainly help you to learn the art of proper belly breathing. Even if you think you breathe mainly from the diaphragm, the following exercise is likely to help you make your breathing even more complete and efficient.

> Breathe gently in and out through your nose. Breathe out all the air from your lungs, pause briefly, and begin to breathe in again. Concentrate on taking long, smooth, unhurried breaths.
>
> As you breathe in push your belly out, as this will ensure you are filling the whole of your lungs with air. When your lungs feel comfortably full, pause briefly again, and then breathe out through your nose. Repeat this cycle always making sure that your belly is moving in and out as you breathe.

If you're not used to deep breathing exercises, and particularly if you tend to chest breathe, you might be pleasantly surprised at just how quick and effective this is for reviving your energy and clearing your head. Just ten breaths are all that it normally takes for the benefits of deep breathing to be felt.

Although belly breathing takes some conscious effort to begin with, practice usually makes perfect. In time, you may well find that deep, diaphragmatic breathing becomes second nature to you.

I generally recommend that individuals who are learning belly breathing start with ten good breaths, three times a day. In most cases, this really does seem to be enough to get things started. Within a couple of weeks, individuals normally feel like they've got the hang of diaphragmatic breathing, and may be extending their ten breaths to twenty or more at a time without even thinking about it. From time to time, it's a good idea to do the hand test to see whether or not you tend to belly or chest breathe at rest. You may be surprised to find that your old chest-breathing habits give way to healthier and invigorating belly breathing in time.

More breathing exercises

There are a couple of breathing exercises which I quite like myself and often teach to clients. They are based on belly breathing, but use pauses between inhalation and expiration to maximize the effect.

Breathing in threes

Take a good long belly breath and count 'one thousand, two thousand' etc. in your head while you do this. Once you have inhaled fully, hold your breath for the same number of counts as it took you to inhale, and then exhale completely over the same number of counts again. For instance, if you inhale to the count of six, hold your breath for six counts, exhale for six counts and then repeat this cycle. I generally recommend ten to fifteen cycles, repeated three times a day.

To begin with, you may need to adjust your count until you find a length of time you are comfortable with. If you go too slowly to begin with, you may find that you start to run out of breath and are unable to complete the exercise. If your breaths are too quick, you are unlikely to get the maximum benefit from them.

Breathing in fours

Breathing in fours is very similar to breathing in threes. The only difference is that after exhalation, the breath is held for the same count as the other components of the cycle. As an example, breathe in over six counts, hold for six counts, breathe out for six counts, hold for six counts and repeat. Breathing in fours is a little more challenging than breathing in threes, and is something to progress on to once you're comfortable with the easier exercise. I recommend ten to fifteen cycles, repeated three times a day, once you're proficient.

Summary

- Oxygen is an essential ingredient in the reactions which convert food into energy

- Insufficient oxygen or inefficient breathing may stall the metabolism and lead to problems with low energy and reduced vitality

- Inadequate oxygen might also impair the function of any of the body's cells

- Inefficient breathers tend to breathe into the upper chest, while efficient breathers tend to breathe into the lower reaches of the lungs using the diaphragm

- Hyperventilation and problems associated with it including asthma can often be helped by a specific breathing technique known as the Buteyko method

- Learning diaphragmatic or belly breathing is a good first step in developing healthy breathing habits

- Once belly breathing is mastered, moving on to more ambitious exercises such as breathing in threes and breathing in fours can help maximize the effect

- Good breathing habits can be an effective way to enhance health and vitality, and may also be beneficial in harmonizing body and mind

2. Give Your Body Water

The body is about 70 per cent water. Just that fact alone tends to suggest that water is an important component in health and well-being. However, while water plays a multitude of roles in the body and is essential to life, it very rarely gets the attention it deserves. I am convinced that drinking more water is one of the simplest, cheapest and most effective ways of improving health and vitality. In this chapter, we'll be exploring the benefits that water has to offer, how much water we need each day, and what types of water are the best for our health.

What, precisely, does water do in the body?

Every second of every day countless reactions and processes that are integral to life are taking place in the body. Nerve impulses from the brain stimulate movement and control unconscious actions such as the speed at which the heart beats. Acid and digestive enzymes are secreted into the intestinal tract to break down food ready for absorption. Hormones are secreted in various organs around the body and travel in the bloodstream to tissues where they have their effects. The circulation pumps blood around the system delivering oxygen and nutrients to the body's cells. Blood is filtered in the kidneys, allowing impurities to be eliminated from the body. The one thing that these and all other processes in the body have in common is water.

Water is absolutely essential for the maintenance of optimum health and efficiency in all the body's systems. Nerves simply do not transmit their messages efficiently if they are not properly hydrated. If the circulation is lacking in volume, it simply does not deliver oxygen, nutrients and other essential substances to the tissues as well as it might. Poor circulation to the kidneys means that toxins are less readily removed from the system. Dehydration jeopardizes all of the most basic processes and systems in the body.

The effects of dehydration

It doesn't take much fluid loss from the body for it to impact on our well-being. There is evidence that as little as 1 per cent dehydration (about 500 mls of fluid for a 70 kg adult) can impair the body's physiological and biochemical processes. In the short term, even mild dehydration can provoke problems with a diverse array of symptoms including headache, fatigue, loss of appetite, heat intolerance, light-headedness and dry mouth and eyes.

Dehydration generally causes the urine to be more concentrated. There is a theory that concentrated urine is more likely to lead to the development of kidney or bladder stones (urinary calculi). Research shows that kidney stones are more common in populations where urine volume is low (*refs* 1–9). Not only this, but the research has also shown that increasing urine volume to about 2 to 2.5 litres a day reduces the risk of kidney stones (*refs* 1, 4, 5, 7). Anyone wanting to protect themselves from kidney stones should therefore ensure a good fluid intake, and this is particularly important for individuals who have a history of this condition.

There is good evidence that a reduced intake of fluid can increase the risk of certain cancers. One study found an increased risk of cancers of the kidney, bladder, prostate and testes in individuals who consumed relatively low levels of fluid (*ref* 10). Other research has found that increasing fluid intake seems to reduce the risk of cancer of the bladder (*ref* 11). More research has found a link between water consumption and cancer of the colon. One study found that women consuming five or more glasses of water per day had about half the risk of developing cancer of the colon compared with women consuming two or fewer glasses of water per day (*ref* 12). There is even evidence that water can protect against breast cancer. A pilot study found that water consumption was associated with about an 80 per cent reduction in risk of breast cancer in women after the time of menopause. Risk for pre-menopausal women was reduced by a third (*ref* 13).

Cancer is a condition which is rapidly becoming more common in the Western world. It seems incredible that doing something as simple as drinking more water might help significantly reduce our risk of this condition. Good hydration is likely to dilute and speed the elimination of toxic, 'cancer-inducing' substances within the body. Dehydration may also impair the activity of key enzymes involved in the regulation of important detoxification and immune-system related processes. Quite how water reduces cancer risk is not known for sure, but the evidence that it does is there!

How much water do we need?

Water is clearly fundamental to health, the question is, how much do we need? Water in the body is in a state of constant renewal. Water is lost from the body via the urine, faeces, breath and sweat. Each day an adult loses the equivalent of about 4 per cent of body weight in water. For a 70 kg person this equates to about 2,500 to 3,000 mls (2.5 to 3 litres) of water. Clearly, to prevent dehydration, this quantity of fluid must be replenished in the body.

Water is essentially obtained by eating and drinking. Our diet will provide us with about 1 litre of fluid per day. The rest has to come from drinks. This means, that as a *minimum*, we need to consume between 1.5 and 2 litres of water per day. This rough approximation can be fine-tuned according to weight. For average day-to-day needs, we should aim to consume about 30 mls of water for each kilogramme of our body weight (this equates to about half an ounce of water for each pound of body weight). A 70 kg adult should drink just over 2 litres ($30 \times 70 = 2100$ mls $= 2.1$ litres). A 100 kg adult would need 3 litres per day as a minimum requirement.

How do we know if we are getting enough?

Some people use thirst as a sign that they need to drink more. However, it does seem that by the time we're thirsty, the body is about 1 to 2 per cent dehydrated (*refs* 14, 15). Bearing in mind that at 1 per cent dehydration we may already be feeling the effects, it seems as though thirst is not to be relied upon to tell us when it's time to drink.

The degree of the body's hydration can be gauged by measuring the concentration of the blood or urine in the laboratory. Clearly, this is not practical for day-to-day use. Fortunately, a simple and cost-free method for gauging hydrations does exist; it appears that we can assess our state of hydration quite simply and accurately from the colour of our urine (*ref* 16). Essentially, the paler in colour our urine, the better our state of hydration. Our aim is to keep our urine colour very pale yellow or pale yellow throughout the day. If our urine colour strays into darker tones, particularly if this is accompanied by a pungent smell, then we know it's time to step up our water intake.

Does it have to be water?

Now we know why we need water, and have a pretty good idea of how much we need. Does it really have to be water or will other types of fluid do?

Let's have a look at some alternative drinks and their effects on hydration and health. Coffee and tea and some soft drinks contain caffeine. Caffeine is what is known as a 'diuretic'. This means it stimulates the production of urine, dehydrating the body in the process. Another substance that has a diuretic effect is alcohol. Both caffeine and alcohol tend to induce toxicity in the body (more about this in chapter 3). So, in summary, caffeine and alcohol contribute to the body's toxicity, but also reduce the body's capacity to eliminate those toxins. Not ideal.

Clearly, drinks containing caffeine or alcohol cannot be substituted for water. In fact, for each caffeinated or alcoholic drink, it makes sense to consume a glass of water on top of the normal recommended amount. This helps to dilute and eliminate toxicity from the body, and obviously also helps to keep the body hydrated. The other thing about balancing caffeinated or alcoholic drinks with water is that it generally leads to a reduction in the consumption of these drinks anyway (there's only so much we can drink, after all!).

Perhaps decaffeinated drinks are better? Because decaffeinated drinks have little or no caffeine they tend not to be diuretic in nature, and therefore are better than their caffeinated versions in terms of body hydration. However, it is interesting to note that in some studies, water, and only water, seems to be associated with health-giving properties. For instance, in the study mentioned above that found increased fluid consumption reduced the risk of colon cancer in women, this association was only true for water: not even fruit juice appeared to have a protective effect.

Sugar-laden soft drinks should generally be avoided. Not only can they upset blood sugar control, but they may also suppress the immune system, reduce levels of 'healthy' HDL cholesterol, and increase levels of uric acid in the body (which may increase the risk of gout). Sugared soft drinks have also been found to be linked to childhood obesity (*ref* 17). One study found that for each additional can or glass of sugar-sweetened soft drink consumed each day, risk of obesity rose 60 per cent. Perhaps 'diet' drinks are a viable alternative. It turns out that artificial sweeteners are not without hazards of their own. These are discussed in chapter 4.

There really is no getting away from the fact that there is no better fluid than water. Don't forget, for pretty much all of our evolution, we drank nothing but water. These days there is a bewildering array of beverages which are readily available and sometimes very enticing. Unfortunately, from a health perspective it's difficult to make a case for any of them.

What form of water?

There are three main forms of water – *tap*, *distilled* and *mineral*. Let's look at each of these and discuss their pros and cons in turn.

Tap water

A common theme in nutrition is that processed foods should be generally avoided. What about processed water? After all, that's what tap water is. Not only that, but water in some countries is not processed just once, but again and again. Many of us are basically drinking sanitized water that comes from dishwashers, washing machines, baths and showers.

For water to be made 'fit to drink' it is first allowed to sit so that some of the impurities can settle. After this, the water is treated chemically to encourage the sedimentation of some of the lighter impurities in the water. Next, the water is filtered, after which it is disinfected. Disinfection generally involves chlorine, although ozone and ultraviolet light radiation are other more expensive options.

There is concern about the presence of chlorine in tap water and its possible role in causing cancer. Chlorine is what is known as an 'oxidizing' agent, and can induce chemical changes which, at least in theory, should increase cancer risk. Water may also contain related compounds which are by-products of the chlorination process known as 'trihalomethanes'. These are also thought to have cancer-inducing potential. A review of ten studies that examined the link between chlorine and its by-products found that exposure to these harmful chemicals increased the risk of bladder cancer by 21 per cent and rectal cancer by 38 per cent (*ref* 18). Another study found that exposure to chlorine or trihalomethanes was associated with an increased risk of brain tumour (*ref* 19).

Another substance which is used in the purification of water is aluminium sulphate. There is some concern that aluminium may have some role to play in Alzheimer's Disease. While the evidence here is far from clear-cut, it is known that aluminium is a potentially toxic substance, and there does seem to be at least enough evidence to suggest it should be viewed with suspicion.

And what of fluoride? This substance is added to the water in some countries because it is believed to protect teeth from decay. The most recent study to look at this association – often referred to as the 'York study' – did indeed confirm this to be the case (*ref* 20). However, the York study also found that the protection offered by fluoride is much lower than previously thought. In fact, just one in six people drinking fluoridated water benefits from this practice. However, drinking fluoridated water was also found to cause 'dental fluorosis' (a condition in which the teeth become mottled due to excess fluoride) in half of individuals drinking fluoridated water. One might question the wisdom in preventing dental disease in one in six while at the same time causing dental disease in one in two!

Also, because dental fluorosis is a sign of fluoride toxicity, could it be that fluoride might also lead to more sinister health effects? There is at least some evidence which suggests, for instance, that fluoride exposure may increase the risk of bone fracture. Not only all this, but there is a wealth of scientific evidence that fluoride may have toxic effects in many parts of the body including the brain, pineal gland and thyroid. More information about the potential hazards of fluoride can be found on the website www.fluoridealert.org.

What can be done to improve tap water quality?

My advice is to avoid tap water. At the very least, I recommend that it is treated to reduce some of its potentially harmful qualities. A simple and relatively inexpensive way to do this is to use a jug which has an integrated carbon filter. These filters help to get rid of much of the chlorine and other chemicals that may be in your tap water, but will allow most of the healthy minerals in water (see below) to get through. Bacteria are not removed either. It is important to remember to change the filter frequently (most are good for 50 to 200 litres of water).

A step up from jug filters are filters which are plumbed into the water supply. These generally contain carbon filters, though some also include fine clay particles to help filter out bacteria. These are more expensive than the jug filters (expect to pay about £200) and cartridges do need replacing from time to time (usually annually). However, they are very convenient and generally do a good job.

Another form of 'in-house' water purification is known as the 'reverse osmosis system'. This is good for removing impurities including bacteria, but may also filter out healthy minerals. The systems are on the expensive side, quite costly to run, slow, and discard about 80 per cent of the water they treat. Overall, I prefer the plumbed-in carbon and ceramic filters.

Distilled water

Distilled water is 'pure' water. One of the major advantages that distilled water has over other forms of water is that it is free from impurities and potentially hazardous elements such as lead, fluoride, chlorine and pesticides. Personally, I'm not convinced that distilled water is actually the best water for the human body. For a start, I always think it is a good idea to stick quite closely to the sort of diet we evolved on, because it stands to reason that this is the diet we are best adapted to. We did not drink distilled water during evolution, and this casts some doubt about its suitability for us as human beings. Another factor against distilled water is that there is some evidence to suggest that the minerals found in other forms of water may actually have some health-giving properties.

Water hardness and health

Tap and mineral waters contain elements such as calcium and magnesium. The 'hardness' of a water refers to the concentration of calcium carbonate in the water. 'Hard' waters are classified as having 75 mg or more of calcium carbonate per litre, while 'soft' waters have less than this. The forms of nutrients such as calcium and magnesium found in water are known as 'inorganic' salts. These compounds are not thought to be easily used by the body in its physiological and biochemical processes, and have traditionally been believed to have little in the way of health-giving properties. However, there is some evidence that hard water may protect against certain conditions, particularly heart disease and stroke.

Dozens of studies in several countries (particularly the UK, the United States and Canada) have examined the link between water hardness and health. Not all the results of these studies have been consistent, but there has certainly been a strong trend to suggest that hard water can protect against cardiovascular conditions such as heart disease, stroke, high blood pressure, and other conditions. Studies in the United States and Canada have reported that cardiovascular mortality rates are about 15 to 20 per cent higher in populations using very soft water compared with those consuming hard water.

There are two main theories which have been put forward to explain why hard water might protect against cardiovascular disease. The two main nutrients in water are calcium and magnesium. There has been some research which has suggested that these minerals have a beneficial effect on health. In one study, calcium and magnesium in drinking water was found to protect women from heart attack (*ref* 21). Another study found that low levels of magnesium in drinking water appeared to increase the risk of death due to stroke (*ref* 22). Other research has found that individuals consuming water containing 13.5 mg or more of magnesium per litre, had a 40 per cent reduction in risk of stroke (*ref* 23). Magnesium in drinking water has also been found to be associated with a reduced risk of diabetes (*ref* 24) and prostate cancer (*ref* 25).

Soft water tends to be more corrosive than hard water. As a result, certain potentially harmful metals in plumbing materials are more likely to leach into soft water and contaminate. Two of the metals that have been linked to an increased risk of disease include cadmium and lead. Cadmium has been shown to produce high blood pressure in rats. Other studies show that cadmium can damage the human kidneys, which may lead to an increase in blood pressure. While research here is lacking, it is likely that cadmium has an adverse effect on human health. The same is true of lead, high levels of which have been found in individuals living in homes served by lead pipes.

Mineral water

As their name suggests, mineral waters can supply the body with minerals such as calcium and magnesium. According to European law, mineral waters must emerge from the ground in a state fit to drink, and must be bottled at source. The water must also be protected from pollution to ensure its purity. Natural mineral waters have nothing added, and nothing taken away. I'm a fan!

Are all bottled waters good to drink?

In a word – no. Bottled waters may be labelled in a variety of ways. Commonly used terms are 'natural mineral water', 'mineral water', 'spring water' and 'table water'. In Europe, only one of these terms (natural mineral water) refers to proper mineral water which has not been processed except by, perhaps, the addition of some carbon dioxide bubbles. The other terms are used to label waters from other sources, including rivers, lakes and municipal water supplies. The quality of these bottled waters is not assured in the same way as natural mineral waters and I would therefore avoid them.

In the United States, as in Europe, proper mineral water can be found labelled as 'natural mineral water'; however, the term 'natural spring water' is also used to describe this premium water. 'Natural spring water' is generally used to describe waters of lower mineral content, while higher mineral content water is usually labelled 'natural mineral water'. However, just to confuse matters there is some overlap. My advice is to opt for waters labelled 'natural mineral water', or to study the label for mineral content if you are looking for specific mineral quantities.

What about mineral content then?

Bearing in mind the potential benefit of 'hard' water over 'soft', I like waters with a high mineral content. While a lot has been made of the benefits of calcium, there is good evidence to suggest that magnesium is very important for health. Some of the evidence supporting magnesium's role in disease protection was discussed above. In general, I think calcium is a somewhat overrated mineral, while magnesium appears to be quite underrated. When I look at mineral waters, I look at the magnesium content first. After this, I check the calcium (I'm less concerned about this), and then I look at the sodium content. Because of concerns about sodium raising blood pressure in some people, and the fact that we appear to get far too much sodium in our diets than we need, I tend to avoid it wherever possible. My all-time favourite mineral water in the UK is called Ashbourne. It has a very high level of magnesium, a good level of calcium, and very little sodium. Other waters with a high magnesium content include Apollinaris, Badoit and San Pelligrino.

Sparkling or still?

I generally advise people to drink still rather than sparkling mineral waters. Why? Well, first of all, carbon dioxide is acidic. There is a concept in natural medicine that many of us are prone to acidity in the body, and this can predispose us to disease, including inflammatory conditions such as arthritis. Does putting carbon dioxide into the body via water add to this acidity? I don't think anybody knows for sure but it stands to reason that it might. Remember also that carbon dioxide is a gas that the body is generally trying to rid itself of.

Another qualm I have over fizzy water concerns digestion. The bubbles in carbonated water can coat food in the stomach, which may impair acid and other digestive secretions from penetrating the food. This is quite likely to impair digestion, and that's not good. If you have a particular penchant for carbonated mineral water, I suggest you keep the balance of your consumption towards still water. Some people find it acceptable to drink still water most of the time, migrating to sparkling water on occasions such as when eating in a restaurant.

Keep water around!

For many people, drinking 2 litres of water a day seems quite a feat. However, if we assume we are awake for 16 hours a day, then 2 litres a day equates to 125 millilitres per hour. Put that way, 2 litres a day doesn't seem quite so daunting.

The one big piece of advice I can give about getting 2 litres of water into the body each day is this – *keep water by you*. Water is something that we don't tend to seek out. For this reason, I suggest it is kept readily to hand. If you're doing the gardening, keep a bottle of water with you. Put a bottle of water on your desk at work. Make sure there is water available in meetings. Put a half-litre bottle of water in the car and carry one in your handbag or briefcase when you are out and about. My experience with clients has led me to conclude that if we keep water by us we generally get through decent quantities of the stuff, but if we don't – we won't.

Summary

- Water is essential to all the body's most basic physiological and biochemical processes

- Even mild dehydration can provoke symptoms such as fatigue, headache and loss of appetite

- Long-term dehydration can increase the risk of important conditions such as kidney stones and certain forms of cancer

- We should aim to consume about 30 mls of water for each kg of body weight (about half an ounce of water per lb of body weight)

- Thirst is a relatively late indicator of the need to drink

- We can tell how well hydrated we are from the colour of our urine – aim to ensure your urine is very pale yellow or pale yellow throughout the day

- Tap water should be avoided as there is concern over some of its common constituents, including aluminium, chlorine and fluoride

- If tap water is drunk, it is best to filter it first

- Distilled water lacks minerals that have proven value for health including calcium and magnesium

- Natural mineral water is probably the best form of water for regular consumption

- To ensure you get through your water quota each day – keep it by you!

3. Detoxify the System

Our body is constantly exposed to a stream of substances which can lead to toxicity within it. Some of these, such as the pollutants we breathe and the herbicides and pesticides that lace many of the foods we eat, come from the outside. Others are the result of the metabolic and physiological processes that go on within our bodies every day. Fortunately, the body has evolved ways to process and eliminate unwanted substances from the body. Unfortunately, sometimes our body cleansing processes can't keep up.

If the toxic load on the system is large, and/or if there is some problem with the body's detoxification processes, then toxins may build up. This toxic accumulation effectively poisons the body, and may give rise to a range of health issues including fatigue, lethargy, weight gain, headache, joint and muscle aches and pains, acne, bad breath, and cellulite. Ensuring efficient elimination of toxins from the system is a fundamental and important aspect of health and well-being.

In order to understand how toxicity in the body comes about, we must first understand the systems designed to keep the body pollutant free. Central to these processes is an organ called the liver.

The liver and its role in detoxification

The liver sits in the upper right-hand side of the abdomen, and is the primary organ of detoxification in the body. It takes blood directly from the digestive tract and also the general circulation. In this way the liver is exposed to a bewildering array of potential toxins from the diet, from the processes of metabolism, and also pollutants from the air absorbed via the lungs. One of the liver's chief jobs is to process these toxins, so that they can be removed harmlessly from the body.

This involves a two-stage process known as Phase 1 and Phase 2 detoxification. Phase 1 detoxification treats toxins in a way that makes it easier for them to be attached to other molecules for elimination from the body. Once complete, Phase 2 detoxification actually joins the toxins together with one of four basic 'carrier' molecules for elimination from the body mainly via the urine, bile, or faeces. Detoxification in the liver is dependent on certain nutrients which will be covered later in this chapter.

If for any reason either Phase 1 or Phase 2 detoxification is faulty, or if the liver is simply overwhelmed, then problems with toxicity may arise.

Is toxicity your problem?

The following questionnaire is designed to help you assess if toxicity is a problem for you. Score each question as indicated, and then add up your total score.

Do you suffer from:

1. Bad breath

No	0 points
Occasional or mild problems	2 points
Frequent or severe problems	4 points

2. Abdominal bloating

No	0 points
Occasional or mild problems	2 points
Frequent or severe problems	4 points

3. Constipation

No	0 points
Occasional or mild problems	2 points
Frequent or severe problems	4 points

4. Fatigue

No	0 points
Occasional or mild problems	1 point
Frequent or severe problems	2 points

5. Intolerance to rich/fatty food

No	0 points

Occasional or mild problems   2 points
Frequent or severe problems   4 points

6. **Food sensitivities**
   No   0 points
   Occasional or mild problems   2 points
   Frequent or severe problems   4 points

7. **Sensitivities to perfumes, paint fumes, traffic fumes or detergents**
   No   0 points
   Occasional or mild problems   2 points
   Frequent or severe problems   4 points

8. **Headaches**
   No   0 points
   Occasional or mild problems   1 point
   Frequent or severe problems   2 points

9. **Acne or spots**
   No   0 points
   Occasional or mild problems   3 points
   Frequent or severe problems   5 points

10. **Cellulite.**
    No   0 points
    Occasional or mild problems   3 points
    Frequent or severe problems   5 points

11. **Gallstones or episodes of gallbladder inflammation.**
    No   0 points
    Yes   4 points

12. **Have you ever suffered from hepatitis?**
    No   0 points
    Yes   4 points

13. **Are you frequently exposed to industrial or agricultural chemicals such as solvents, paint fumes, plant sprays and fertilizers?**
    No   0 points
    Yes   4 points

14. How many caffeinated drinks will you have in a day?

0	0 points
1–3	3 points
4 or more	6 points

15. How many units of alcohol do you consume each day on average?

0–1	0 points
2–3	3 points
4 or more	6 points

Interpreting your score

0–9: body toxicity is very unlikely

10–19: body toxicity should be considered as a possibility

20–29: body toxicity is quite likely, and steps taken to reduce this may well be beneficial

30 and above: body toxicity very likely, and steps taken to reduce this will almost certainly be beneficial

Optimizing the body's detoxification processes

While liver function may be somewhat sluggish from time to time, the good news is that it has enormous capacity for regeneration. The cornerstone of a liver-friendly programme is a healthy diet. The essentials of a liver-supporting diet are:

1. The diet should contain an abundance of fresh fruits and vegetables. Not only do these foods tend not to tax and stress the liver, they also contain an abundance of nutrients such as vitamin C and carotenoids (e.g. beta-carotene) which can support liver function.
2. Foods which contain a lot of either fat or protein should be downplayed in the diet, as they require quite a lot of chemical processing in the liver. The main foods to avoid are fatty meats such as beef, lamb and duck, dairy products and unhealthy hydrogenated vegetable oils present in most margarines and many processed, baked and fast foods.
3. Foods which contain artificial additives such as sweeteners, colour-

ings, flavourings and preservatives should be minimized in the diet.

4. Just about everyone will be aware of alcohol's ability to stress the liver. For this reason, alcohol should be moderated, and preferably eliminated during the initial phase of any detoxification regime.

5. Caffeine should also be moderated in the diet, as it too stresses the liver.

6. Water helps detoxification. About 1.5 to 2 litres of water (mineral water is best) each day is right for most people. More details about water requirements can be found in chapter 2.

Constipation and liver toxicity

One of the main functions of the large bowel is to eliminate waste material from the gut. Sometimes, bowel function is sluggish, leading to a problem with constipation. Constipation increases the likelihood that toxins in the waste material within the large bowel are reabsorbed into the system, giving the liver more work to do. Overcoming any degree of constipation is therefore important if the liver and the system generally are to be kept as toxin-free as possible.

One quite common but under-recognized medical cause of consti-pation is low thyroid function. Anyone who has other symptoms of this such as weight gain, fatigue, sensitivity to cold, dry skin and cold hands and feet would do well to read chapter 5 for more details about how to diagnose and treat this condition. Constipation can be a side-effect of certain medications including antacids, iron, and pain-killers based on codeine. Occasionally, constipation can be related to a tumour in the large bowel (colon). Often, the constipation will alternate with diarrhoea. Sometimes there may be blood in the bowel motion. Anyone over the age of forty who has had a persistent change in bowel habit should have this investigated by his or her doctor.

Combating constipation

Bowel regularity is very important for health. Many individuals use laxa-tives based on substances such as sennakot to ensure regular bowel movements. While these may temporarily relieve a constipation problem, many people find that they can become reliant on laxatives. As much as possible, any problem with constipation should be relieved naturally and the use of laxatives, especially in the long term, should be avoided.

1. **Increase your intake of fibre**

   One essential ingredient for healthy bowel function is fibre. High-fibre breakfast cereals based on wheat bran are often advised for people suffering from constipation. However, the fibre in these cereals is quite hard and scratchy and may actually irritate the delicate lining of the gut. Plus, wheat is one of the most common foods to trigger food sensitivity problems (see later in this chapter for more details about this). The fibre found in oats, fresh fruits and vegetables is generally much kinder to the gut and is preferred. Aim to eat at least five servings of fruit or vegetables a day.

2. **Use natural bulking agents**

   An effective and convenient way to increase your fibre intake is to add a natural bulking agent to your diet. These can really help to improve bowel regularity. Take 1 to 2 dessert spoonfuls of either psyllium husks or ground linseeds with water each day. These can be sprinkled over cereals, soups or salads.

3. **Drink more water**

   Apart from fibre, the other essential ingredient for bowel regularity is fluid. However, some alcohol and drinks that contain alcohol can dehydrate the body and therefore worsen constipation. The best form of fluid for bowel health is water. Again, 1.5 to 2 litres of mineral water is enough for most people.

4. **Take exercise**

   Exercise can help relieve constipation. Aim to take thirty minutes worth of aerobic exercise (e.g. brisk walking, light jogging, cycling, rowing, aerobics, aqua-aerobics) at least three or four times a week.

5. **Always respond to the call of nature**

   In the long term, failing to respond to the urge to open your bowels may cause a suppression of processes essential for defecation to take place.

Other detoxifying methods

Sometimes a good way to give the detoxification system a good shove in the right direction is to fast. While some people opt for nothing but water during a fast, I think this is simply too strenuous for most people. A good alternative is the one-week-rice-and-vegetable fast – nothing but brown rice and raw and steamed vegetables for one week. The only fluids to be drunk are still mineral or filtered water, herb teas free from additives, and freshly prepared vegetable juices. The benefits of this fast are that it does not encourage yeast overgrowth (more about this later in the chapter), is unlikely to include foods such as wheat and dairy products to which there may be a sensitivity (more about this too later on), and excludes foods and drinks that tend to stress the liver. However, the diet is nonetheless sustaining. If possible, the rice and vegetables should be organic, but this is not critical. If the food is not organic, then make sure you give it a good, thorough washing before cooking.

Once you come off this modified fast, it is generally a good idea to introduce food gently back into the diet. Perhaps some fish and fruit for the first few days followed by a little meat if you eat this. Gradual reintroduction of foods allows your liver to become gradually accustomed to a more varied and challenging diet once more.

A word of caution

During the initial stages of any detoxifying regime, it is not uncommon for individuals to feel worse, rather than better. The theory is that once the body has the opportunity, it may throw off toxins which might have been building up for a long time. Such a large outpouring of toxins from the body's cells can be too much for the liver, and the spillover may give rise to symptoms such as headache, lethargy, achiness and mild flu-like symptoms. Detoxification reactions of this nature normally only last a few days, but if the system is very toxic or if the liver function is very compromised, symptoms may persist for two weeks or more. To help minimize the adverse effects of a fast or cleansing regime, it is important to ensure that plenty of fluids (these help flush toxins out through the urine) and liver-supporting nutrients are taken (see pages 31–2).

Other methods of detoxification

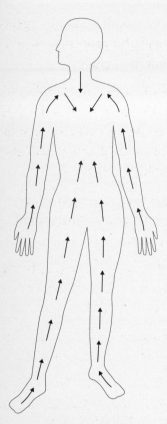

Direction of Skin Brushing

Elimination of toxins from the body can be speeded up in a number of ways, including steam baths, saunas and colonic irrigation. These approaches have their merits. However, for convenience and simplicity I recommend skin brushing.

Toxins in the body tend to accumulate in the fat cells and in the lymphatic system. The lymphatic system is made up of a network of vessels, along which are stationed collections of immune cells called 'lymph nodes'. The lymphatic vessels take tissue debris and many of the end products of cell metabolism and shunt these to the lymph nodes where immune cells may process and deactivate them before they are dumped into the body's circulation. It is thought that lymph fluid can become somewhat sluggish, causing toxins to accumulate. Incidentally, accumulation of toxins in the lymph system and fat cells at the back of the thighs is probably a major factor in the development of cellulite. Skin brushing can be used to help shift lymph fluid and the toxins contained within it, and can be a useful technique in combating cellulite and promoting detoxification.

Skin brushes made of natural fibre can usually be found for sale in health food stores. Ideally, skin brushing should be performed on dry skin, for about five minutes, twice a day. The brush should be used quite vigorously on the legs and arms, and the direction of brushing should always be towards the heart (see diagram). If cellulite is a problem, particular attention should be given to the back of the legs.

Supporting the liver with supplements

The world of natural medicine throws up a wide range of agents which may help support liver function and the process of detox-ification. Some of the more important nutrients include:

Milk thistle – this herb contains a complex of bioflavonoid molecules known collectively as silymarin. Silymarin appears to protect the liver cells by reducing the take-up and enhancing the removal of harmful toxins (*refs* 1, 2). Silymarin also has powerful antioxidant activity (*ref* 3) and can help in the regeneration of injured liver cells (*ref* 4).

Choline and Inositol – these nutrients are generally classified as part of the B-vitamin complex and help in the breakdown and utilization of fat and cholesterol, reducing fatty build-up in the liver.

Biotin – generally regarded as one of the B-complex vitamins, biotin participates in fat metabolism and can therefore help in the processing of fat in the liver.

Lipase – lipase is a fat-digesting enzyme. Lipase helps reduce the fatty load on the liver and may help to keep the liver cells free from fat.

Alpha lipoic acid – this nutrient is itself a powerful antioxidant which has the power to protect the liver from free radical damage. It also participates in the recycling and regeneration of other liver protective antioxidants.

Green tea extract – green tea is a rich source of substances called polyphenols which have potent antioxidant activity. Like alpha lipoic acid, it can also participate in maintaining the activity of other liver protective substances.

Hepranol is a combination supplement which contains a range of liver-supporting and detoxifying ingredients including choline, inositol, lipase, biotin, alpha lipoic acid, and green tea extract. Long-term supplementation with Hepranol may assist liver function and reduce body toxicity. The normal recommended dose is 1 capsule, twice a day with food. Details of how to obtain Hepranol can be found in the section at the back of the book entitled Useful Information, under the name 'VitaTech'.

Toxicity and food sensitivity

It is easy to imagine how toxicity in the body can be the result of 'alien' substances such as pollutants and chemical ingredients in food. However, experience has shown that many even commonly eaten foodstuffs such as wheat and milk can create toxicity in the body through a mechanism known as 'food sensitivity'. Food sensitivity is a broad term which is used to describe unwanted reactions to food in the body. To understand how this comes about, and also what to do about it, we need first to understand the concept of digestion.

Digestion

Digestion takes place in the digestive tract, that begins at the mouth and runs to the anus at the other end (see diagram). The parts of the digestive tract which are actively involved in the process of digestion are the mouth, stomach and small intestine.

In the mouth, the very act of chewing stimulates the secretion of digestive juices lower down in the gut. Chewing also mixes food with an enzyme which starts the digestion of starchy foods such as bread, potatoes, rice and pasta. By breaking food up, chewing also increases the surface area available for contact with the digestive juices, allowing them to penetrate the food and do their digestive work. Once food is

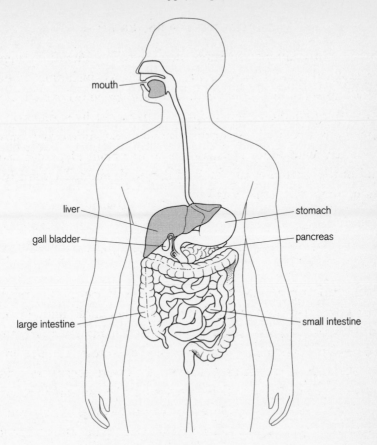

The Digestive Tract

swallowed it passes to the stomach. In health, the stomach contains concentrated acid which is important for digestion, especially of protein-based foods such as meat, fish and dairy products. Once food leaves the stomach, it passes into the small intestine. Here it is subjected to the action of digestive enzymes that continue the digestive process. Some of these are found in the wall of the gut itself, while some of these are secreted by a gland called the pancreas. Bile, secreted by the gallbladder, also works on the food and helps with the digestion of fat.

Conventional medical wisdom dictates that before food is absorbed through the gut wall into the bloodstream, it is first broken down to its smallest molecular constituents. In other words, fats are broken down into fatty acids, starches are broken down into individual sugar molecules, and proteins are broken down into amino acids. If this were the case, then the reality is there would be very limited potential for foods to cause adverse reactions in the body. The basic molecular constituents of food are simply too small to be seen as foreign by the body.

However, it is now known that partially digested food can indeed be absorbed into the body. Poor digestion often plays a role here, as does a degree of 'leakiness' in the gut wall. Gut leakiness is discussed in more detail on page 48). When undigested food is absorbed into the system there is enormous potential for unwanted reactions.

For instance, adverse food reactions can occur when partially digested food comes into contact with the immune system, triggering it into action. These immune reactions are believed to have the potential to give rise to a wide variety of symptoms and conditions, including fatigue, eczema, weight gain, fluid retention and arthritis. Other conditions which appear to be related to these food reactions include irritable bowel syndrome, migraine headaches, Crohn's disease, rheumatoid arthritis, infantile colic and childhood ear infections. For many individuals, identifying the foods to which they are sensitive is a critical step in bringing about vibrant health.

Is food intolerance your problem?

The following questionnaire is designed to help you ascertain whether food sensitivity is a problem in you. Score each question as indicated, and then add up your total score.

1. Do you feel lethargic soon after eating?

No	0 points
Occasional or mild problems	2 points
Frequent or severe problems	4 points

2. Do you often feel better if you don't eat?

No	0 points
Marginally better	2 points
Much better	4 points

3. Did you have problems such as colic, glue ear, ear infections, eczema, asthma or recurrent tonsillitis as a child?

No	0 points
Yes, occasional problems	3 points
Yes, frequent and/or severe problems	5 points

4. Do you have recurrent, unexplained symptoms?

No	0 points
Occasional or mild problems	2 points
Frequent or severe problems	4 points

5. Do you suffer from excess mucus or catarrh formation in the throat, nose or sinuses?

No	0 points
Occasional or mild problems	2 points
Frequent or severe problems	4 points

6. Do you feel particularly drawn to certain foods such as bread or cheese?

No	0 points
Occasionally	2 points
Frequently	4 points

7. Do you have dark circles under your eyes?

No	0 points
Yes	2 points
Frequent or severe problems	4 points

8. Do you suffer from fluid retention? (tight rings, puffy face or ankles and a weight which fluctuates by two or more pounds from day to day are classic signs)

No	0 points
Occasional or mild problems	2 points
Frequent or severe problems	4 points

9. Do you suffer from irritable bowel syndrome?

No	0 points
Occasional or mild problems	1 point
Frequent or severe problems	2 points

10. Do you suffer from eczema, hives (urticaria) or undiagnosed rash?

No	0 points
Occasional or mild problems	2 points
Frequent or severe problems	4 points

Interpreting your score

0–9: food sensitivity is unlikely

10–25: food sensitivity should be considered as a possibility and testing (see below) is recommended

26 and above: food sensitivity is very likely, and testing is highly recommended

Testing for food sensitivity

There are a number of methods that can be used to find out which foods you may be sensitive to. These include:

Scratch testing and IgE blood testing

The scratch test, also known as the prick test or patch test, involves scratching the outer layer of the skin, and introducing a tiny amount of the food or other substance (e.g. animal hair, pollen) to be tested. Redness and swelling at the site of the test indicates a sensitivity to whatever is being tested. Blood tests also exist which detect immune substances called antibodies to specific foods. One type of antibodies which can be measured in the laboratory are known as IgE antibodies. These are responsible for obvious allergic conditions such as hay fever, and peanut allergy; however, they almost certainly have no bearing on the sort of health issues that concern us here.

The cytotoxic test

This test is performed by mixing immune cells with individual food extracts and then looking for a reaction in the immune cells. Usually a technician uses a microscope to assess whether the immune cells have reacted and to what degree. In this sense, the test may be affected by human error, and there is much doubt about the reproducibility and consistency of these tests. I don't generally recommend them.

The ALCAT test

ALCAT stands for the antigen leucocyte cellular antibody test. It is quite similar to the cytotoxic test, except that the white cells' reaction to foodstuffs is measured by a sophisticated piece of laboratory equipment rather than a technician. It is possible that ALCAT is more accurate than cytotoxic testing, but ALCAT is usually more expensive.

IgG testing

Antibodies come in different forms, and there is some evidence that a type known as IgG antibodies are involved in many food sensitivity reactions. It is possible to detect IgG antibodies to specific foods using sophisticated biochemical techniques. There are two basic techniques used, RAST (radioallergosorbent test) and ELISA (enzyme-linked immunoserological assay). These tests are thought to be quite reliable indicators of food sensitivity. It is believed that ELISA is more sensitive than RAST, and is cheaper too. This is probably the best test if you like blood tests!

Electro-dermal testing

Practitioners of Chinese medicine believe that energy flows down tracts in the body known as meridians. In the 1950s a German doctor by the name of Reinholdt Voll discovered that you could find out much about the health status of the body by measuring the electrical current flowing through the acupuncture points. Electro-dermal testing involves measuring the electrical current that flows through an acupuncture point, and then detecting any changes in this as the body is challenged with individual foods. In this form of testing, foods are often tested by having extracts of those foods put in the same circuit as the subject being tested. If adding the food changes the electrical current flowing through the acupuncture point, then this suggests that there is a problem with the food. Some more sophisticated devices have foods stored on a computer in the form of the electromagnetic 'fingerprint' of that food.

In skilled hands, this method seems to give good results which are instantaneous. Electro-dermal testing is relatively cheap compared with the blood tests that are available. Because it is economical and instantaneous, I have to say I like this form of testing, but I think it helps to find a practitioner who has had plenty of testing experience.

Applied kinesiology

This is similar to electro-dermal testing except that the practitioner measures muscle strength in response to foods rather than the electrical current flowing through the body. Typically, muscle strength is first ascertained by the practitioner pressing down on the subject's out-stretched arm. This is repeated while challenging the subject with foods, either by having them hold the food close to the body or by putting samples of food under the tongue. Like electro-dermal testing the results are thought to be relatively accurate in skilled hands and the results are instantaneous. Again, testing tends to be inexpensive compared with blood tests.

The elimination diet

The elimination diet is regarded by many practitioners of nutritional medicine as the most accurate way of testing for food sensitivity. The concept is simple: all likely problem foods are removed from the diet for a period of time. Once the symptoms or condition being treated alleviate, foods are added back into the diet, one at a time, and a note is made of which foods cause a recurrence of the symptoms.

Knowing which foods to eliminate from the diet is an art in itself. To help you, here is some guidance:

1. Eliminate all sources of wheat (a very common problem food) from the diet. These include most breads, pasta, pastry, pizza,

biscuits, cakes, wheat-based breakfast cereals, wheat crackers, breaded food, battered food and anything containing wheat flour.

2. Eliminate milk, cheese and yoghurt from the diet (dairy products are very common problems, especially milk and cheese).

3. Eliminate foods and drinks which you consume repeatedly, say on four or more days each week (the more of a food you eat, the more likely it is to be a problem).

4. Eliminate the foods and drinks which you crave and think you might not be able to do without (we can often end up feeling we 'need' the very foodstuffs to which we are sensitive).

5. Eliminate the foods and drinks which you suspect make you feel bad.

All these foods should be eliminated for two weeks.

Taking a food out of the diet is one thing, finding something to replace it with is another. The table overleaf includes a list of the most common food sensitivities, and some viable alternatives.

Generally speaking, the sort of meals which most food-intolerant individuals settle on are based on the following theme:

Meat, fish, eggs (e.g. omelette or hard-boiled eggs) or tofu
Vegetables
Rice or potato

Typical combinations may include:
Roast chicken with steamed broccoli and carrots and roast potatoes
Tuna salad with new potatoes
Grilled salmon with salad and rice
Omelette and salad
Tofu casserole with rice and salad
Tofu and vegetable kebabs and brown rice

If you do indeed suffer from food sensitivity, you may well be feeling much better after a week or two on this regime. Many individuals whose health issues are linked with food sensitivity find that they experience a sudden improvement in their condition, along with increased energy, enhanced mental clarity and less problematic digestive function.

Problem foodstuff	Alternative
wheat-based bread	100 per cent rye bread
	rye crackers
	rye pumpernickel bread
	rice cakes
	oat cakes
wheat-based breakfast cereals	oat muesli
	porridge (oatmeal)
	cornflakes
	puffed rice
	multi-grain cereals based on non-wheat grains such as amaranth, millet and rice
	vegetable, rice and corn-based pasta
egg noodles	rice noodles
gluten-containing food (wheat, oats, rye and barley)	rice cakes
	rice
	rice noodles
	vegetable, rice and corn-based pasta
	potato
	polenta (corn meal)
cow's milk	sheep's milk
	goat's milk
	soya milk
	rice milk
cow's cheese	goat's cheese
	sheep's cheese (e.g. feta)
cow's yoghurt	sheep's yoghurt
	goat's yoghurt
	soya yoghurt
coffee and tea	herb and fruit teas
	dandelion coffee
	chicory/barley-based coffee substitutes

As is the case with general detoxification, it is not uncommon for sensitive individuals to experience withdrawal reactions during the initial phase of an elimination diet. A gnawing hunger, nasal stuffiness, inability to concentrate, fatigue, insomnia and nervousness are not uncommon symptoms of this. These reactions normally last for a few days, and very rarely longer than a week. The symptoms can be lessened by taking 1 g of vitamin C every couple of hours or so.

Re-testing foods

If you are feeling better after a couple of weeks on the elimination diet, it's time to start testing foods. Take one of the foods you have eliminated, and have a substantial portion of it one morning. A glass of milk at breakfast is an example. Over the next few hours, you will need to look out for any symptoms which suggest food sensitivity. These include headache, itching, depression, fatigue, irritability and foggy thinking. If you get any reaction, make a note that the provoking food is one of your sensitivities, and eliminate it again from your diet. If you have no reaction to your first exposure to the food, try it again at lunch and dinner. If by the following morning you are totally free of symptoms, add it provisionally to your safe list of foods.

For the next three days, re-eliminate the food and keep a watchful eye out for any symptoms that suggest a food reaction. It is possible that the symptoms of a reaction can come on two or three days after a food or drink is consumed. If such a reaction occurs, then you should suspect this food. If you still feel well after the three-day break, you can be pretty sure the foodstuff you are testing is fine for you.

In this way, proceed through the major foods you have eliminated, making a note of safe and unsafe foods as you go.

What if the elimination diet outlined above didn't help?

If the elimination diet outlined above doesn't help your situation, then there are two main possible explanations:

1. The foods to which you are sensitive were not eliminated from the diet.
2. You don't have a food sensitivity problem.

To find out which of these is the case, it might be worthwhile eliminating more foods than the ones outlined above on pages 38–9. A useful diet which you can employ is what is known as the 'Stone Age' or 'caveman' diet.

The Stone Age diet

In this diet, all foods which were introduced after the advent of farming and animal domestication practices are eliminated from the diet. This means no grains (wheat, oats, rye, barley, rice and corn), dairy products (butter, milk, cheese, yoghurt), refined sugar, alcohol, food additives including sweeteners and margarine. Eggs are often permitted on such a diet, but I prefer to eliminate them because in practice they are quite often a problem. Permitted foods include meat, fowl, fish, root vegetables and other vegetables, fruit, nuts, seeds, filtered or mineral water, herb teas and sea salt. This diet is very limited, but usually unearths food sensitivities if they are there. It is normal for individuals to feel the benefit from this elimination diet after only five to ten days.

Overcoming food sensitivities

The first step in overcoming food sensitivities is to avoid the problem foodstuff(s). In normal circumstances, it is wise for problem foods to be excluded from the diet for at least a month. Two months is better if you can manage it. Abstaining from a food for a period of time can make the body more tolerant to the food in the long term. However, with regard to food reintroduction, there are a few things that need to be borne in mind:

1. **Initially, food reactions can be worse, not better, than before**
For some time (often a month or two) after the point of exclusion, it is common for an adverse reaction to a foodstuff to be worse than it was before. This is often referred to as 'hypersensitivity'. Care needs to be taken, therefore, when dealing with potentially serious medical conditions such as asthma. Elimination and reintroduction of foods is sometimes better done under the supervision of a nutritionally oriented doctor for this reason.

2. **When a food is reintroduced, it is best not to eat too much of it, too frequently**
It is usually possible to reintroduce a problem food back into the diet, and not have problems with it. However, if that food is eaten in relatively large quantities and/or is eaten quite frequently, then this increases the risk of the original problems recurring. It is a good idea when reintroducing problem foods to eat them in 'rotation'. This means only eating the food once every few days, often three or four days. So, toast for breakfast on Sunday followed by a pasta supper on Wednesday but no other wheat in between is unlikely to re-ignite the original symptoms which led you to exclude wheat in the first place.

    As a general piece of advice about putting foods back into the diet, I say, avoid it when you can and don't worry when you can't. In other words, avoid buying the foodstuffs which have been found to be a problem, and opt for something else if choosing from a menu. However, if you're with friends for dinner and pasta is being served, my advice is to eat it. Even if you don't feel great afterwards, at least you know why.

3. **In the long term, food sensitivities can be reduced by improving digestion and healing the lining of the gut**
Earlier in this chapter we discussed how poor digestion and leakiness in the intestinal wall can underlie a food sensitivity problem. Discerning whether or not these factors are a problem, and combating them if they are, can really help to reduce the likelihood of old sensitivities returning or new ones developing.

Improving digestion in the stomach

While acid-suppressing medication is often prescribed for individuals with indigestion, their problem is often not too much acid, but too *little*. A low level of acid in the stomach stalls the digestion of food, causing it to ferment. Common symptoms of this include bloating or belching immediately after meals, or a feeling that food tends to 'get stuck'. Individuals with low stomach acid often find that they feel full after only a relatively small amount of food.

Low stomach acid can also lead to the poor absorption of certain nutrients, including minerals such as iron and vitamins such as B12 and folic acid. All of these nutrients are essential for healthy red blood cell formation. As a result, long-standing low acid secretion can lead to a problem with anaemia. Poor mineral absorption can also lead to weak nails (this is quite a common symptom in women but I've rarely seen it in men). Another common symptom in women is hair that is thin, brittle and tends not to grow well. In men and women, a red complexion on the face, or dilated/broken capillaries on the cheeks can be a sign of low stomach acid secretion.

Low stomach acidity has also been associated with other illnesses, particularly those in which the body's immune system has turned against its own tissues (auto-immune diseases) such as rheumatoid arthritis, vitiligo (de-pigmentation of the skin), and systemic lupus erythematosus. Other conditions that seem to be commonly associated with low stomach acid secretion include eczema, asthma, gallbladder problems, osteoporosis, chronic urticaria (hives) and rosacea (a facial skin disorder).

Conventional medical tests for stomach acidity

Probably the most accurate test for stomach acidity uses something called 'radiotelemetry'. Here, the subject swallows a capsule on a thin piece of string. The capsule, known as a Heidelberg capsule, contains a pH sensitive electrode. Once in the stomach, the capsule transmits a reading of the stomach acidity which can then be detected by a sensing device held over the stomach on the skin surface. This test is good and relatively inexpensive. However, this test is not considered to be part of mainstream medicine, and your doctor is unlikely to have heard of it. For details about relevant testing facilities, see the section entitled Useful Information at the back of the book.

A simple home test for low stomach acid

While the test described above can be a very good way to diagnose a low acid problem, a simple home test can help to identify this condition. Take a level teaspoon of bicarbonate of soda and dissolve in some water. Drink this mixture on an empty stomach. If sufficient quantities of acid are present in the stomach, bicarbonate of soda is converted into gas, producing significant bloating and belching within five or ten minutes of drinking the mix. Little or no belching is suspicious and could mean low stomach acid.

Problems with digestive enzymes

Another potential cause of poor digestion and food sensitivity is a lack of the digestive enzymes normally present in the small intestine. Low levels of digestive enzymes can provoke feelings of fullness after meals, along with symptoms such as indigestion, bloating, belching and wind. However, whereas individuals with low stomach acidity tend to get their symptoms immediately after meals, individuals with an enzyme problem will only normally start to get symptoms one to three hours after the meal.

Natural methods for improving digestion

Certain supplements can be used to improve digestion, and we will cover these at the end of the chapter. However, there's an enormous amount that can be done to rev-up the digestion before you reach for the supplement bottle.

1. Chew your food thoroughly

Proper chewing is essential for proper digestion. As mentioned earlier in this chapter, chewing stimulates the secretion of acid and digestive enzymes. Chewing also mixes food with saliva, which contains an enzyme that starts the digestion of starchy foods such as bread, potatoes, rice and pasta. And perhaps most importantly of all, chewing breaks food up, massively increasing the surface area available for contact with the digestive juices. This increases the efficiency of digestion by giving digestive enzymes the opportunity to penetrate the food and do the work of digestion. Each mouthful should be chewed to a cream before swallowing.

2. Avoid big meals

The larger the meal, the larger the load on the digestive system. Small, frequent meals ease the burden on the digestive system and reduce the risk of indigestion.

3. Avoid drinking with meals

Some people tend to drink quite a lot of fluid with meals and believe that this can only help to 'wash food down'. The reality is quite the reverse. Drinking with meals dilutes the acid and enzymes which do the digestive work, and does nothing to help the process of digestion. In the main part, drinking should be done between meals, not at meal times.

4. Consider food combining

Foods are made up of several chemical constituents including protein and carbohydrates (sugars and starches). Proteins and starches are very different chemically, and are digested by different enzymes in the gut. In addition, proteins are initially digested in acid, while starches are digested in alkali (quite the opposite). Food combining is designed to make digestion easier by separating protein and starch at the same meal. This means eating either protein or starch, and combining it with a food which is classified as 'neutral' (neither protein nor starch). Eating to this pattern can bring tremendous relief to sufferers of indigestion and increase the chances of complete and rapid food breakdown.

The following list includes all the common protein, starch and neutral foods:

Protein	Neutral	Starch
Meats	*All green and root*	bread
beef	*vegetables apart*	potatoes
lamb	*from the potato*	rice
chicken	asparagus	pasta
turkey	aubergines	cereal
veal	broccoli	oats
venison	Brussels sprouts	
pork	cabbage	*Food made with flour*
bacon	carrots	pastries and pies
	cauliflower	cakes
Fish	celery	biscuits
mackerel	courgettes	
herring	green beans	*Dried fruits*
trout	leeks	dates
salmon	mushrooms	figs
tuna	onions	currants
cod	parsnips	sultanas
plaice	peas	raisins
skate	spinach	
	turnips	*Other fruit*
Shellfish		bananas
prawns	*Salad vegetables*	mangoes
cockles	avocado	
mussels	cucumber	*Sweeteners*
oysters	tomatoes	sugar
crab	lettuce	maple syrup
lobster	spring onions	honey
	red and green peppers	
Dairy products	radishes	
cheese		
eggs	*Nuts and seeds*	
milk		
yoghurt	*Fats and oils*	
	cream	
Vegetable proteins	butter	
soya beans	extra virgin olive oil	
soya bean curd (tofu)	other vegetable oils	

So, according to the principles of food combining, examples of healthy meals include:

Meat or fish with salad or vegetables other than potato
Pasta with tomato-based sauce (no meat) and salad
Vegetable curry and rice
Baked potato, ratatouille and salad
Meat stew with vegetables
Avocado salad sandwich
Omelette and salad

Leakiness in the gut wall and toxicity

Leakiness in the gut wall is a common feature in food sensitivity and toxicity issues. This can be assessed with a laboratory test. Here, the subject drinks a fluid containing molecules of a range of sizes. The urine is then collected and analysed for these molecules. If large molecules are found in the urine, this suggests leakiness in the gut.

Leaky gut tests (called 'tests for intestinal permeability' in the trade) are available via specialist laboratories. For details about how to go about getting one of these tests, see the section entitled Useful Information at the back of the book. It is important to remember that leakiness in the gut is itself usually related to other factors such as food sensitivity and candida overgrowth (see below), and considering these factors is therefore important. It is often advisable to work with a practitioner who is skilled at diagnosing gut and liver imbalance, and may therefore help you pinpoint the underlying nature of your symptoms.

Supplements for overcoming food sensitivity

Acid supplements

Supplements of hydrochloric acid taken in capsule form can certainly assist in the digestive process in individuals who have low or no stomach acid. Part of the action of hydrochloric acid is to convert an inactive substance called pepsinogen into an active enzyme called pepsin. The function of pepsin is to start the digestion of protein food molecules. Acid supplements are therefore best combined with pepsin for maximum potency. Acid supplements should be taken before meals.

CAUTION:

Acid supplements should not be used if there is a present or past history of peptic ulcers (stomach and duodenal) or stomach inflammation (gastritis) unless under the instruction of a nutritionally oriented doctor.

Suggested supplement: Acidol and Pepsin contains betaine hydrochloride (the type of acid used most commonly to acidify the stomach), along with pepsin. The normal recommended dose is one capsule, to be taken before each main meal. Acidol and Pepsin may be very effective in improving digestion, and can often help to reduce the tendency to food sensitivity in time. Details of how to obtain Acidol and Pepsin can be found in the section entitled Useful Information at the back of the book under the name 'VitaTech'.

Digestive enzymes

Digestive enzyme supplements may help to make up for inadequate or sub-optimal digestion in the small intestine. A good digestive enzyme supplement will normally contain a range of enzymes, each of which is responsible for digesting a certain food type. Examples of such enzymes include protease and bromelain (for the digestion of protein), amylase (for the digestion of starch), sucrase (for the digestion of sugar), lactase (for the digestion of the milk sugar lactose), and lipase (for the digestion of fat).

Suggested supplement: Enzyme Forte is a combination supplement which contains all the above enzymes. One capsule should be taken after each meal. By helping to ensure the complete digestion of food, Enzyme Forte may help to combat food sensitivities in the long term.

Contraindications: Enzyme Forte should not be used in individuals suffering from gastritis (inflammation of the stomach lining) or stomach/duodenal ulceration.

Details of how to obtain Enzyme Forte can be found in the section entitled Useful Information at the back of the book under the name 'VitaTech'.

Gut healing nutrients

Certain nutrients have an important role to play in healing the gut lining. Some of the important ones include:

Glutamine – an essential fuel for the cells which make up the lining of the small intestine, glutamine can help to promote healing in the gut.

N-acetyl glucosamine (NAG) – N-acetyl glucosamine provides a sort of tissue 'cement' to help bind gut cells together.

Gamma Oryzanol – actually an extract of rice bran, gamma oryzanol has anti-inflammatory and healing properties within the gut.

Vitamin E and Vitamin A – both of these nutrients play an important role in healing the gut lining.

Suggested supplement: Permaguard is a combination supplement which contains L-glutamine, N-acetyl glucosamine, gamma oryzanol, vitamin E, vitamin A and the healthy gut organism L. acidophilus. Long-term supplementation with Permaguard may promote healing in the lining of the digestive tract, reducing the risk of food sensitivity. The recommended dose is 1 capsule, three times a day. Details of how to obtain Permaguard can be found in the section entitled Useful Information at the back of the book under the name 'VitaTech'.

Case Study

Veronica, a 37-year-old shop manager, originally came to me complaining of fatigue and fluid retention. She found her energy level was quite unpredictable, though it was noticeably worse about an hour after lunch. She felt 'puffy', often had swollen ankles after working in the shop all day, and sometimes found her rings difficult to get on and off her fingers. Fluid retention was a particular problem before her period when she would gain 3–4 lbs in weight.

Veronica suffered from eczema as a child. Eczema in children is usually caused by food sensitivity, and her symptom of fatigue within an hour or so of a meal also suggested this. Food sensitivity testing (electro-dermal testing) revealed sensitivities to wheat, milk and cheese. Looking at Veronica's diet it was not surprising that she was feeling tired a lot of the day: her breakfast was a wheat-based cereal and milk, lunch was a sandwich, and supper was usually a pasta dish.

Because Veronica was very attached to wheat products, we discussed a range of alternative foods including corn and rice-based cereals, rye bread and wheat-free (corn) pasta. Cow's milk was swapped for rice milk. It was suggested that during elimination of her problem foods she also take a supplement of healthy gut bacteria (see below) to help restore general digestive health, a supplement to support her liver (Hepranol), and a digestive enzyme supplement (Enzyme Forte – one with each main meal) to improve digestion.

Veronica returned a month later. She had been quite strict with the diet and had taken her supplements. Breakfast had been cornflakes or puffed rice with rice milk. For lunch she was mainly taking a rye bread sandwich into work. Sometimes she would have a salad (chicken or tuna) supplemented with rye crackers. Supper was usually a piece of meat or fish with vegetables including some potato. Occasionally, she had wheat-free pasta. For the first few days she had felt more tired than usual, but by the end of the first week felt she had much more energy than usual. Her fluid retention had also resolved very quickly. She had had a period since the last consultation and had noticed no significant increase in weight.

A week before the consultation she had eaten pasta at a friend's house, and had noticed how lethargic she felt after this. Although Veronica had had some initial cravings for wheat, she was now over these and was happy to stay off wheat the majority of the time. Later on, she went on to have occasional slices of bread or wheat-pasta, but found that these did not provoke symptoms as long as she did not eat them too frequently or in large amounts.

Yeast overgrowth and toxicity

So far, we have looked at general toxicity in the body, and also at specific factors that may contribute to this, namely food sensitivity, poor digestion, and leakiness in the gut wall. Before we leave the subject of toxicity, there is just one more factor which warrants discussion – *yeast*.

Within the gut reside about three or four pounds of healthy bacteria which have a variety of roles in the body, including assisting in digestion, keeping unhealthy organisms at bay and ensuring that the lining of the gut remains healthy. The gut also contains the yeast organism Candida albicans. Under certain circumstances candida can overgrow in the gut, and this can lead to a number of symptoms including abdominal bloating, wind, fatigue, sweet or starch cravings and thrush (vaginal yeast infection). Candida is well known to produce a range of potential toxins which are believed to have the capacity to get into the system by breaching the gut wall.

What causes yeast overgrowth?

Antibiotics are a major, perhaps *the* major factor, in candida overgrowth. Designed to kill harmful bacteria in the body, they can kill healthy bacteria too. Yet, they do not kill yeast. As a result, antibiotics can lead to a predominance of yeast in the gut (*ref 5*). Some women find that they can be prone to vaginal yeast infection (thrush) if they take antibiotics. The killing of healthy gut bacteria by antibiotics and subsequent yeast overgrowth explains this phenomenon.

Other common underlying factors in yeast overgrowth include stress (it can suppress the immune system), the consumption of yeast-encouraging foods such as sugar, bread, cheese and alcohol, and the taking of the pill or hormone replacement therapy.

Is candida your problem?

The following questionnaire is designed to help you ascertain whether yeast overgrowth is a factor in you. Score each question as indicated, and then add up your total score.

1. Do you find that your bowel habit can be somewhat erratic, perhaps constipated some of the time, and on the loose side at others?

No	0 points
Occasional or mild problems	2 points
Frequent or severe problems	4 points

2. Do you tend to suffer from excessive wind and flatulence?

No	0 points
Occasional or mild problems	2 points
Frequent or severe problems	4 points

3. Do you suffer from significant abdominal bloating?

No	0 points
Occasional or mild problems	2 points
Frequent or severe problems	4 points

4. Do you suffer from anal itching?

No	0 points
Occasional or mild problems	2 points
Frequent or severe problems	4 points

5. Do you suffer from thrush (vaginal yeast infection) from time to time?

No	0 points
Occasional or mild problems	3 points
Frequent or severe problems	6 points

6. Do you suffer from pre-menstrual syndrome, or painful or irregular periods?

No	0 points
Occasional or mild problems	1 point
Frequent or severe problems	2 points

7. **Do you suffer from episodes of mental confusion, mental fatigue, loss of concentration, low mood or irritability?**

No   0 points

Occasional or mild problems   2 points

Frequent or severe problems   4 points

8. **Do you suffer from periodic skin problems such as urticaria (hives), athlete's foot, generalized itching or a rash between your buttocks or in your groin?**

No   0 points

Occasional or mild problems   3 points

Frequent or severe problems   6 points

9. **Do you suffer from recurrent bouts of cystitis and/or problems with vaginal irritation?**

No   0 points

Occasional or mild problems   3 points

Frequent or severe problems   5 points

10. **Do you crave sugar, sugary foods such as chocolate, biscuits or cakes, or yeasty foods such as cheese, bread, alcohol or vinegar?**

No   0 points

Occasional or mild problems   2 points

Frequent or severe problems   4 points

11. **Do you suffer from multiple allergies, and react to chemicals in the environment such as petrol and diesel fumes, cleaning fluids and perfumes?**

No   0 points

Occasional or mild problems   2 points

Frequent or severe problems   4 points

12. **How would you describe your antibiotic consumption in the past, including childhood?**

Very few antibiotics generally   0 points

Moderate use for occasional infections such as winter
    infections, chest infections etc.   5 points

Frequent and/or extended use for problems such as acne,
  recurrent urinary tract infections, chronic sinusitis,
  tonsillitis etc.   10 points

13. **Have you currently been taking the oral contraceptive pill for more than six months, or did you take it in the past for more than a year?**
Yes   3 points
No   0 points

14. **Have you had steroid drugs such as prednisolone, dexamethasone or betamethasone by mouth or cortisone injections?**
Yes   4 points
No   0 points

15. **Have you ever had inhaled steroids (usually for asthma) such as Becotide for three months or more?**
Yes   4 points
No   0 points

16. **Do you have a number of vague health problems which no one has been able to explain?**
Yes   4 points
No   0 points

Interpreting your score
0–9: yeast overgrowth is unlikely
10–24: yeast overgrowth should be considered as a possibility and further testing or a trial of the anti-candida regime is likely to be worthwhile
25–39: yeast overgrowth is likely, and steps taken to combat yeast are very likely to help improve weight loss and general health
40 and above: yeast overgrowth is very likely, and steps taken to combat this are almost certainly going to improve weight loss and general health

If you have scored highly or moderately on the questionnaire, you may wish to confirm whether or not you have a yeast problem with some form of testing. Several types of tests are available, and the most commonly available are listed below.

Tests for candida

1. Stool tests

Stool samples can be sent to a microbiological laboratory for yeast analysis. These tests generally need to be administrated by a doctor, and are by no means foolproof. I don't think it's uncommon for someone with a genuine yeast problem (as indicated by their symptoms and response to treatment) for culture tests to come up as clear. One potential problem is that if yeast is stuck to the bowel wall, it simply may not appear in the stool. Plus, yeast may be found, but it's difficult to determine sometimes how much is too much.

2. Candida antigen in the blood

An antigen is a particle which stimulates the immune system. There is a specific blood test for candida antigen, and if this is positive, it probably indicates an ongoing yeast infection. Not only that, but it suggests that the yeast has escaped from the gut itself, and made its way into the bloodstream. Antigen tests are thought to provide pretty hard evidence of a candida infection, but there is always the possibility that if candida is confined to the gut, the blood test will be negative.

3. Candida antibodies in the blood

Antibodies are what the immune system produces in response to antigens. Two types of antibody, IgG and IgM, are usually measured. If the level of antibodies specific for candida is raised, this may indicate infection.

4. Candida antibodies in the gut

A type of antibody known as secretory IgA is produced within the gut. Measuring the amount of secretory IgA made specifically against candida can be a good guide to the presence of yeast in the gut. The higher the value, the more likely there is to be a yeast overgrowth in the intestine.

5. The gut fermentation test

Yeast tends to metabolize sugar into alcohol. The gut fermentation test is based on this principle. A blood sample is taken, and the subject is then given a measured dose of sugar. An hour later, another sample of blood is taken. Both blood samples are analysed for various fermentation products. The presence of these substances in significant quantity can point to the presence of excess yeast in the gut.

6. Other tests

It is possible to diagnose yeast overgrowth through a number of non-laboratory tests including iridology, electro-dermal testing (e.g. Vega, BEST system, Eclosion), dowsing and applied kinesiology. All of these forms of testing have their own merits, especially if the assessment is being carried out by an experienced and skilled practitioner. Assessment is usually relatively cheap and the results are immediate. Another advantage with these forms of testing is that they invariably allow contact with a practitioner who is likely to be able to guide you through the intricacies of an anti-candida programme, if testing shows this to be a problem.

How important is testing for candida?

The short answer to this is, in my opinion, not much. I think it is usually possible to diagnose candida by looking carefully for the symptoms and underlying factors that are typical in the condition. Occasionally, I may perform a test where the diagnosis really is questionable, but usually the patient's story gives it away.

The anti-candida diet

The cornerstone of the anti-candida approach is a diet which helps starve yeast out of the system. This means no foods which feed yeast directly, or encourage yeast by being yeasty, mouldy or fermented in their own right.

Yeast-feeding foods to avoid

Sugar

Sweetening agents such as maple syrup, molasses, honey and malt syrup

Sugar-containing foods such as biscuits, cakes, confectionery, ice cream, pastries, sugared breakfast cereals, soft drinks and fruit juice

White flour products including white bread, crackers, pizza and pasta

Yeasty, mouldy, or fermented foods to avoid

Bread and other yeast-raised items

Alcoholic drinks, particularly beer and wine which are very yeasty

Gravy mixes (most contain brewer's yeast)

Vinegar and vinegar-containing foods such as ketchup (which also contains sugar), mustard, mayonnaise and many prepared salad dressings

Pickles, miso, tempeh and soy sauce (all fermented)

Aged cheeses including Cheddar, Stilton, Swiss, Brie and Camembert (cheese is inherently mouldy)

Peanuts (and peanut butter) and pistachios (tend to harbour yeast)

Mushrooms (mushrooms *are* mould!)

Dried fruit (are intensely sugary and tend to harbour mould)

Yeast-containing foods such as soups and pre-packaged foods

Individuals who have a candida problem are likely to have food sensitivities, particularly to wheat and/or dairy products (see above).

The safest bet, therefore, is also to avoid these foods, at least for a month or two.

Foods to eat freely

The foods which are generally very safe to eat on an anti-candida regime are listed below.

Protein foods	celery
eggs	cabbage
fish, including naturally	broccoli
smoked fish	cauliflower
shellfish	spinach
chicken	chard
turkey	kale
lamb	watercress
beef	Brussels sprouts
pork	asparagus
duck	onions
tofu (soya bean curd)	leeks
	green beans
Vegetables	parsnips
lettuce	aubergines
tomato	artichokes
cucumber	avocado

Foods to be eaten in moderation

Certain foods such as grains, high-starch vegetables, legumes or pulses can be eaten on an anti-candida regime, but it's best not to eat masses of them because they tend to have some fermentation potential. The bulk of the diet should be based around the foods which can be eaten freely, supplemented with more limited amounts of the foods that follow in this list:

High-starch vegetables	*Grains*
potatoes	yeast-free rye bread
sweet potatoes	rye crackers
squash (e.g. butternut)	brown rice
	wild rice
Legumes	rice cakes
lentils	barley
split peas	millet
kidney beans	corn
navy beans	rye
lima beans	oats, oat cakes and
black beans	oat-based breakfast
adzuki beans	cereals
	buckwheat
	quinoa
	spelt
	brown rice cakes

What about fruit?

Whether or not fruit is advisable on an anti-candida regime is a real moot point. Some practitioners say it can be eaten freely, others say it should be completely excluded, at least to begin with. I have to say, I take the middle ground. My experience is that one or two pieces of fruit a day are generally very well tolerated, though I'm no fan of grapes that are intensely sugary and usually are covered in a mouldy bloom. All fruit that you're not going to peel prior to eating should be washed thoroughly. The best fruits are those that contain the least sugar (raspberries, blueberries, grapefruit and fresh figs). Dried fruits, as mentioned before, are out.

Candida and blood sugar balance

Candida sufferers tend to be prone to fluctuations in blood sugar levels. This can lead to symptoms such as fluctuating energy, cravings for sweet or starchy foods and problems with low mood, irritability or mood swings. The food cravings associated with blood sugar imbalance can be very intense, so getting on top of a blood sugar problem is of prime importance if the anti-candida diet is to be adhered to without too much angst. More details about how to stabilize blood sugar levels can be found in chapter 4. In particular, the chapter also includes details of nutrients and supplements which may really help to counter this problem.

The anti-candida diet – quite a lot to think about

Just to recap, the main principles of the anti-candida diet are:

1. To avoid foods and drinks which feed yeast (sugar and refined carbohydrates).
2. To avoid food and drinks which encourage yeast (yeasty, mouldy or fermented foods).
3. To avoid wheat, milk and cheese because these foods are common sensitivities in candida sufferers (cheese also tends to encourage yeast overgrowth).
4. To eat a diet based around foods which release sugar slowly into the bloodstream.

You might be asking what this leaves? What I've outlined below is a few menu suggestions to help you get on your way. In my experience, just about everyone will find foods within these suggestions that they find practical and palatable.

Breakfast

- Oats (soaked overnight in water or milk substitute) with chopped almonds and hazelnuts, pumpkin and sunflower seeds, rice or soya milk, natural, live unsweetened yoghurt and some chopped fresh fruit

- Oat porridge made with water, soya or rice milk sweetened with banana

- Puffed brown rice cereal, or non-wheat multi-grain cereal, with rice or soya milk, natural yoghurt, nuts, seeds and some fruit

- Poached egg on yeast-free rye bread toast
- Kipper or haddock with poached egg, grilled tomatoes and yeast-free rye toast

Lunch

- Brown rice salad (brown rice with a variety of added ingredients such as tuna, chicken, chick peas, tomato, bell pepper, cucumber, spring onion, garlic, herbs and dressing made from extra virgin olive oil and lemon juice
- Chicken or tuna salad sandwich made with yeast-free rye bread
- Chicken, tuna or prawn salad (extra virgin olive oil and lemon juice dressing) with rye crackers or brown rice cakes
- Spanish omelette (without cheese) and salad
- Poached salmon, steamed vegetables with a few boiled new potatoes
- Grilled chicken and roast vegetables including some potato
- Chicken, turkey or fish with brown rice and salad
- Stir-fried tofu and vegetables with brown rice or rice noodles

The supplements

I can't stress strongly enough how important the anti-candida diet is to overcoming a candida problem. However, in conjunction with a good diet, certain supplements really do seem to be able to speed recovery and restore health to the gut and the body. The basic nutritional supplements which are often used to accompany an anti-candida programme include the following:

1. Healthy gut bacteria supplements to restore the intestinal ecosystem
2. Liver supporting agents to protect the liver and body from the toxins that can be released during the initial phase of an anti-candida regime
3. Nutrients to support blood sugar stability
4. Supplements to kill yeast
5. Supplements to help heal the gut lining

Not all of these need to be used in every individual. In my experience, the first three play a big role in the management of the vast majority of sufferers, while the last two types of supplements are less important generally.

Healthy gut bacteria supplements

Healthy gut bacteria supplements are also known as 'probiotics'. They have been given this name because they put bacteria back into the body, quite the opposite of antibiotics which take them away. Probiotic supplements have attracted a lot of criticism from certain quarters who claim that often the supplements that are bought off the shelf in health food stores do not contain what they say they contain on the label. There is some evidence that supplements do indeed exist which do not contain the quantities of living organisms declared on the label, and some even seem to contain organisms which just shouldn't be there. I've included here probiotics which are independently validated.

Suggested supplements

Replant – Replant is a probiotic supplement which contains massive numbers of healthy gut bacteria. It is particularly useful in the initial stages of an anti-candida regime. Taken at this time, I have found that this product usually significantly speeds recovery from yeast and re-establishment of healthy gut organisms. Replant contains three organisms: Lactobacillus acidophilus (the predominant organism in the small intestine); Bifidobacterium bifudus (the predominant organism in the large intestine); Lactobacillus bulgaricus (an organism which has been linked with health and well-being in individuals who consume yoghurt rich in this organism).

Replant comes in sachets, each of which provides a massive 30 billion organisms (10 billion of each organism). The supplement should be taken for a week, and I generally recommend that half a sachet is taken twice a day.

Replant very often causes increased bloating and wind, and very occasionally discomfort. These symptoms may be caused by a war which is going on between the healthy gut bacteria and less healthy organisms including yeast. The symptoms normally only last for three or four days, and are usually very manageable.

Acidophilus Forte is a probiotic supplement suitable for continued use, and contains the following organisms: Lactobacillus acidophilus (the predominant organism in the small intestine); Bifidobacterium bifidus (the predominant organism in the large intestine).

The total dose of organisms per capsule is 6 billion organisms. This gives a good dose of healthy gut bacteria in the initial stages of an anti-candida regime if taken twice a day.

Details of how to obtain Replant and Acidophilus Forte can be found in Useful Information at the back of the book under the name 'VitaTech'.

Liver support

During the initial phases of an anti-candida regime, it is quite common for individuals to experience a worsening in their condition. Symptoms such as lethargy, fuzzy-headedness, and flu-like symptoms can start a day or so after the regime starts, and generally last from between a few days to a couple of weeks. This reaction is sometimes referred to as 'die-off', and is thought to be due to an increase in candida-derived toxins in the system. If yeast cells die, they will tend to liberate toxic substances which pass from the gut to the liver. Often, the liver does not cope adequately with them, which can allow the toxins to escape into the general circulation, where they may give rise to the sort of symptoms listed above.

One way to help reduce the effects of die-off is to use liver-supporting agents. Hepranol, a supplement designed to protect and strengthen liver function, is a good option. More details about Hepranol's ingredients can be found earlier in this chapter.

Blood sugar control

If you do exhibit symptoms of blood sugar imbalance, and particularly if food cravings are a problem, you may well benefit from taking nutrients that play a role in maintaining blood sugar levels. These nutrients and a suitable combination supplement (Glucoguard) are covered at the end of chapter 4.

Anti-fungal supplements

Some of the natural agents which may be useful in combating yeast in the body include:

Oregano – this herb contains a number of active ingredients, probably the two most important of which are carvacrol and thymol. Studies have shown that oregano has anti-fungal properties and can inhibit the growth of candida.

Garlic – garlic has the ability to kill a range of organisms including bacteria, viruses, parasites and fungi. In natural medicine, garlic is a widely used substance in the control and eradication of candida.

Grapefruit seed extract – extracts of grapefruit seed are thought to have the ability to kill candida in the body. Many candida sufferers report that taking grapefruit seed extract has helped them control their symptoms and conquer their yeast-related problems.

Suggested supplement – Canditrol is a combination supplement which has been specifically formulated to combat yeast in the body. It contains garlic, oregano oil and grapefruit seed extract. If I do recommend an anti-fungal supplement, I normally advise that it is taken for three or four months, starting a month after the anti-candida diet is commenced. The normal recommended dose for Canditrol is one capsule with food, twice a day.

Note: Canditrol capsules should not be chewed or opened.

Contraindications: Canditrol should not be used during pregnancy or if pregnancy is planned. The use of Canditrol should also be avoided in cases of gastritis (inflammation of the stomach lining) and stomach/duodenal ulceration. Details of how to obtain Canditrol can be found in Useful Information at the back of the book under the name 'VitaTech'.

Gut healing nutrients

These have been covered already in this chapter (see page 50).

Case Study

Tina, a 29-year-old personal assistant, came to see me complaining of a number of problems. Her main issues were 'irritable bowel syndrome' and weight gain. She suffered from abdominal bloating and wind, and a bowel habit that alternated between constipation and diarrhoea. She also suffered from vaginal thrush, about two bouts per year. In between she often found her vagina to be somewhat 'irritated'. Tina had taken several courses of antibiotics during childhood for ear infections, and had a six-month course of antibiotics in her early twenties for acne. This history, along with the thrush, made the diagnosis of yeast overgrowth easy.

We started Tina on an anti-candida diet with plenty of probiotics (Replant followed by Acidophilus Forte) and a liver-supporting supplement (Hepranol). Tina also had evidence of blood sugar imbalance including carbohydrate cravings and an energy crash in the late afternoon, so we incorporated dietary changes to help with this. We also added a supplement designed to improve blood sugar control (Glucoguard – see chapter 4 for more details about this). Food sensitivity assessment by electro-dermal testing revealed sensitivities to wheat, oats, and all dairy products other than butter. These changes were also incorporated into Tina's dietary regime.

Tina came back six weeks later. She had already made substantial improvement, had very little bloating, and no wind to speak of. Her bowel habit was now very regular, with no constipation, but occasional loose-ish stools. She had no vaginal symptoms at all. Her weight loss had been quite satisfying – a drop from about 155 lbs down to 142 lbs. Tina felt generally much better too, was needing less sleep and waking much more refreshed. The afternoon slump had gone, and her carbohydrate cravings were under control.

I suggested that, if she could manage it, Tina should continue as we had been doing for a further two months, and then review. In the meantime, I suggested she take a yeast-killing supplement (Canditrol).

When she returned again, she was still feeling very well, and had lost another 8 lbs in weight. We agreed that she would put occasional wheat-containing foods into her diet, like the odd pasta dish. I suggested she avoided yeasty, wheat-based bread if she could, and go easy on wine. I suggested she halve the doses of supplements for her liver and blood sugar control, but stay on full doses of the probiotics and yeast-killer for a further two months and then tail down.

By the time Tina came back for her final visit, she was well. Her energy, both mentally and physically, was high, and her digestive function seemed entirely normal. She had lost a few more pounds in weight and was feeling very comfortable with her shape. We agreed that she should move on to a diet somewhere between the new diet and the diet she had been on when she first came to see me. She did not feel well when reintroducing wheat into her diet, so we resolved that she would avoid this whenever possible. Tina was happy with rice milk as an alternative to cow's, and to eat cheese only occasionally. Now that her carbohydrate cravings had gone, she confessed to having no interest in chocolate, sweets and puddings. The major food issue was around alcohol. Tina loved white wine. I suggested that she have this occasionally, but to make sure that she drank plenty of water when she did so. Tina remained well on this regime.

Summary

- Toxicity is an important cause of health problems such as low energy, weight gain, bad breath, poor skin and headache

- The function of the liver is key to the elimination of potentially toxic substances

- A liver-supporting diet is one that includes easily digested food such as fruit, vegetables and grains, and is low in liver-taxing foods such as fatty foods, dairy products, processed foods, alcohol and caffeine

- Certain nutrients and herbs such as milk thistle, choline, inositol, green tea extract and alpha lipoic acid can be very effective in improving liver function and reducing toxicity in the long term

- Food sensitivity is an important and often undiagnosed cause of ill-health and reduced vitality

- Food sensitivity is often related to problems with poor digestion or leakiness in the digestive tract

- Foodstuffs identified as a problem should be eliminated from the diet for one to two months, after which time they can often be reintroduced in small amounts without causing a recurrence of the original symptoms

- Acid and/or digestive enzyme supplements may be very useful for improving digestion and reducing a tendency to food sensitivity in time

- Candida albicans overgrowth in the gut can lead to a wide range of health problems, including weight gain, irritable bowel syndrome, mood disturbance, fatigue and food cravings

- Factors which encourage candida overgrowth include antibiotic use, stress, hormonal treatments and a diet containing foods that encourage yeast growth, including sugar, refined carbohydrates, bread and alcohol

- The cornerstone of the anti-candida regime is a diet based on foods that do not encourage candida growth such as meat, fish, eggs and vegetables

- Supplements that help restore healthy gut bacteria can be very useful in the management of candida

- Other supplements useful in managing candida are those that support the liver and help to stabilize the blood sugar level

- Natural anti-fungal supplements and those that help heal the lining of the gut may also be of benefit

- Overcoming issues with internal toxicity can often bring about a profound improvement in both physical and mental well-being

4. Balance Your Blood Sugar

Every moment of every day the body adjusts its internal mechanisms to keep it in balance. The name given to this principle of internal balance is 'homeostasis'. One very important component of homeostasis is the regulation of the level of sugar in the bloodstream. However, the mechanisms designed to keep blood sugar on an even keel can fail. To start with, imbalance in the blood sugar level can give rise to symptoms such as fluctuating energy, mood swings, and cravings for sweet and starchy foods. Over time problems such as weight gain, high cholesterol and diabetes can develop. Experience shows that blood sugar imbalance is common. It is also true that correcting this problem almost invariably leads to a significant improvement in health and well-being.

Blood sugar balance in the body

For most of us, a significant proportion of our diet comes in the form of carbohydrates such as sugars (e.g. fruit, fruit juices, confectionery, cake, biscuits, desserts) and starches (e.g. bread, potatoes, rice, pasta, cereals). Starches actually consist of very long chains of sugar molecules which are too long to be absorbed through the gut into the bloodstream. Consequently, in order to absorb starches we must first break them down into their single sugar components through the processes of digestion.

When we eat carbohydrate the blood sugar level rises (see figure overleaf). When this happens, a hormone called 'insulin' is secreted by the pancreas. One of the chief effects of insulin is to transport sugar out of the bloodstream and into the body's cells. In this way, blood sugar is lowered again, preventing the accumulation of sugar in the bloodstream. In general, the body copes well with foods which release sugar quite slowly into the bloodstream. However, if the blood sugar level rises very quickly, the body tends to secrete a lot of insulin in

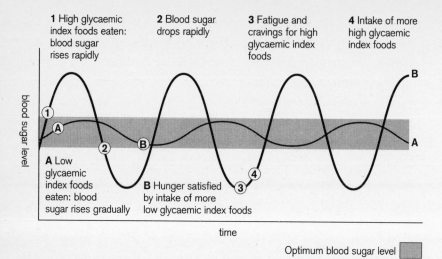

1 High glycaemic index foods eaten: blood sugar rises rapidly

2 Blood sugar drops rapidly

3 Fatigue and cravings for high glycaemic index foods

4 Intake of more high glycaemic index foods

A Low glycaemic index foods eaten: blood sugar rises gradually

B Hunger satisfied by intake of more low glycaemic index foods

blood sugar level

time

Optimum blood sugar level

response. The problem here is that this may drive blood sugar levels lower than normal, a condition which is referred to as 'hypoglycaemia'. Hypoglycaemia can induce some pretty unwelcome symptoms. These include:

1. Fatigue

Sugar is *the* main fuel in the body, and if the level of sugar in the blood drops, fatigue is inevitable. Individuals with blood sugar imbalance tend to experience peaks and troughs of energy as a result of the rise and fall of blood sugar levels.

2. The mid-afternoon slump

A classic time for the fatigue associated with hypoglycaemia is the mid/late afternoon. The big rise in blood sugar which may follow lunch can trigger an insulin surge, leading to low blood sugar (and sleepiness) later on.

3. Morning grogginess

The fatigue associated with hypoglycaemia is often at its worst first thing in the morning. People prone to blood sugar imbalance tend not to maintain blood sugar levels unless they eat. For this reason, blood sugar can fall during the night, leading to fatigue and grogginess in the morning.

4. Poor concentration, low mood or irritability

Although the brain makes up only about 2 per cent of our weight, at rest it uses roughly half the sugar circulating in our bloodstream. What is more, while most of the body can use other foods to generate energy, the brain is almost entirely reliant on sugar for its normal and healthy function. Blood sugar imbalance quite commonly causes problems with poor concentration, depression, irritability and mood swings as a result.

5. **Waking in the night**
When blood sugar levels drop during the night, the body may attempt to correct this by secreting hormones which stimulate the release of sugar from the liver. The main hormone which the body uses for this is adrenaline which increases arousal and may trigger feelings of anxiety and even panic. Not ideal for restful sleep! Hypoglycaemia is a very common cause of waking in the night.

6. **Food cravings**
Another common symptom of hypoglycaemia is food cravings. If our blood sugar level drops it is natural for our body to crave foods it knows will restore the blood sugar level quickly. This commonly manifests as cravings for sweet and/or starchy foods.

The symptoms of blood sugar imbalance are most manifest when sugar levels are low. However, in response to a high blood sugar level, the body secrets insulin. While insulin is important for keeping blood sugar in check, excess amounts of this hormone can have significant hazards in the body.

The effects of excess insulin

Some of the effects of excess insulin include:

1. **Fat production**
Insulin stimulates the conversion of sugar into a starch-like substance called 'glycogen' in the liver and muscle. However, when the glycogen stores in the body are full, insulin stimulates the production of substances called 'triglycerides', which is actually fancy language for *fat*. People with blood sugar imbalance tend to put on weight for this reason. Excess insulin tends to predispose

toward the deposition of fat around the middle, which may give rise to what is colloquially referred to as a 'spare tyre'.

2. High blood pressure and fluid retention

Many of the mechanisms the body uses to balance the amount of fluid it contains, along with the levels of key substances such as sodium, potassium and chloride, take place in the kidneys. In the kidneys, insulin causes the body to hang on to sodium (sodium retention), and this can predispose to high blood pressure (hypertension) and fluid retention in time.

3. Raised cholesterol

While much is made of the need to cut down on fats in the diet, to control cholesterol, carbohydrates are rarely mentioned. However, most of the cholesterol in the bloodstream doesn't come from the diet, it is made in the liver. Insulin actually stimulates the liver to make more cholesterol, and this is likely to increase the risk of both heart disease and stroke.

4. Type II diabetes

High levels of insulin in the body can increase the risk of diabetes. If the body secretes a lot of insulin over many years, then it can become increasingly less sensitive to the effect of that insulin. This may lead to a condition known as type II diabetes (also known as non-insulin dependent diabetes). Taking steps to improve blood sugar control is likely to reduce your risk of developing diabetes in the long term.

Is blood sugar imbalance your problem?

The following questionnaire is designed to help you assess whether you have a blood sugar imbalance. Score each question as indicated, and then add up your total score.

1. Does your energy tend to fluctuate during the day?

No	0 points
Occasional or mild symptoms	2 points
Frequent or severe problems	4 points

2. Do you find that eating something can often pick up your energy level?

No	0 points
Occasionally	2 points
Frequently	4 points

3. Do you often feel tired or unable to concentrate in the mid to late afternoon?

No	0 points
Occasional or mild problems	2 points
Frequent or severe problems	4 points

4. Do you feel tired or groggy on waking, despite sleeping for eight or more hours?

No	0 points
Occasional or mild problems	2 points
Frequent or severe problems	4 points

5. Do you tend to wake in the middle of the night, sometimes feeling anxious or nervy?

No	0 points
Occasional or mild problems	3 points
Frequent or severe problems	5 points

6. Are you prone to mood swings and/or irritability, especially if a meal is skipped?

No	0 points
Occasional or mild problems	2 points
Frequent or severe problems	4 points

7. Can you crave sweet or starchy foods from time to time?

No	0 points
Occasional or mild symptoms	3 points
Frequent or severe symptoms	5 points

8. Do you feel you need to eat very regularly?

No	0 points
Occasional or mild problems	2 points
Frequent or severe problems	4 points

9. Can you find yourself craving alcohol in the early evening?

No	0 points
Occasional or mild problems	1 point
Frequent or severe problems	2 points

10. Do you have a history of type II (mature-onset) diabetes in your family? (see page 72)

No	0 points
Yes	4 points

Interpreting your score

0–9: blood sugar imbalance is unlikely

10–19: blood sugar imbalance is quite likely and measures taken to stabilize blood sugar are likely to be of benefit

20 and above: blood sugar imbalance is likely, and measures taken to stabilize blood sugar are highly recommended

Blood tests for blood sugar balance

The symptoms of impaired blood sugar balance are usually clear-cut enough to enable a diagnosis to be made without the need for testing. However, if you decide a test is appropriate for you, several are available. The relative merits or otherwise of these tests is discussed here:

The Random Blood Glucose Test

The most commonly performed test for hypoglycaemia is the random blood glucose test. Here, a sample of blood is drawn and analysed for its glucose (sugar) concentration. However, this test only provides a snapshot in time of the level of sugar in the bloodstream. As blood sugar levels can vary greatly during the day, this test is virtually useless.

The Glucose Tolerance Test

A more useful test in the diagnosis of blood sugar imbalance, is the Glucose Tolerance Test (GTT). Here, a sample of blood is drawn, after which a measured dose of glucose is administered to the test subject in the form of a sugary drink. Blood samples taken at usually hourly intervals for five hours are then analysed for glucose. In individuals who have a problem regulating blood sugar, the test may reveal a rapid rise in blood sugar that often peaks at a level higher than we would like. In addition, this initial rise is often followed by a lower than normal blood sugar level some time later. While it has its place, some doctors and scientists believe that even the GTT is not the best test for blood sugar imbalance (*ref* 1). It is now thought that measuring insulin levels during the GTT is critical to the accuracy of this test. This test, known as the glucose-insulin tolerance test, is increasingly becoming regarded as the most relevant test for blood sugar imbalance.

The Glucose-Insulin Tolerance Test

In a glucose-insulin tolerance test (GITT), insulin levels are measured, along with sugar levels, for up to five hours. This test may reveal elevated insulin levels in subjects who have normal blood sugar levels (*ref* 2). Because of this, the GITT is thought to be a much more sensitive indicator of blood sugar balance than the GTT. The GITT can be a very useful test because of its ability to pick up elevated insulin levels.

Getting blood sugar back in balance

One important factor in getting blood sugar back in balance is to eat a diet based on foods which give a controlled release of sugar into the body. The speed and extent to which a food increases blood sugar can be quantified using something called the 'Glycaemic Index Scale'. Here, the speed and extent of a food's sugar release into the bloodstream is compared with glucose which is given a value of 100. The higher a food's glycaemic index, the faster it releases sugar into the bloodstream, and the worse it is for you. This is a list of the commonly eaten carbohydrates and their respective glycaemic indices:

High Glycaemic Index Foods (with glycaemic indices greater than 50)

glucose	100	cantaloupe melon	65
French baguette	95	high-fibre rye crispbread	65
Lucozade	95	couscous	65
baked potato	85	bread – rye	64
cornflakes	83	muffin	62
Rice Crispies	82	muesli bar	61
pretzels	81	ice cream	61
rice cakes	77	pizza – cheese	60
Cocopops	77	rice – white	58
doughnut	76	pitta bread – white	57
French fries	75	potato – new	57
corn chips	74	muesli	56
potato – mashed	73	popcorn	55
bagel – white	72	rice – brown	55
Sultana Bran	71	spaghetti – durum wheat	55
bread – wheat, white	71	sweetcorn	55
Shredded Wheat	69	sweet potato	54
bread – wheat, wholemeal	69	banana	54
croissant	67	Special K	45
gnocchi	67	kiwi fruit	53
pineapple	66	orange juice	52

Low Glycaemic Index Foods (with glycaemic indices up to 50)

pumpernickel	50	pear	37
porridge	49	chick peas	33
baked beans	48	butter beans	31
instant noodles	47	apricots – dried	31
grape	46	soya milk	30
orange	44	kidney beans	29
All-bran	42	lentils	29
apple juice	41	grapefruit	25
apple	38	cherries	22
spaghetti – wholemeal	37		

(Adapted from *The Glucose Revolution* by Jennie Brand-Miller and Thomas Wolever.)

The glycaemic indices have a few surprises in store

For a long time, traditional nutritional wisdom dictated that simple sugars produce rapid rises in blood sugar, while starches, because they need to be broken down to sugar prior to absorption, release more slowly into the bloodstream. However, we can see from the glycaemic index list that this is far from the truth! While some starches, e.g. oat porridge, release sugar relatively slowly, others, notably pasta, potato, bread, rice and sweetcorn, do not.

The key to establishing better blood sugar control is to base the diet around foods which truly release sugar slowly into the bloodstream. Some of the best foods for this include beans and pulses and most fresh fruits and vegetables (not potatoes though!). Protein-based foods such as meat, fish and tofu contain little or no carbohydrate and therefore do not upset blood sugar control. In fact, better than that, they can actually *help* to stabilize it. Here's why:

Protein and blood sugar control

We know that insulin lowers blood sugar levels. However, there is another important hormone called 'glucagon' which has the opposite effect. Also secreted by the pancreas, glucagon works in concert with insulin, balancing its effect. One of the major triggers for the release of glucagon is dietary protein, so in addition to cutting back on fast-releasing carbohydrates, upping our intake of protein may also help to stabilize blood sugar levels. (This theory is a central theme in the book entitled *The Zone* by Dr Barry Sears.)

I have to say I have found the addition of significant amounts of protein in the diets of my hypoglycaemic clients to be very beneficial in the great majority of cases. The question is, how much protein? It's not so much the amount of protein, but the protein to carbohydrate ratio that seems to be important here. If you want to get into the nitty-gritty of this and feel compelled to start calculating the protein and carbohydrate contents of some of your favourite foods, then you'd better invest in a copy of *The Zone*. If, however, you want a simple, low-tech guide to using protein to balance blood sugar, then you really need to know only two things.

1. If you are eating fast-releasing carbohydrate (white bread, white rice, white pasta, potato) then you need approximately the same volume of protein (meat, fish, egg, tofu) to maintain blood sugar levels. In other words, if you are eating a small baked potato you're going to need a leg of chicken or a whole 200 g (7 oz) can of tuna to balance this.
2. If you are eating slow-releasing carbohydrate (wholemeal pasta, pumpernickel, baked beans, porridge) then you need about half as much in the way of protein to keep blood sugar on an even keel.

To these meals you can add all the green and leafy vegetables you want.

A moderate amount of fast-releasing food may be OK

You might be wondering whether you need to completely exclude the high glycaemic index foods from your diet. The answer is, no, not necessarily. While the glycaemic index scores are a good guide to the tendency of a food to upset blood sugar, they actually represent the effect of a standard amount of that food eaten on its own. Basically, if we eat a lot of a high glycaemic index food, the chances are we'll get a massive rise in blood sugar and a huge surge of insulin to go with it. A much smaller amount of the same food is obviously going to be much less disruptive. There's a world of difference, for example, between eating a huge baked potato and a couple of new potatoes or a handful of chips or crisps.

Mixing meals for better balance

One way to ensure our diet is generally slow releasing is to mix foods in a way which 'dilutes' the effects of the faster releasing foods. Protein helps here, as we have already discussed. Another way would be, say, to add plenty of slow-releasing vegetables to a meal. For example, let's say you're going to eat a meal which contains white rice. White rice has a high glycaemic index and is therefore not ideal from a blood-sugar balance point of view. However, if that white rice is eaten as part of a meal which also contains some fish or lean meat, or beans and pulses with plenty of fresh, steamed vegetables such as broccoli and French beans, then it is much more likely that there will be a controlled release of sugar into the bloodstream. Studies show that the overall glycaemic index of a meal comes from a balance of the speed of sugar release of its components and their relative amounts.

Regular meals are essential to overcoming hypoglycaemia

Many hypoglycaemics do not maintain blood sugar levels at all well if a meal is skipped or delayed significantly. This is often connected to weakness in organs known as the 'adrenal glands'. This problem is discussed in more depth later on in the chapter. Obviously, though, to give our body a fighting chance of keeping blood sugar levels stable it is important to eat regular meals. Breakfast does seem to be especially important. I have very rarely seen a person with blood sugar imbalance get stability in this area without eating a breakfast of some sort or other. Also, at least in the initial stages of re-establishing better blood sugar control, it is almost always beneficial for healthy snacks to be had between meals too.

The afternoon is usually a real danger time for people with blood sugar imbalance. The insulin surge that comes after lunch can drive blood sugar levels down in the mid/late afternoon causing problems with lethargy, drowsiness and cravings for something sweet such as chocolate or biscuits. If we succumb, blood sugar levels may rise quickly which can get us out of the hole. But the body's response to this generally drives blood sugar levels back down again, putting us back at square one.

Tactical eating

If you do tend to get a problem with hypoglycaemia it can be useful to employ the principle of tactical eating. What this means is having something to eat in anticipation of low blood sugar later on, even when you don't feel hungry. Eating something before your blood sugar level drops into your boots can stop it happening at all. So, if you tend to fall to bits around 4.00 p.m., why not eat a piece or two of fruit and some raw cashew nuts around 3.00 p.m.? This will generally save a lot of grief later on.

A snack before bedtime

As we discussed earlier, hypoglycaemia in the night can cause a surge of adrenaline which can disrupt sleep. Eating a snack before bedtime can give your body 'something to chew on' while you're asleep, which can help maintain blood sugar levels (and sleep!) throughout the night. We don't want to overtax the digestive system though, so keep it light. Again, some fresh fruit and a handful of raw nuts should do the trick.

Caffeine and blood sugar control

Caffeine is a favourite energy prop of many people with blood sugar imbalance. However, caffeinated drinks such as coffee, tea, and cola are a bit of a disaster for those with unstable blood sugar levels. This is because caffeine stimulates the secretion of insulin, effectively destabilizing the blood sugar system. Caffeine, because it has stimulant effects in the body, will almost certainly pick up flagging energy levels, but its effect on blood sugar generally leads to a slump in energy later on. Another downside to caffeine is that it appears to worsen the symptoms of hypoglycaemia. This means that for a given level of blood sugar, hypoglycaemic symptoms are more likely and generally more pronounced if there is caffeine in the system.

Coming off caffeine

If you habitually take caffeine in your diet, either in coffee, tea or caffeinated soft drinks, then you would do well to kick or at least moderate this habit. One way to get off caffeine is the 'cold turkey' method, which means just stopping caffeine dead. This method is quick, but there's usually a price to pay. Anyone with a half-decent caffeine intake is likely to get caffeine withdrawal, which normally manifests itself as general fatigue accompanied by a horrendous headache. These symptoms generally last a couple of days, after which a state of calm returns pretty briskly to the system.

Another way of coming off caffeine is to gradually reduce your intake. This takes longer than the cold turkey method, but is much less painful. I generally advise my clients to reduce their intake of caffeine by a drink per day every three or four days. This means that if they drink five cups of coffee a day, then for three or four days they drink four cups per day, reducing this to three cups per day and so on until they're drinking nothing at all. Another tactic is to swap caffeinated drinks for their decaffeinated versions. Look out for coffee which has been decaffeinated using the water (also known as the 'Swiss' method) or carbon dioxide methods. These methods of decaffeination avoid the potentially hazardous solvents which are often used in the extraction process.

Artificial sweeteners

People who are quite wedded to sugar may look forward to reducing their intake of this foodstuff with some trepidation. The natural tendency may be, therefore, to opt for artificial sweeteners instead. However, there is emerging evidence that sweeteners such as aspartame (Nutrasweet, Equal) and saccharin are not necessarily the healthy alternatives to sugar they're made out to be. Aspartame may reduce levels of the brain chemical serotonin, which in turn can lead to mood and sleep disturbances (*ref* 3). Large amounts of aspartame may provoke headaches, fainting, seizures, memory loss, mood swings, depression and nausea. Small doses can cause itching and rashes in susceptible people.

And, if that isn't enough, there is some scientific evidence to suggest that artificial sweeteners may actually encourage us to eat more in the long term (*ref* 4). In one study, researchers found that subjects were inclined to eat more after eating yoghurt sweetened with saccharin than those who had eaten yoghurt sweetened with sugar (*ref* 5). One study showed that saccharin induced hypoglycaemia in test subjects, even if it was only tasted and not swallowed (*ref* 6). It looks as though the body just can't be fooled into feeling satisfied by mimicking more natural sources of sweetness.

Menu suggestions for stabilizing blood sugar levels

With the theory behind us, what does all this mean in practical terms? Here are some meal ideas based on the fundamental principles outlined in this chapter:

Breakfast

- Poached egg on whole, rye toast with grilled tomato

- Poached egg and grilled haddock or kipper with grilled tomato, mushrooms and wholewheat or whole rye toast

- Unsweetened muesli with milk (cow's, goat's, rice, soya), live natural yoghurt (this is slow-releasing), seeds and fresh fruit

- Oat porridge (oatmeal) topped with live natural yoghurt and flaked almonds

Lunch/Dinner

- Grilled trout or chicken with fresh steamed vegetables and a few boiled new potatoes

- Brown rice salad made with chicken or fish, chopped vegetables (e.g. tomato, cucumber), beans and pulses

- Spanish omelette and salad

- Smoked salmon on pumpernickel bread with salad

- Wholewheat pasta with meat or fish sauce and salad

- Chicken or fish with brown rice and steamed vegetables

In-between meal snacks

- Raw nuts and seeds

- Fresh fruit

- Rye cracker with chicken and tomato topping

Nutrients for blood sugar balance

The processes which regulate the level of sugar in the bloodstream are dependent on hormones and enzymes. The function of these hormones and enzymes is, at least in part, dependent on the availability of certain nutrients. What follows is a guide to the most important nutrients which can help combat hypoglycaemia and return you to a state of well-being.

Chromium polynicotinate – the trace mineral chromium has a very important part to play in the regulation of blood sugar levels, and can be effective in combating hypoglycaemia (*refs* 7, 8). It seems to have the capacity to regulate the action of insulin in the body, and in so doing helps to ensure efficient handling and metabolism of sugar.

Manganese – this trace mineral plays an important part in activating the enzymes which are involved in sugar metabolism in the body (*ref* 9).

Magnesium – this mineral is very important for blood sugar regulation. One of its key actions is to activate the enzymes which mediate the conversion of glycogen (a storage carbohydrate) in the body to sugar and vice versa. Magnesium supplementation has been shown to improve the action of insulin and stabilize blood sugar (*ref* 10).

There are several different forms of available magnesium. Some of the most useful forms of magnesium for blood sugar balance include:

Magnesium ascorbate – actually a buffered (non-acidic) form of vitamin C, this nutrient can also help support adrenal gland function which is often weakened in cases of sugar imbalance.

Magnesium pantothenate – also known as vitamin B5, this nutrient also supports adrenal gland function.

Magnesium malate and magnesium fumarate – both these forms of magnesium feed an energy-producing system in the body known as the Kreb's cycle.

Vitamins B1, B2 and B3 – all of these nutrients have a critical role to play in the metabolism of carbohydrate sources of energy in the body.

Suggested supplement: Glucoguard is a supplement which has been specifically formulated for improved blood sugar stability. Its chief ingredients are chromium polynicotinate, magnesium (in ascorbate, malate, fumarate and pantothenate forms), vitamins B1, B2 and B3 and manganese. For individuals who suffer from blood sugar imbalance, regular supplementation with Glucoguard is very likely to help improve energy levels, enhance mental function and reduce the tendency for food cravings.

    Dosage: 1 capsule should be taken with breakfast and supper.

    Contraindications: Glucoguard is not to be used by those who have diabetes unless under medical supervision.

    Availability: details of how to obtain Glucoguard can be found in the Useful Information section at the back of the book under the name 'VitaTech'.

Glutamine: Glutamine is an amino acid (basic building block in protein). Glutamine can be used as fuel for the brain, and can therefore be very effective in reducing the carbohydrate cravings caused by hypoglycaemia. This supplement is useful in the initial stages of the rebalancing process when food cravings are most likely to strike.

    Recommended dosage: 500 to 1,000 mg, three or four times a day.

    Availability: Glutamine is widely available in health food stores.

Case Study

Sue, a 31-year-old charity worker, was troubled by fatigue and food cravings. She woke up in the morning and, no matter how much sleep she had had, still felt tired. She also often felt tired around four o'clock in the afternoon. Sue often had 'terrible' cravings for chocolate and would generally eat a chocolate bar or two in the afternoon. She sometimes had cravings for sweet foods after supper and was quite partial to shop-bought chocolate mousse. Sue had some concern about her weight which was gradually increasing. She wanted to lose 7 lbs in weight and was keen to get control of her eating habits.

Sue's symptoms were absolutely classic of blood sugar imbalance. I asked her what she ate. Breakfast was a muffin and a cup of milky coffee. Lunch was a sandwich or a baked potato with cheese or baked beans. Supper was usually pasta or something quick from the freezer such as pizza. We discussed blood sugar balance, and I went on to recommend a diet which would be better for blood sugar control. I suggested that she make a little more time for breakfast and have a piece of 100 per cent wholemeal toast with a poached egg. If she was really short of time I suggested she eat some fresh fruit (e.g. apple, pear, orange) and some raw nuts.

For lunch I suggested that she take a salad (smoked salmon, tuna, chicken or prawn) into work and have this with one or two rye crackers. Supper was to be a piece of meat or fish with vegetables and some potato or brown rice. I also suggested she have some healthy snacks (fresh fruit and raw nuts) between meals, particularly in the middle of the afternoon. In addition I suggested she take a supplement designed to help balance blood sugar levels (Glucoguard – one capsule, twice a day).

Sue came back a month later. Already she was feeling much better. Her energy levels were much more stable. Sue was waking up feeling much more refreshed and was not getting any noticeable dip in energy in the afternoon. Although she had not mentioned a problem with mood swings at the first consultation, Sue felt these had improved considerably since changing her diet. Best of all, she was no longer craving chocolate or other sweet foods like before; there was still the occasional pang, but these were very manageable. She had also lost 4 lbs in weight and felt much happier about herself. Sue was happy to continue with her new diet and I suggested that she continue her blood sugar stabilizing supplement for another three or four months and then tail off.

The adrenal glands and their role in health

Some people just don't do well on the standard measures typically used to stabilize blood sugar levels. Despite eating regular meals and snacks based around slow sugar-releasing foods, they can still have continued problems with fluctuating energy, food cravings and a need to eat very regularly. In my experience, what is usually underlying such a problem is weakness in the adrenal glands. In recent years, there has been growing interest in the role of these in the maintenance of health and well-being. Weakness in this area may not only impair blood sugar balance, but can have profound effects in many other areas including immune function and energy.

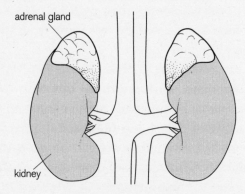

The Adrenal Glands

There are two adrenal glands, one on the top of each kidney. Each one is about the size of an apricot (see figure). The adrenal glands secrete a variety of hormones which play important roles in maintaining homeostasis, or balance, in the body. They are also the body's chief glands responsible for dealing with stress. Some of the most important hormones secreted by the adrenal glands include:

1. Adrenaline

Adrenaline is one of the main hormones secreted by the adrenal glands in response to stress. It is this hormone which is involved in what is known as the 'flight or fight' response. Among other things, adrenaline increases the heart rate and increases blood pressure. As was mentioned earlier, adrenaline can increase blood sugar levels by stimulating the conversion of glycogen into glucose.

2. Cortisol

The other main stress hormone secreted by the adrenal glands is cortisol. However, while adrenaline has a relatively short duration of action in the body, cortisol is chiefly involved in the body's handling of longer-term stress. Like adrenaline, cortisol tends to increase blood sugar levels, partly through its ability to stimulate the conversion of non-carbohydrate fuels such as amino acids (the building blocks of protein) into glucose. It also has very important roles in the regulation of various body systems including the immune system and the control of inflammation in the body. Cortisol is absolutely essential to life, but like anything else, you can get too much of a good thing. Prolonged stress can cause higher than normal levels of cortisol, which may in turn lead to problems such as impairment of the immune system, insomnia and depression.

3. Dihydroepiandrosterone (DHEA)

DHEA has a number of regulating roles in the body such as helping in the growth and repair of proteins in body tissues, especially muscle. This hormone also plays a part in the processes that heal tissues after injury or infection. In addition, DHEA can be converted into other hormones, principally testosterone and oestrogen, which themselves have important actions in the body.

4. Aldosterone

Aldosterone is what is referred to as a 'mineralocorticoid' – essentially meaning that it participates in the regulation of minerals in the body. Aldosterone helps to preserve sodium levels in the body, and encourages loss of potassium. These actions help to maintain fluid levels and blood pressure.

Adrenal weakness

In some individuals, adrenal function may be somewhat weakened. This condition is sometimes referred to as 'hypoadrenalism', 'adrenal exhaustion' or 'adrenal weakness'. Some of the most prominent symptoms of adrenal weakness include:

1. Fatigue

Adrenally weakened individuals tend to be tired. They often lack the get up and go they once took for granted. They quite often have to force themselves through the day, and may prop themselves up with caffeine to give themselves the energy they need. As time goes on, these individuals tend to need more and more sleep. However, despite taking more sleep, they very often feel very tired on waking.

2. 'Fatigueability'

Adrenally weakened individuals often have little in the way of energy 'reserve'. Not only do they generally feel tired, but they often get tired out quite easily. I use the term 'fatigueability' to describe this feature of the condition. For people with adrenal weakness, any additional stress (of a physiological and/or emotional nature) on the body can cause real energy lows. A busy week at work, the stress associated with a child's illness, or a couple of late nights can be all it takes to bring energy crashing down.

One activity which tends to bring this concept to the fore is exercise. People with good adrenal function tend to feel buoyed up and energized by exercise. While adrenally weakened individuals may feel emotionally satisfied to have taken exercise, the fact is it can lead them to feel tired and 'wiped out'. Some are so compromised that even orgasm leaves them feeling drained and physically weak.

Fatigue and 'fatigueability' are two very common features of the condition 'chronic fatigue syndrome'. In my experience, adrenal weakness is a common underlying feature in this condition. What is more, many cases of chronic fatigue syndrome tend to respond to measures designed to support adrenal gland function.

3. Low blood pressure

Low blood pressure (hypotension) is quite a common feature in people who have weak adrenal function. The normal blood pressure is usually around 120–130/70–80 mmHg. Adrenally weakened individuals often have a blood pressure of 110/70 mmHg or less. Their blood pressure also tends to drop on standing from a seated or lying position. This condition, the medical term for which is 'postural hypotension', can cause occasional dizziness on standing.

There is a theory that the hypotension characteristic of adrenal weakness is caused by a failure of the adrenal glands to secrete sufficient quantities of the hormone aldosterone. A lack of aldosterone can lead to the body losing sodium, lowering blood pressure as it does this.

4. Salt craving

Some individuals with adrenal weakness will crave salt. Probably what is going on here is that the body is looking to salt to help replenish sodium, which is not being retained due to a lack of aldosterone or other hormones.

5. The need to eat regularly

People with adrenal weakness tend to need to eat regularly to keep them from feeling weak and light-headed. If the body is not being fuelled from the outside (by eating), the body needs to generate sugar from the breakdown of stored fuels in the body such as glycogen in the liver. If the adrenal glands are weakened, it is possible that the stress hormones, such as cortisol, are not made in sufficient quantities to enable adequate amounts of sugar to be mobilized in this way.

Is adrenal weakness your problem?

1. Do you sometimes feel dizzy on standing from sitting or lying down?

No	0 points
Occasional or mild problems	2 points
Frequent or severe problems	4 points

2. **Do you ever crave salt or salty foods such as salted peanuts or crisps?**

No	0 points
Occasional or mild problems	2 points
Frequent or severe problems	4 points

3. **Do you suffer from persistent fatigue which does not appear to have any identifiable cause?**

No	0 points
Occasional or mild problems	2 points
Frequent or severe problems	4 points

4. **Can you feel 'wiped out' after strenuous exercise?**

No	0 points
Occasional or mild problems	2 points
Frequent or severe problems	4 points

5. **Are you prone to mood swings and/or irritability if a meal is skipped?**

No	0 points
Occasional or mild problems	2 points
Frequent or severe problems	4 points

6. **Do you feel the need to eat very regularly?**

No	0 points
Occasional or mild problems	2 points
Frequent or severe problems	4 points

7. **Do you feel tired or groggy on waking, despite sleeping for eight or more hours?**

No	0 points
Occasional or mild problems	2 points
Frequent or severe problems	4 points

8. **Are you generally slight in stature and find it difficult to gain weight?**

Yes	4 points
No	0 points

9. **Do you tend to 'feel the cold' but also find yourself intolerant of heat too?**

Yes	4 points
No	0 points

10. Do you tend to be prone to allergic conditions such as hay fever, asthma, or sensitivity to perfumes, paint fumes and cigarette smoke?

Yes	4 points
No	0 points

Interpreting your score

0–15: adrenal weakness is unlikely

16–28: adrenal weakness is quite likely and measures taken to strengthen adrenal function are likely to be of benefit

29 and above: adrenal weakness is very likely, and measures taken to strengthen adrenal function are highly recommended

What causes the adrenal glands to weaken?

The adrenal glands are only really designed to cope with relatively defined periods of stress. During our evolution, the adrenal glands were adapted to coping with relatively short and defined periods of stress. However, these days, the frenetic pace of life and the challenges brought by modern-day living can cause the adrenal glands to weaken in time. Almost incessant stimulation of the adrenal glands can eventually take their toll.

In my experience, adrenal weakness almost always manifests in individuals who are 'doers'. Usually from an early age, these people have been used to packing a lot into the day. As children, they are often quite academic and competitive, possibly with a sporty bent too. They often progress to busy jobs with long working hours. If they are women and have opted for a family, usually they are juggling a number of different commitments. Some describe themselves as chronically 'stressed', and are often consumed with personal, financial and/or work-related pressures.

It is also possible that the adrenal glands may malfunction as a result of something known as 'auto-immune disease'. Auto-immune diseases are those in which the immune system reacts against the body's own tissues. Addison's disease (adrenal insufficiency) is known in many cases to be an auto-immune disease, where the immune system is reacting to adrenal tissue. It is entirely possible that the cause of low adrenal function in some individuals is due to this.

Laboratory tests for adrenal function

At this stage, it is probably useful to distinguish adrenal weakness from another condition – 'adrenal insufficiency' or Addison's disease. This is characterized by extreme adrenal weakness to the extent that regular doses of steroids (such as cortisol) and perhaps other drugs are necessary to maintain health. This condition is severe, but thankfully rare.

To understand the laboratory tests for adrenal function, we need to know a little more about the physiology of the adrenal glands. The secretion of stress hormones is governed by another hormone known as adrenocorticotrophic hormone (ACTH for short). ACTH is secreted by the pituitary gland, a small organ at the base of the brain. When we become stressed, the pituitary gland makes more ACTH, which stimulates the adrenal glands to make stress hormones such as cortisol. When the stress goes away, ACTH levels decline and so does the production of stress hormones from the adrenal glands.

The main conventional medical test used is something called the 'short ACTH stimulation test' – also known as the 'Synacthen® test'. Here a blood sample is taken, after which an injection of ACTH is given. Half an hour later a second sample of blood is taken. The cortisol levels are measured in both samples. If the first sample shows a low level of cortisol, and/or if there is not a sufficient rise in the cortisol level in response to ACTH, further testing is usually advised.

The next test which is commonly used is the 'prolonged ACTH stimulation test'. Here, ACTH is given on three consecutive days. If the cortisol level has failed to reach a certain level six hours after the last injection, Addison's disease is diagnosed.

Many doctors do not believe in the concept of adrenal weakness. The attitude here is that if blood tests do not show Addison's disease, then the adrenal gland function is fine. However, is it not possible that between fabulous adrenal function and Addison's disease there are many shades of grey in between? The fact is, the conventional criteria used to diagnose adrenal problems tell us only whether or not someone has Addison's disease. Unfortunately, most individuals with evidence of adrenal weakness are simply labelled as 'normal'.

Someone who did a lot of pioneering work on adrenal health is the

American doctor William McK Jefferies. In his book *Safe Uses of Cortisol Acetate*, he describes his own version of the short ACTH test. Here, cortisol levels are compared before and half to one hour after an injection of ACTH. According to Dr McK Jefferies, if the second sample does not show a doubling of the original cortisol level, this signifies adrenal weakness.

Adrenal hormones can also be measured using saliva samples. One of the most commonly used tests is known as the adrenal stress index (ASI) test. Here four saliva samples taken at intervals during the day are measured. The test aims to detect any abnormality in the 'normal' levels of cortisol, which are generally high in the morning, and gradually decline during the day. In addition, one of these samples is also analysed for levels of DHEA.

Any disruption of the cortisol rhythm and either high (rare) or low (common) DHEA suggests adrenal weakness. One of the reservations I have with this test is that, like most tests, it really only provides a snapshot of adrenal function on a given day. Also, even though the test takes several measures of cortisol in that day, it does not measure the adrenal *response*. Plus, there is much controversy about whether it is possible to measure adrenal hormones accurately in the saliva, particularly the active form of DHEA known as DHEA-sulphate.

If your symptoms suggest adrenal weakness, then by all means seek out a practitioner who can give you access to these tests. All tests have some use and validity. However, remember also that no test will always tell us what is really going on in the body.

Blood pressure, adrenal weakness and chronic fatigue

In practice, if an individual's symptoms suggest low adrenal function, I will want to take their blood pressure. I am suspicious if this is on the low side (110/70 mmHg or less). Even more telling is if the blood pressure tends to drop on standing (the medical term for which is 'postural hypotension').

Clinically, many individuals with adrenal weakness have been diagnosed as having a condition known as chronic fatigue syndrome (CFS). The official line on the cause of CFS is that it remains a mystery. However, in my experience there are many different factors which can underlie CFS, including food sensitivity, nutrient deficiency, inefficient breathing and low thyroid function. However, I see adrenal weakness as a very common and under-diagnosed problem too.

It comes as no surprise that while postural hypotension is a common feature in adrenal weakness, research suggests that it is also a common feature in CFS (*ref* 11). Another study which suggests a link between CFS and adrenal weakness is one in which it was found that CFS sufferers had less than half the amount of adrenal tissue compared to healthy subjects (*ref* 12). Work in animals has shown that stress initially causes the glands to enlarge. However, in long term stress, glands have been shown to reduce in size or 'atrophy'.

Restoring adrenal health

I'll say from the outset, restoring health to the adrenals is not always easy, and doesn't generally happen overnight. However, if successful, adrenal enhancement almost always leads to a significant and sustained improvement in an individual's well-being and vitality. There are a number of different approaches which can be taken, including the use of natural substances.

Supplements for supporting the adrenal glands

There are a range of nutrients and herbs which appear to help support adrenal function and restore health to the area. Some of the most widely used natural agents are:

VITAMIN C
In the whole body, the place where vitamin C is found in highest concentration is the adrenal gland. Vitamin C is thought to play an important part in adrenal gland function, which is why practitioners of natural medicine often advise supplements with this nutrient in

cases of adrenal weakness. A good dose would be 1 g of vitamin C, twice a day.

VITAMIN B5

Vitamin B5, also known as pantothenic acid, is believed to be important for adrenal gland function. A dose of 500 mg taken twice a day provides a good level of vitamin B5.

GINSENG

One of the most popular agents for treating adrenal weakness is Siberian ginseng (*Eleutherococcus senticosus*). Siberian ginseng has been shown to have a number of beneficial effects on the physiology of both animals and humans. One of this herb's most important effects appears to be an ability to protect the adrenal glands, increasing their capacity to withstand prolonged stress. In animals, Siberian ginseng has been shown to protect against the effects of a wide range of potential stresses, including heat, cold, surgery, blood loss and infection. Numerous studies have shown that Siberian ginseng can be of benefit in a diverse array of individuals including explorers, sailors, deep sea divers, rescue workers, truck drivers, pilots and factory workers.

Siberian ginseng is widely available in health food stores. The normal dose is 1–4 g of dried herb per day, or 2–8 ml per day of a liquid extract. Sometimes, Siberian ginseng products will be standardized to the content of one of its active ingredients, a compound known as eleutheroside E. As an example, 1.25 g tablets containing 0.7 mg of eleutheroside E should be taken 1–3 times a day. Traditionally, it is recommended that Siberian ginseng be taken for periods of six weeks, interspersed with breaks of two weeks. Siberian ginseng appears to be safe to take in the long term.

LICORICE

Another natural substance which is commonly used in natural medicine to treat adrenal weakness is licorice. Licorice contains a compound called glycyrrhizin. In the body, glycyrrhizin breaks down to glycyrrhetinic acid. Glycyrrhetinic acid has anti-inflammatory actions in the body, and also slows down the breakdown of cortisol in the

Ultimate Health

body. In this way, licorice can enhance the effects of cortisol, and
may help to 'take the strain off' the adrenal glands.

The normal recommended dose is 5–6 g of whole licorice root
taken in two or three divided doses during the day. Alternatively 250
to 500 mg of concentrated extract can be taken three times a day.
High doses of licorice can lead to sodium accumulation and a loss of
the mineral potassium in the body. These changes may increase blood
pressure. Even though this may have positive benefit for someone
suffering from hypotension, it does pose a small risk. For this reason,
it is best that licorice is taken under the supervision of a practitioner
experienced in its use.

Suggested supplement: Adrenol is a supplement which has been specifically formulated to improve adrenal gland health. Its chief ingredients
are vitamin C, vitamin B5, licorice and Siberian ginseng. Details of
how to obtain Adrenol can be found in the Useful Information section
at the back of the book under the name 'VitaTech'.

Dosage: 1 capsule should be taken with breakfast and supper.

Medications

Cortisol

If the adrenal glands are weak, and there is evidence that they are not
producing sufficient quantities of cortisol, then it makes sense that
supplementing with cortisol might help. This concept is explored in
Safe Uses of Cortisol Acetate, by Dr McK Jefferies who writes about the
use of low-dose cortisone in the treatment of many health conditions,
including chronic fatigue. The dosing regime he recommends is 5 mg
of hydroxycortisone, four times a day (one dose with each meal and
then again before bed). He reported impressive results for many
individuals with evidence of adrenal weakness using this regime.

There is some support for the use of low-dose hydrocortisone in
medical literature. One study found that 5–10 mg of hydrocortisone
given each day for just a month significantly reduced fatigue and
disability in a group of individuals with CFS (*ref* 13). Another trial
found benefits from 25–35 mg of hydrocortisone a day, although this

dose also seemed to suppress the adrenal glands' own output of cortisol.

While hydrocortisone may offer benefit to adrenally weakened individuals, particularly those with CFS, it needs to be used with caution. My advice is generally that no more than 15 mg should be taken each day (as 5 mg taken three times each day) as any more may suppress the adrenal function. I recommend working closely with a practitioner who is experienced in the use of low-dose cortisol.

DHEA

As with cortisol, DHEA may be used to supplement inadequate levels of this hormone due to adrenal weakness. Useful doses are in the range of 5–15 mg for women and 10–30 mg for men. While DHEA is available over the counter in some countries (notably the USA), my feeling is that it should not be used unless under the guidance of a practitioner.

Adrenal glandulars

In the next chapter I talk about how the use of preparations of thyroid tissue (also known as 'thyroid glandulars') may help individuals who have low thyroid function. It is also true that adrenal glandulars can help some sufferers of adrenal weakness. Again, adrenal glandulars are best taken under the supervision of a practitioner experienced in their use.

Case Study

Alan, a 24-year-old self-employed systems analyst, came to see me complaining of 'fainting spells'. Increasingly frequently Alan would suddenly find himself feeling light-headed and 'woozy', to the extent that he would sometimes need to lie down. After several minutes he would usually feel well enough to stand up again, although he might feel quite drowsy for several hours after the event. Alan had had a number of conventional medical tests including an EEG (an electrical trace of the brain) and a brain scan. All test results were normal.

Because fainting is associated with low blood pressure, and this can be a sign of adrenal weakness, I asked about other symptoms that would suggest this. Alan said that his energy was 'fine', but did confess to needing to consume several cups of coffee and often a couple of cans of diet cola to keep him going through the day. I asked how he felt in the evening, at the weekend, and when he was on holiday. 'Pretty shattered' was the reply. I wondered whether there might be a degree of blood sugar imbalance too. Alan did not have sweet cravings, but he did feel the need to eat very regularly. He had the impression that his fainting spells were more likely to come on if he had not eaten for some time. He also said that he could also feel tired in the late afternoon which is when he tended to want coffee or diet cola.

I took his blood pressure which was 110/70 mmHg (low) when he was sitting, dropping to 100/66 mmHg when he stood up. We discussed adrenal weakness and blood sugar balance. I made some recommendations about how he might adjust his lifestyle, and in particular his work practices, to reduce the stress he was under. I suggested he see a clinical psychologist specializing in work/life balance to get expert help in this area. I recommended a diet designed to improve blood sugar control and a supplement designed to help with this. I also recommended a combination supplement to help enhance adrenal function (Adrenol).

I asked Alan to return in two months. He had adjusted his working hours, and was certainly working less hard. He was no longer working in the evenings or weekends, which he had been prior to his visit. He had adhered well to a blood sugar stabilizing diet, and in particular was eating regularly, including healthy snacks such as raw nuts in between meals. His caffeine consumption had dropped: no diet cola and just two cups of coffee per day.

His fainting spells, which had been once or twice each week, were now about every two weeks. His blood pressure was slightly higher (115/70 mmHg dropping to 110/65 on standing). He felt more energetic, though fatigue was still a factor in the evenings and at weekends. I suggested that he continue his current regime and come back in three months.

Between his second and third visit Alan continued to improve. In the last month he had only one fainting spell, the day after a particularly stressful event at work. He felt much stronger in himself, and seemed a lot happier. With continued adrenal support and the lasting changes in his working practices, Alan continued to be well and remained free of the fainting spells that once plagued him.

Summary

- The body likes to keep the level of sugar in the bloodstream within relatively narrow limits

- Blood sugar instability is a major underlying factor in obesity and other health problems including fatigue and diabetes

- In most cases, blood sugar instability can be diagnosed on the basis of symptoms. The best laboratory test is the glucose insulin tolerance test

- Individuals who suffer from hypoglycaemia should base their diet around foods which release sugar slowly into the bloodstream including beans, pulses, vegetables (other than the potato) and fresh fruit. Protein in the diet (e.g. natural yoghurt, eggs, meat, fish and tofu) can also help to stabilize blood sugar levels

- Regular meals should be taken (including breakfast) with healthy snacks such as fruit and raw nuts in between

- Supplements of certain nutrients such as chromium, vitamin B3 and magnesium can help improve blood sugar stability and control the symptoms of hypoglycaemia

- Weakness in the adrenal glands can underlie a problem with blood sugar imbalance and may cause significant health issues

- Common problems associated with adrenal weakness include fatigue, fatigue after exercise, the need for regular meals, salt craving and low blood pressure

- Nutrients and herbs which can help restore adrenal health include vitamin C, vitamin B5, Siberian ginseng and licorice

- Other agents which may help to restore adrenal health and improve health include cortisol, DHEA and adrenal glandulars

- Better blood sugar balance and restoration of adrenal gland health can often lead to very significant improvements in energy, general health and well-being

5. Maintain Thyroid Function

The thyroid is a gland, about the size and shape of a bow tie, which sits in the front of the neck just above the top of the breastbone and collarbones (see diagram overleaf). The thyroid is essentially the body's thermostat, and determines its temperature and the speed at which it burns fuel. Each cell in the body burns fuel for energy, some of which is released as heat. The speed at which the cells do this, also known as the 'metabolism', is regulated by the thyroid. If, for any reason, thyroid function should falter, *all* the cells in the body tend not to function as well as they should. The problems associated with low thyroid function are incredibly diverse and include a tendency to feel the cold, fatigue, mental lethargy, frequent infections, depression, and dry skin and hair. Ensuring proper thyroid function has important implications for physical and mental health.

The physiology of the thyroid

The thyroid produces a variety of hormones, the most important of which is thyroxine (also known as 'T4'). Outside the thyroid, T4 is converted into T3 (tri-iodothyronine), which is the active form of the hormone. In normal circumstances T3 travels in the bloodstream to all the body's tissues, entering each of the body's cells. T3 stimulates cells to burn fuel with oxygen to release energy, some of this being released as heat. Essentially, the more T3 there is around, the faster the metabolism, the less tendency there is for weight gain and the warmer the body is.

The thyroid's production of hormones is itself regulated by another gland, the pituitary, which sits underneath the front of the brain. One of the pituitary's jobs is to monitor and control the level of thyroid hormones in the blood. If the pituitary senses that thyroid hormone levels are dropping, it increases its own production of a substance

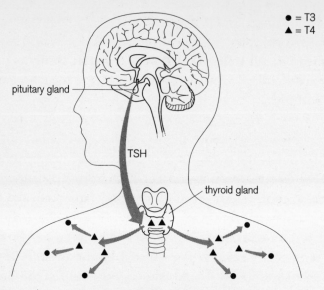

● = T3
▲ = T4

pituitary gland

TSH

thyroid gland

Location of the Thyroid Gland

known as 'thyroid stimulating hormone' (TSH). This hormone instructs the thyroid to produce more thyroid hormones, thereby up-regulating the metabolism. As the thyroid hormone levels rise, the production of TSH is down-regulated, bringing thyroid hormone levels back down again. This mechanism is designed to ensure stable levels of thyroid hormones in the body.

The thyroid and health

The effect of thyroid hormones on the body is far-reaching. A lack of thyroid hormones, referred to by the medical profession as hypothyroidism, can bring about a whole host of symptoms and conditions. We have already touched on the tendency for a sluggish thyroid to lead to weight gain. In addition, with low levels of thyroid hormones the body tends to retain water, salt and protein. Blood cholesterol levels also tend to rise when thyroid hormones are deficient. The growth of the skin, hair and nails all tend to be slower when thyroid hormones are in short supply. Thyroid hormones are essential for the normal functioning of the nervous system, and mental fatigue and sluggishness are common in individuals who suffer from low thyroid function. The thyroid is intimately woven with other elements of the hormone system, such as glands which control sexual function. As a result, men often manifest low thyroid function as impotence while women may suffer from menstrual problems including heavy or irregular periods.

Is low thyroid function your problem?

The following questionnaire is designed to help you identify a potential thyroid problem. Score each question as indicated, and then add up your total score.

1. Do you suffer from unexplained fatigue or lethargy?

No	0 points
Occasional or mild problems	2 points
Frequent or severe problems	4 points

2. Do you find that your energy can be low in the morning even after a good night's sleep?

No	0 points
Occasional or mild problems	3 points
Frequent or severe problems	5 points

3. Do you feel the cold, and have to wrap up more than other people?

No	0 points
Occasional or mild problems	3 points
Frequent or severe problems	5 points

4. Do you suffer from cold hands and feet?

No	0 points
Occasional or mild problems	2 points
Frequent or severe problems	4 points

5. Do you suffer from dry skin?

No	0 points
Occasional or mild problems	1 point
Frequent or severe problems	2 points

6. **Do you suffer from dry or brittle hair?**

No	0 points
Occasional or mild problems	2 points
Frequent or severe problems	4 points

7. **Do you find that you do not sweat much even when you exercise?**

No	0 points
Yes	4 points

8. **Do you suffer from constipation?**

No	0 points
Occasional or mild problems	2 points
Frequent or severe problems	4 points

9. **Do you find it very difficult to lose weight, despite eating less or exercising more?**

No	0 points
Yes	5 points

10. **Do you suffer from swelling in the face?**

No	0 points
Occasional or mild problems	2 points
Frequent or severe problems	4 points

11. **Do you find that your eyelids tend to be swollen and puffy?**

No	0 points
Occasional or mild problems	2 points
Frequent or severe problems	4 points

12. **Do you find that you suffer from bags under your eyes?**

No	0 points
Occasional or mild problems	2 points
Frequent or severe problems	4 points

13. **Do you feel that your memory is not what it used to be?**

No	0 points
Occasional or mild problems	1 point
Frequent or severe problems	2 points

14. Do you have yellowing of the skin, particularly in the palms of the hand and soles of the feet?

No	0 points
Occasional or mild problems	2 points
Frequent or severe problems	4 points

15. Do you suffer from depression?

No	0 points
Occasional or mild problems	2 points
Frequent or severe problems	4 points

16. Do you suffer from ankle swelling?

No	0 points
Occasional or mild problems	2 points
Frequent or severe problems	4 points

17. Do you feel that your movements are somewhat slow?

No	0 points
Occasional or mild problems	3 points
Frequent or severe problems	5 points

18. Do you suffer from a hoarse voice which is not connected to throat infection?

No	0 points
Occasional or mild problems	3 points
Frequent or severe problems	5 points

19. Do you think that you are less mentally sharp than you used to be?

No	0 points
Occasional or mild problems	2 points
Frequent or severe problems	4 points

20. Do you feel that your eyebrows are not as thick as they used to be?

No	0 points
Yes	5 points

Interpreting your score

0–9: low thyroid function is very unlikely

10–24: low thyroid function should be considered as a possibility and testing (see below) is recommended

25–39: low thyroid function is quite likely, testing is highly recommended
40 and above: low thyroid function is very likely, testing is highly recommended (see below), and thyroid support is likely to be of benefit

Testing for low thyroid function

If answering the questionnaire above has aroused your suspicions about your thyroid, you may consider having your thyroid status assessed with a conventional blood test. My feeling is that while conventional blood testing may pick up some individuals with low thyroid function, it misses a lot of others. Let me explain why:

T4 and TSH – good in theory but not necessarily in practice

The conventional medical test for hypothyroidism involves drawing a blood sample and having this measured for TSH (thyroid stimulating hormone) and T4 (thyroxine). In theory, if thyroid function is low, then we should see this reflected in a low T4 level. As TSH tends to rise as T4 falls, the low T4 should be accompanied by a high TSH level. Some individuals with hypothyroidism do indeed have low T4 and high TSH levels. However, many people who have clear symptoms and signs of low thyroid function, have a 'normal' blood test. Why is this?

The normal ranges of thyroid hormones are determined by measuring the hormone levels of a group of people deemed to have normal thyroid function. The question is, how can we be sure that the sample of the population used to assess what is 'normal' is actually representative of good thyroid function? Assessing thyroid function clinically is notoriously difficult, and this certainly opens up the possibility that the population whose hormone levels were used to set the normal range actually included individuals with sub-optimal thyroid function.

Another potential deficiency of conventional thyroid testing is that while it may show the level of hormones in the bloodstream, it does not tell us how active and effective those hormones are. It is now well recognized, for instance, that individuals can become resistant to the hormone insulin (known as 'insulin resistance'), which may eventually lead to a problem with diabetes. It is possible, therefore, that individuals may have perfectly normal levels of thyroid hormones in their systems, but that their bodies are failing to respond.

Assessing thyroid function using a simple home test

Last century, an American doctor called Broda Barnes became very interested in the thyroid. After years of research, he came to the conclusion that it is possible to get a very good idea of thyroid function by measuring an individual's temperature first thing in the morning (*ref* 1). The theory behind this is that in the absence of an infection the body's temperature is essentially determined by thyroid function. Low thyroid function is therefore often reflected in a low body temperature.

To assess body temperature, Barnes developed the following test, which is usually referred to as the Barnes test.

Take a mercury thermometer and before you go to sleep shake it down and leave it by the bed. On waking, before getting up, place the bulb of the thermometer in your armpit and wait for a full ten minutes. Record the temperature.

A mercury thermometer should be used as these seem to be more accurate than the newer digital models currently available. The ten minute 'cooking time' is important because it is essential to make sure the mercury has risen to its maximum value before the reading is taken. Men and post-menopausal women can take the temperature on any day, as long as they don't have an infection. Because pre-menopausal women's temperatures tend to fluctuate with the hormonal cycle, Barnes suggested that the most accurate time to assess temperature was on the second, third and fourth day of the period. The normal body temperature in the morning is between 36.6 and 36.8 °C (97.8 to 98.2 °F). A temperature which is 36.4 °C (97.4 °F) or less strongly suggests low thyroid function.

What could be causing low thyroid function?

A few theories have been put forward to explain the apparent prevalence of thyroid-related problems in the population. These are:

1. **Iodine deficiency**
   Iodine is an essential nutrient for thyroid function. Without it the thyroid gland tends to malfunction and enlarge, creating what is known as a goitre. Goitres, and other symptoms of hypothyroidism, are rare in Japan, a country with a population having a very high intake of iodine. Iodine deficiencies, and therefore goitres, are common in mountainous or inland areas far from the sea, such as the Alps and Pyrenees in Europe, the Andes in South America and the Himalayas of Asia.

    Another theory relating to iodine is that it may not be able to do its job, even though it is available in adequate amounts to the body. Iodine comes from the same chemical group as fluorine, chlorine and bromine. These substances are becoming increasingly more common in the environment, and some scientists think that they may interfere with the way iodine is utilized by the body.

2. **Chemical pollutants**
   There is some evidence that goitres can occur as a result of poisoning by chemical substances. The increasing prevalence of pollutants in the environment might therefore be a factor in problems with hypothyroidism.

3. **Genetic factors**
   Hypothyroidism can lead to increased susceptibility to infection and reduced sexual functioning. In the past, because of these factors, many sufferers of hypothyroidism did not get the opportunity to pass their genes on to future generations. With the advent of antibiotics and effective thyroid treatments, this has all changed, meaning that the genes which may increase the likelihood of thyroid disease are now likely to be much more prevalent.

Treating a sluggish thyroid

There are several options for treating a low thyroid function. From a physiological point of view, the main treatments are:
1. Nutrients and herbs
2. Thyroxine
3. Thyroid extracts

1. Nutrients and herbs

There are several herbs and nutrients which may be of benefit in supporting thyroid function. These are the best of the bunch:

IODINE

As discussed earlier in the chapter, iodine is an essential component of the thyroid hormones, and without it, the thyroid simply cannot make these hormones in sufficient quantity. Supplementing with iodine, for instance in the form of kelp or dulse, may therefore help to improve thyroid function.

Caution: Iodine is one of those nutrients for which too much can be a bad thing. High levels of iodine may in fact suppress thyroid function. Do not exceed 500 microgrammes (mcg) per day unless under the instruction of a doctor with an interest in this area.

SELENIUM

Low selenium may reduce the effectiveness of the thyroid hormones. Selenium participates in the conversion of T_4 into T_3, and a deficiency of selenium may stall this process. Other studies have also linked low levels of selenium with hypothyroidism.

Caution: Very high levels of selenium may actually lower levels of T_3. It is important, therefore, not to exceed 300 mcg per day unless under the advice of a doctor.

VITAMIN A

Vitamin A has a very important role to play in thyroid function, and a deficiency of this does seem to significantly affect thyroid output.

Caution: Women who are pregnant or are planning pregnancy should not take more than 10,000 IU (international units) of vitamin A per day in supplement form.

CALCIUM AND MAGNESIUM

Calcium and magnesium are important minerals which help in the regulation of the function of the thyroid and parathyroid glands.

L-TYROSINE

L-Tyrosine is an amino acid which has an essential role in the formation of thyroid hormones. Tyrosine has also been found to help in the treatment of hypothyroidism.

L-GLUTAMINE AND L-GLYCINE

These two amino acids are required for normal functioning of the thyroid gland.

SPECIFIC SUPPLEMENTS

Thyranol is a supplement specifically formulated to support thyroid function. Its principle ingredients are dulse (a source of iodine), selenium, vitamin A, calcium, magnesium, tyrosine, glutamine and glycine. Thyranol also contains Siberian ginseng (which can help in the regulation of body temperature) and licorice (which can give general support to the body's hormonal system). Long-term supplementation with Thyranol can help to stimulate thyroid function, and reverse symptoms of hypothyroidism, including sensitivity to cold, fatigue and weight gain.

Contraindications: Thyranol should not be used during pregnancy or if pregnancy is being planned. Advice should be sought from a doctor if conventional thyroid medication is being taken.

Details of how to obtain Thyranol can be found in the section entitled Useful Information at the back of the book under the name 'VitaTech'.

2. *Thyroxine*

The conventional medical approach to hypothyroidism is centred around the use of a synthetic version of the hormone thyroxine (T4). This is normally administered at a dose of 50 to 100 mcg per day, and increased in doses of 50 mcg every three or four weeks until blood results come into the normal range. The usual maintenance dose is between 100 and 200 mcg.

Certainly, some hypothyroid individuals feel significant benefit from taking thyroxine in the right dose. However, there are also many others who do not. Often, people who have been diagnosed hypothyroid feel little or no better on thyroxine treatment.

One reason for this may be that some individuals may have a problem converting thyroxine into T3, the active form of the hormone. If you are currently taking thyroxine and feel it is not doing as much for you as you would like, it might be worth adding a selenium supplement to your regime, as this helps in the conversion of thyroxine to T3. Take 200 mcg per day.

Some doctors prescribe T3 for low thyroid function, either with or without thyroxine. This obviously gets round any problem there may be with the conversion of thyroxine into T3. T3 has a much shorter duration of action in the body than thyroxine, and this makes regular dosing quite important. However, T3 can offer significant benefit for people who do not respond to thyroxine.

In addition to thyroxine, the thyroid also secretes a hormone called di-iodotyrosine. Some doctors believe that this hormone has a more important effect than thyroxine in regulating thyroid gland function. This may help to explain why some people fail to feel real benefit from treatment with thyroxine alone.

3. *Thyroid extracts*

Some doctors, usually naturally orientated ones, recommend supplements which contain actual thyroid tissue. These extracts, often referred to as 'thyroid glandulars', are usually made from cow or pig thyroid, and contain not just T4, but T3 also. It is believed that the range of hormones available in a glandular supplement is much more likely to have a beneficial effect on hypothyroid individuals than the single hormone conventional treatment.

Some people who do not do well on thyroxine seem to respond much better to glandular supplements. The most widely used thyroid glandular in the USA is a product called Armour desiccated thyroid. Often, patients are started on a quarter to a half a grain of this product per day, after which the dose is increased by a quarter or a half a grain increments every seven to ten days, until the patient feels well. Adults usually require a maintenance dose of between one and three grains a day.

Apart from containing a range of hormones, rather than just one, are there any other advantages for using a thyroid glandular over thyroxine? People who start on thyroxine usually take it for the rest of their lives. This doesn't seem to be so true for those on thyroid glandulars. It seems that after a period of treatment (between one and two years is typical), it is possible for people to wean themselves off thyroid glandulars without ill-effect. Why this should be is not known for sure, but it is thought that giving glandular products may give the thyroid the opportunity to rest and recover in time. I have a strong suspicion that thyroid recovery of this nature is even more likely if other thyroid supportive measures are taken. I often find that the best results are achieved through using a combination of nutrients, herbs and glandular-based products.

CAUTION:

I strongly recommend that anyone considering using thyroid glandulars should work with a doctor with experience and expertise in this area. Thyroid glandulars must be used with special caution in those with a history of heart disease. They also have the potential for side-effects if taken in excess, such as anxiety, nervousness, palpitations, excessive weight loss and insomnia.

Monitoring your progress

With the appropriate support, thyroid function can improve in time. As it does this, you may start to notice changes in your health that reflect this improved function. You can expect general improvements in your levels of energy, both physical and mental, and less tendency to depression if this is a feature in you. In my view, the best way to monitor your progress with regard to your thyroid function specifically is the Barnes test. In practice, I have found that symptoms of low thyroid function do not resolve unless the temperature approaches normal, and that the temperature correlates very well with the overall functioning of the thyroid.

Case Study

Helen, a 39-year-old magazine editor, came to see me complaining of an inability to lose weight. She weighed 151 lbs, but she felt most comfortable at round 130 lbs. However, despite eating a very meagre diet, she was unable to lose any weight at all. She was not exercising, but a stint of gym sessions three times a week and a spartan diet a few months previously had had practically no effect. Another of Helen's problems was that she was tired. Getting out of bed was difficult, and she would often collapse in the evening. On questioning, she also confessed to having cold hands and feet, undue sensitivity to cold, and dry hair.

I suspected that Helen's thyroid function was low so I asked her to do the Barnes test. I also took a sample of blood for thyroid function testing. Helen's TSH level was normal, but her T4 and T3 levels were on the low side. Plus, her Barnes test revealed a body temperature of just 35.9 °C. Helen started on a blend of nutrients and herbs designed for the thyroid (Thyranol).

When Helen returned in two months she was quite a lot happier. The weight loss had not been dramatic (6 lbs), but she was at least satisfied that something had started to shift. She also had more energy and felt warmer. She returned in another two months. Between visits she had made continued improvement. She had lost more weight (another 5 lbs), and again her energy was better. She said that her mood was also brighter, and she had a better outlook on life. Helen continued to do well on this regime, and got down to the weight she felt suited her in a total of about seven months.

Summary

- Undiagnosed low thyroid function plays a major role in problems with health and vitality

- Common symptoms of low thyroid function include sensitivity to cold, weight gain, cold hands and feet, dry skin and hair, puffiness around the eyes, low mood and lethargy

- The conventional blood tests designed to diagnose low thyroid function may miss a significant proportion of sufferers

- Diagnosing hypothyroidism may be better done on the basis of an individual's symptoms and the Barnes temperature test

- The treatment options for a sluggish thyroid include thyroxine (conventional treatment), herbs and nutrients, and thyroid glandulars

- The Barnes test is generally a good guide to how well the thyroid is responding to treatment

- Supporting the thyroid with appropriate agents often leads to significant enhancement in general health and well-being

6. Take Exercise

During exercise the circulation pumps the blood more forcefully into the tissues, supplying them with increasing amounts of oxygen and nutrients. It comes as no surprise that most people find exercise energizing and exhilarating. Exercise has also been shown to benefit the body and mind in a myriad of ways. Research has shown that a number of health benefits can be attributed to regular exercise. It is known to improve muscular strength and mobility, reducing the risk of disability in the long term. Several studies now show that weight-bearing exercise can increase bone density and reduce the risk of osteoporosis. Regular exercise and activity is also associated with a reduced risk of chronic illnesses such as heart disease, stroke, diabetes and obesity. Those who exercise can generally look forward to a longer life. There is also research supporting the use of exercise in the treatment of psychological conditions such as anxiety and depression. In this chapter we shall be exploring exercise, how much we need to take, and how to go about taking it!

Some general guidelines about exercise

If you haven't exercised for a while, and even if you have, it may be worthwhile taking note of the following general points.

1. **Get checked out**

   If you suffer from a significant illness such as heart disease, high blood pressure or an arthritic condition, it is a good idea to check with your doctor that you are fit to exercise.

2. **Get in gear**

   You might need to invest in some suitable exercise clothing. I would suggest that the only piece of clothing you really need is a good pair of running shoes or trainers. These will help ensure that you do not jar your body during exercise, reducing the risk of muscular and joint injury.

3. Keep hydrated
Get into the habit of drinking plenty of water on a daily basis. Having water on board before you exercise is well known to enhance performance. Keeping a small bottle of water with you when you exercise and taking sips from this is a good idea too. More information about how to keep up adequate fluid levels in the body can be found in chapter 2.

4. Get planning
If you have a busy life, don't expect exercise slots to just pop up in your diary. Part of the secret to getting more exercise into your life is to schedule activity sessions in advance. As a rule, it helps to put exercise sessions in your diary just as you might schedule meetings, or lunches or what have you.

5. Warm up
Any exercise session is best preceded by a five-minute warm-up. Taking some very gentle exercise to begin with prepares the body for the more strenuous activity ahead. During a warm-up, you will get the heart rate up a bit, increase muscle temperature, activate cooling mechanisms in the body and mobilize the joints. Brisk walking or light jogging is an ideal way to warm up. Straight after the warm-up, take a few minutes to stretch (see below).

6. Cool down
Just as the body should be started up slowly, it should be turned down slowly as well. What this means is that after each session, it's a good idea to go through a period of cooling down. One of the main benefits of cooling down is that it can help in the elimination of waste products from the muscles, which reduces the risk of soreness setting in a day or two later. So, if you started your session with five minutes of brisk walking or light jogging, repeat this at the end of the session. After the cool down, stretch again.

7. Listen to your body

If at any point during exercise you feel faint, dizzy, develop chest pain, have unusual difficulty breathing or experience severe muscular or joint discomfort, stop immediately and if symptoms persist, seek medical attention. Individuals with a history of high blood pressure or heart disease should be especially suspicious of symptoms such as unusual shortness of breath or chest pain.

Stretch it out

Stretching needs to form an integral part of any exercise programme. What stretching does is encourage muscle and joint flexibility. This is important, because even if you are fit and strong, if you lose flexibility, you lose function. Between the ages of twenty and seventy we can expect to lose about 40 per cent of our flexibility, and this has an enormous impact on our ability to do what we want to do in our lives, whether it is gardening, dancing, golf, marathon running or just getting out of bed or a chair without the need for assistance.

The following stretch routine should ideally be performed every day, and at least twice on a day where you take exercise (before and after exercise). Stretching is best performed after a short warm-up as warm muscles are more pliable and less prone to injury than cold ones.

Each stretch should be performed in a slow controlled manner. The muscle group being stretched should be taken to a point where it starts to offer some resistance. At this point a little more tension can be applied, but not so much that the muscle hurts. The stretch should be steady – no bouncing! Hold each stretch for a steady count of twenty, but do remember to keep breathing throughout.

1. Overarm Shoulder Press

Clasp your hands together above your head with your elbows slightly bent. Slowly push your arms backward and hold. Keep looking forward and remember to keep your neck in a comfortable position at all times (avoid craning your head and neck forwards).

2. *Underarm Shoulder Press*

Clasp your hands behind your back with your elbows slightly bent. Slowly, raise your arms and hold. Do not bend forward and remember to keep your neck in a comfortable position throughout.

3. *Hamstring Stretch*

Place your right foot one step in front of the left. Lean forward by bending at the waist, keeping your back straight and your head up. Support both of your hands on the top of your left thigh. Slowly drop your hips and buttocks backward and downward until you can feel mild tension in the back of the right thigh. Keep your right knee slightly bent throughout this exercise. Repeat this stretch on the other side.

4. *Quadricep Stretch*

Face a wall and support your body with your left arm, hand placed against the wall. Hold your right foot in your right hand, slowly easing the heel of your foot toward the buttocks. Hold. Keep your left leg slightly bent throughout this exercise, keep your knees together and keep your back straight. Repeat this stretch on the other side.

5. *Back Stretch*

Lie on your back with your knees bent, and hold the back of your thighs. Slowly pull your knees towards your chest, with your hands clasped behind your thighs. Hold and then relax.

Training programmes

What follows is a guide to some of the exercise sessions which you can incorporate into your life in order to enhance your health. These simple, low-tech programmes do not require you to go to a gym or invest in any fancy equipment. The exercise suggestions here are based around three principal activities:

1. Walking
2. Jogging
3. A home circuit session based around both strength and aerobic based activities

Walking

I rate walking as an excellent form of exercise. It's cheap, convenient, recreational and needs no special equipment other than a decent pair of trainers. Now, if the idea of walking for exercise conjures up images for you of lone individuals in top-to-toe sports gear walking determinedly on treadmills, then you may do well to consider other options. You can don all the gear and join a swanky gym if you want, but there are plenty of other ways. Maybe you want to walk outside, in a local park, for instance. Perhaps you want to take a partner with you – a sort of walking buddy. Maybe the dog wants to come too. The main thing here is that you should do whatever you enjoy the most. And perhaps that will vary from day to day.

A little word of advice about the walking itself: in general, it is better to take quick steps rather than long strides. Longer steps are hard on the joints, especially the knees, and don't allow you to go any faster. Take steps slightly longer than you would normally, landing on your heels and rolling through to your toes.

Although walking is predominantly a lower body exercise, there's no reason why you shouldn't get your upper body involved. Bend your elbows to 90 degrees, relax your shoulders and swing away as you go. This can only help you to use more energy and at the same time give you a better overall workout.

As your fitness improves, you may find that you are able to step up the pace, without getting any more tired. From time to time, you might want to check how long it takes you to get round a set course. Sometimes it helps, especially during the initial stages of a new exercise regime, to get objective proof of your progress. A word of warning here, for goodness sake do not become a slave to the stopwatch. There can be a tendency for individuals who get into timing themselves to get competitive with themselves, often looking to achieve faster and faster times. There will come a point, this happens to everyone (even world class athletes), where you just can't go any faster, and this may turn out to be a bit of a de-motivator. Besides, getting all fussed about times and speeds tends to detract from the enjoyment of the activity, and is completely unnecessary anyway. So, if you're going to time yourself, do it once in a while, and don't let it get in the way of your enjoyment.

You may wish to start your programme with walks of, say, fifteen minutes duration. As you become fitter, you might want to build up gradually to thirty minutes or more. Once you can walk briskly for half an hour at a good, even steady pace, then you may consider progressing to jogging.

Jogging

If, for whatever reason, walking is the only form of exercise you take, that's fine. However, if you find you can progress to jogging without too much aggravation, then you're probably going to lose weight more efficiently in the long term. This is especially important where time is at a premium. If you've only got thirty minutes of exercise time at your disposal, then going just a little bit faster by breaking into a jog is very likely to reap rewards.

If you are new to jogging, then there are a few pointers that should help you get the most from your exercise sessions. First of all, take it easy to begin with. What you should be looking to achieve is a good steady pace throughout the run. There is a tendency for individuals new to running to go off too fast, which may mean they need to stop prematurely. The trick is to start off at a pace which is actually lower than you think you can sustain. If you still feel comfortable after five or ten minutes, then you can step up the pace a little, but not before. As you get more experienced, you will be able to judge your natural pace much more easily, and settle into this very quickly after a warm-up and stretch. Don't forget the warm-up and stretch!

When you begin to jog, you might find that you are unable to keep going for more than a few minutes at a time. That's fine. If you want, you can run for, say, three or four minutes, and then walk for a while. Start running again when you feel you are able to. Gradually, you should be able to build up the amount of time you are able to run for without needing to stop, while gradually reducing the amount of recovery time you need in between. Whatever your ratio of jogging to walking, aim initially to be exercising for a total of about fifteen minutes. Again, you can gradually increase the total exercise time as you get fitter. Build up to sessions lasting about thirty minutes.

Now, if you really get into the running thing, you might want to get a bit more adventurous. Perhaps start jogging in a place which has some inclines and hills. Take small steps and pump those arms up any incline, and hold yourself back a little on your way down – running downhill can be hard on the knees, back and ankles.

Another way to spice up your jog is to vary the pace. Perhaps you can experiment with picking up the pace for thirty seconds or so, going more slowly for a minute and then repeating this cycle. Maybe if you are running in a place which is lined with lampposts or trees, you can use these as markers for your changes of pace.

How much exercise?

To get a real weight loss and health-related benefit, you're probably going to need to set aside enough time to take half an hour's worth of exercise, about four times a week. Five times is better, three will do. These figures are only guides. If you can only grab twenty minutes of exercise, twice a week, then that's clearly much better than none. So, do whatever you can manage, and be satisfied with what you have achieved. If you can do a little more the next week, fine. If you can't, that's fine too.

How hard does the exercise need to be?

Since the 1960s, the heart rate has been used as a measure of the intensity of exercise. It has been established that an exercise effort of between 60 to 80 per cent of maximum heart rate (MHR) is sufficient to gain fitness and health benefits. The MHR is the rate at which the heart rate peaks with maximum effort. The MHR can be estimated using the following formula:

$$\text{Maximum Heart Rate} = 220 - \text{age}$$

The maximum heart rate for a forty-year-old is therefore 180. This equates to a target heart rate between 108 and 144.

To find out whether you are exercising to the correct intensity, stop exercising for a moment to take your pulse. The pulse can be felt on the inside of your wrist close to the base of your thumb. Count the number of beats you feel in 15 seconds. Using the example above, for a forty-year-old individual, the number of beats in 15 seconds should be between 27 and 36.

A more high-tech approach to this would be to invest in something called a 'heart rate monitor'. Essentially, this consists of a band worn around the chest and a watch. The band contains a heartbeat sensing device which is then beamed to the watch for display. Good, basic models are generally inexpensive and can be bought in good sports shops.

The very low-tech guide to assessing exercise intensity is simply to gauge how hard you're working. Generally, if you are taking what is known as an 'aerobic' activity such as brisk walking, jogging, cycling and rowing, you should aim to be so breathless that you can just about snatch a conversation. At this level of intensity you will be working hard enough to get real benefit at a pace you can sustain.

Aerobic – resistance training

So far, this chapter has focused on the benefits of walking and jogging for health. These activities are what are known as 'aerobic' exercises. This means that they are sustainable and demand the body to use a lot of oxygen. Other examples of aerobic activities include rowing, aerobics (of course!), cycling and step-machine exercise. Now, if you have any particular favourites in this bunch, then go for it. They make great substitutes for walking and jogging, their only downside is that they demand special equipment or access to a gym.

Strength training

It's now time to turn our attention to a type of exercise known as 'strength' or 'resistance' training. For many of us, strength training conjures up images of men lifting heavy weights, building big biceps and broad shoulders. However, improving muscle strength doesn't necessarily mean building bigger muscles. Plus, there is good evidence that strength training can have a range of benefits which can be a very powerful adjunct to those we get from aerobic activity. One major boon of strength training is enhanced metabolism.

Muscle metabolism

Muscle is what is termed 'metabolically active'. Muscle burns calories all the time, even at rest. This means that the more muscle you have, the faster your metabolism is and the less likely you are to put on weight. The bad news is that, left to their own devices, muscle tissue tends to dwindle in time. Adults who do not maintain their muscle mass through strength training lose between 5 and 7 lbs of muscle every ten years. Now, because muscles burn calories, this muscle loss leads to an inevitable drop in the body's metabolic rate. In fact, studies indicate that the metabolic rate drops by 2–5 per cent every ten years, and loss of muscle tissue is probably the most important thing here.

The best way to keep the muscle bulk strong and healthy is strength training. It turns out that even relatively small changes in muscle mass can pay big dividends in the long term. Research has showed that just putting on 3 lbs of muscle increases the metabolism by 7 per cent. Individuals who gain muscle burn more calories, even when they're inactive, and are less likely to accumulate fat as a result. To get this extra three pounds of muscle doesn't necessarily take too much effort either. One study showed that this sort of gain could be achieved by both men and women training for twenty-five minutes, three times a week for just eight weeks.

Resistance training for improved muscle strength

Another major benefit of resistance training is that it improves muscle strength. This is important because as we age, the muscles can weaken, and this is a major cause of disability. Studies show that even modest strength training can help maintain and restore mobility, and this obviously has important implications for our quality of life, particularly as we age.

Below is set out an exercise circuit for use in the home. This workout does contain strength-based exercises which are designed to help you maintain and develop your muscle strength and mass, interspersed with aerobic exercises.

The Home Circuit

The home circuit is based on a series of exercises that alternate between resistance and aerobic-focused activities. If you complete the entire circuit three times, this should take about twenty to thirty minutes. If you can manage a couple of such sessions each week, then there's no doubt that you will be ensuring that you will be going a long way to serving your body's exercise needs.

Some technical points about the home circuit session

1. Perform the exercises in order, ensuring that you alternate between resistance and aerobic activities.

2. The exercises should be performed at a slow or moderate pace. Aim at a good consistent pace throughout rather than getting through the session as quickly as possible.

3. Aim to do ten repetitions of each of the resistance-based exercises, followed by thirty seconds of each aerobic exercise. The resistance exercises should be performed with a controlled, smooth action. If you are in the process of getting fit, you might want to restrict the aerobic exercise to something not too strenuous such as actively marching on the spot.

4. Remember to keep breathing! During the resistance exercises it is common for individuals to restrict their breathing.

5. Don't forget to stretch before, and particularly after, the home circuit.

1. Press-Ups

There's a choice of three kinds here:

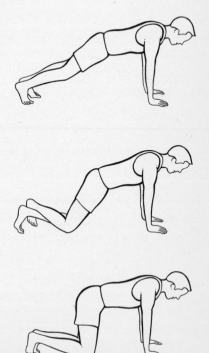

Full – keep your hips and knees straight. Your hands should be directly under your shoulders. Lower your body by bending your elbows until your chest is about 10 cm from the floor. Push up again.

Half – similar to the full press-ups, but the knees are on the ground set behind the hips.

Box – similar to the half, but the knees are directly under the hips.

2. *Active March*

March on the spot, lifting your knees high and pumping your arms.

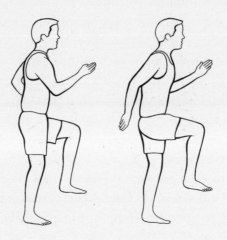

3. *Sit-Ups*

Lie with your back flat on the floor with your knees bent and your feet flat. Place one hand on the thigh of the same side and the other hand behind your neck. Slowly lift your shoulder off the floor by squeezing your abdominal muscles. Curl your upper torso and you move forward towards your knees. Slide your hand along your thigh until your wrist gets to your knee. Hold briefly, and lower yourself back to the ground slowly and in a controlled fashion. Keep your lower back in contact with the floor throughout this exercise, and do not pull your neck and head with the supporting hand.

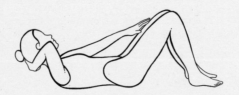

4. Jog on the Spot

Run on the spot keeping upper and lower body relaxed.

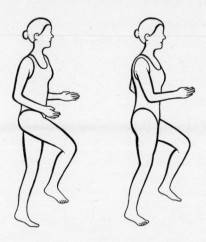

5. Bicep Curls

Take two plastic 1½-litre bottles full of water, one in each hand. Hold the bottles with palms up and forearms parallel to the floor. With your feet shoulder-width apart and knees slightly bent, bend your arms at the elbow, slowly raising your hands towards your chest. Pause briefly at the top and then lower the bottles with an easy, smooth action.

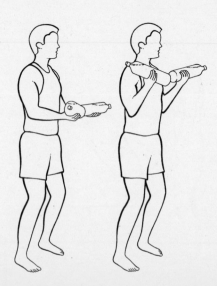

6. *Ski Jumps*

Assume the ski position with feet slightly apart, knees slightly bent, your body slightly forward and your arms out in front. Jump slowly from side to side, cushioning your landing with your knees.

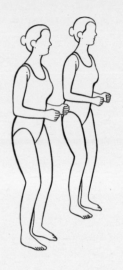

7. *Squats*

Starting with your feet a little more than shoulder-width apart, toes pointed out at about 45 degrees and knees slightly bent, sit back until your thighs are roughly parallel with the floor. Keep your knees over your ankles and swing your arms forward as you sit back to keep your balance. Return to standing but do not lock your knees.

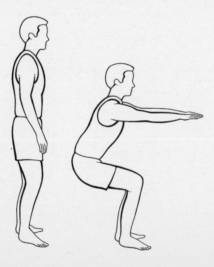

8. Active March

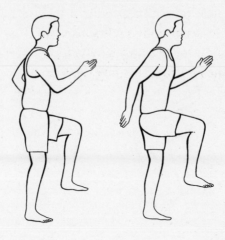

9. Dips

You will need a chair for this. Place the front of the chair behind you. Put your palms on the seat of the chair with your fingers pointing forward. Bend your knees and keep your feet flat on the floor. Take your weight on your arms, and slowly bend your elbows to 90 degrees, lowering your hips towards the floor. Push back up again. Keep your back straight and close to the chair throughout this exercise.

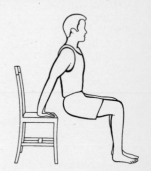

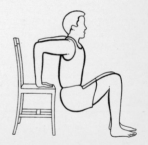

10. *Jog on the Spot*

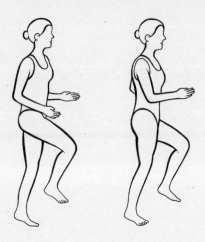

11. *Back Extensions*

Lie face down on the floor, and support your upper body by placing your hands palm down under your chest. Bend your right leg slightly and lift it up off the floor, hold at the top for a count of one or two, and then lower. Repeat with your left leg. Keep the movements slow and rhythmical.

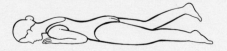

12. *Ski Jumps*

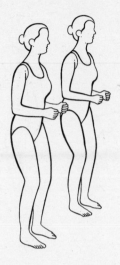

13. *Lateral Raises*

Take two 1½-litre plastic bottles full of water, one in each hand. Stand with your feet shoulder-width apart, and knees slightly bent. With your arms straight, slowly raise them out to the sides until your elbow is in line with your eyes. Pause briefly and slowly return the bottles to your sides.

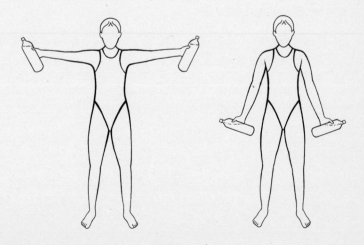

14. Active March

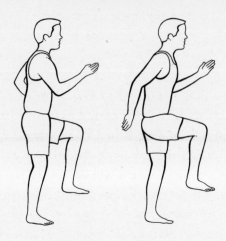

Summary

- Regular exercise has a number of potential benefits for both body and mind

- If you are new to exercise, walking is an ideal way to start your fitness campaign

- If you are able, progressing to jogging is likely to help with both weight loss and health-related benefits

- For significant health-related benefits, aim to take about thirty minutes worth of exercise, four times a week

- Aim to be working at about 60 to 80 per cent of your maximum heart rate (roughly equivalent to 220 minus your age)

- If you can just snatch a conversation during exercise, then you are working hard enough but not too hard

- Resistance exercises can help weight loss by maintaining or developing muscle mass, which in turn impacts positively on the metabolism

- A home exercise session based on both resistance and aerobic exercises offers a great way to get a convenient all-over workout

7. Honour Yourself

It seems incredible that in a world of more than six billion people, no two people look the same. Even identical twins have subtle differences which allow them to be distinguished. Not only do we look different on the outside, we are different on the inside too. Factors such as nutritional needs and the biochemical and physiological workings of the body are known to vary considerably from person to person. Looking even more deeply, another human aspect which is unique and personalized is our emotional make-up. Each of us has a set of beliefs, feelings and motivations which is exclusive to us, and every bit as individual as our fingerprints or facial features. From our basic emotional characteristics come our true needs and desires. How in touch with these we are, and how well we fulfil them, is critical to our sense of happiness and contentment.

To be or not to be, that is the question

Learning to act in harmony with our innate selves is fundamental to our ability to live abundantly. After all, if we don't know what really moves us, or are failing to act on this, how can we ever hope to find life satisfying and fulfilling? In addition, failing to honour ourselves can create emotional disharmony that may take its toll on the body. Let us not forget that the body and mind are inextricably linked. The feelings of disappointment, regret and resentment that may come if we suppress our true selves and live a life of unfulfilled dreams do nothing to support physical health either. Of all the emotionally related issues which are factors in ill-health, I believe not honouring our true selves is perhaps the most common.

How would you know if you are living your life in accordance with your innate self? Start by asking yourself what it is that you *really* want from your life. Do you find yourself hesitating, or that no answer comes at all? Do you feel that there is something missing in your life, but can't seem to put your finger on what it is? Do you find yourself doing things in your life which you don't really *want* to, but feel you *ought* to? If you have answered 'yes' to any of these questions, then this suggests that you are not living your life in tune with your true wishes and desires. In this case, learning the art of honouring yourself could transform both your physical and emotional well-being. The first step is to know who you are.

Who do you think you are?

Ridiculous though this may sound, it seems that many of us simply do not know *who* we are. Beyond obvious things such as our name, where we live and what we do in our day-to-day lives, it is amazing just how little some of us appear to know about our true beliefs, motivations and inspirations. Many of us have issues with making choices and decisions in our lives, often because we feel we just don't know what is best for us. Some of us even struggle to think of something, just *one* thing, which excites us or captures our imagination. Let's be frank, these are not signs of an innate sense of 'self-knowing'. Losing touch with our core beliefs and values is a major cause of the dissatisfaction common in modern-day society.

Losing sight of who we are and what we want appears to be a trait we acquire with age. Newborn babies, for instance, seem to have a very good sense of what they want and don't want in life. If a baby is hungry or feels cold, it cries. Once a baby has what it wants, such as its mother's breast or the warmth that comes from an extra blanket, peace and tranquillity quickly descend. Clearly, when we start out in life it seems we are very in touch with our needs and have no compunction about letting all around us know what they are!

It is as we progress through life that we seem to lose sight of what our individual needs are. One reason for this is that, as we mature, the choices that are available to us seem ever-expanding. Let's face it, our needs when we are born are pretty basic. Love, physical comfort, food and warmth are our main requirements. Yet, by the time we are adult, we are generally faced with a sometimes bewildering array of possibilities on a day-to-day basis. Coupled with this is the fact that, throughout our lives, we can be subject to a myriad of influences which can 'condition' us and pull us away from our innate selves.

Under the influence

Conditioning can start early with the experiences and interactions we have with our parents or guardians. Other important influences may come from relatives, such as grandparents and siblings, and from family friends and acquaintances. In this day and age, we are quite likely to have our beliefs and attitudes shaped, at least in part, by exposure to a variety of different media, including television, radio, the internet, magazines and books. Our schooling and perhaps further education undoubtedly further mould us. Still other important influences may come from religion and social convention. I'm not saying that any of these external factors is inherently 'good' or 'bad'. What I am saying, however, is that problems may come if we end up taking on attitudes, views and behaviours that simply do not reflect who we are.

In my own life, I know there have been times when I have suppressed my true nature, and know the discomfort that this can cause. No more graphically is this demonstrated than in my professional life:

I make no secret of the fact that I am passionate about natural medicine. However, it wasn't always this way. At medical school, I was actually wedded to the principles and practice of orthodox medicine. I believed (or thought I did) that conventional medicine was the only true answer to the ills of the world. I was very into the idea of high-tech, pharmaceutical-based medicine, and for some years courted the idea of becoming a transplant surgeon.

Coupled with this apparent attachment to conventional medicine was my utterly disparaging opinion of complementary medicine. My official position on the forms of natural medicine such as acupuncture, homoeopathy and herbal medicine was that they were a lot of unscientific, unproven mumbo-jumbo. A good friend and colleague when I was at medical school was Jesse Kenton, son of Leslie Kenton. Leslie Kenton was then, and still is, a respected holistic health journalist. In my view she has been instrumental in helping to open many people's consciousness to some important themes in natural medicine and holistic health. I recognize her now as being an important force in helping to push this area forward, and believe she actually helped forge a path for my own work. I'm embarrassed to admit it now, but when I was at medical school, I thought Leslie Kenton was peddling the work of the devil.

While I did not realize it at the time, I see now how some of the attitudes I had to conventional and natural medicine were not really my own. I may have given off the impression that conventional medicine was for me, but deep inside *I had serious reservations. It occurred to me, for instance, that conventional medicine did not seem to address the true underlying causes of illness. What was also apparent, was that the treatments used in orthodox medicine were often ineffective, or worse still, had harmful effects of their own. Another deficiency seemed to be how little emphasis conventional medicine places on the prevention, rather than the treatment, of illness and disease.*

While it is easy for me to articulate these qualms now, during my training I simply chose not to recognize them, preferring instead to proceed through my training led by what can only be described as 'blind faith'. Despite the fact that I thought my future was in conventional medicine, my heart was simply not in it. I was a sporadic attendee at lectures and teaching sessions. The only study I ever undertook was motivated by fear of failing examinations, not through any real interest in the subject matter.

I believe the issues I had when I was studying medicine stemmed from the fact that my 'chosen career' did not truly reflect my true beliefs and interests. From a young age I had been interested in paranormal phenomena such as telepathy, hands-on healing and dowsing. During my teens, I would read about the concepts behind and the practice of natural medicines such as acupuncture and hypnotherapy. When asked during my interviews for medical school what I would do if I were not accepted, I replied that I would take up some form of complementary medicine.

Yet, once I got to medical school I did what I could to 'fit in'. I chose to suppress my interests, and tried to convince myself that conventional medicine was my life's purpose. However, while I clung to the idea of being a doctor, it never really felt right. I was certainly motivated by medicine, but never inspired by it. However much I tried, I felt like a square peg in a round hole. Basically, for a lot of the time I was at medical school, I was struggling.

Finally, around the time that I qualified as a doctor, something clicked. The thought of spending the rest of my working life doing a job which I was not passionate about seemed just too much to bear. I decided that I would not attempt to fulfil my ambition to be a surgeon. In fact, I resolved that I would not work in conventional medicine at all. I decided to leave my chosen career, and look for something else to do.

I did eventually rekindle my interest in natural forms of medicine. Quite how this happened is relevant to the central theme of the next chapter, and I'll pick up this story there. However, what my experience shows is the type of struggle and emotional discomfort that can come when we suppress our true selves, and choose to be something that we are not.

Judge not

You might ask what it is that causes us to dispense with our innate nature in favour of something else. Often at the root of this is the erroneous belief that there is something better for us than what we truly desire for ourselves. Inherent in this belief is that some aspect of our nature is somehow invalid or unworthy. Dropping any judgement about who we are and the worthiness of our true needs is important if we are to really honour ourselves.

Most of us do not like being judged or criticized. Generally, we take it personally to be told that we are arrogant, insensitive, a bad parent, overweight or whatever. However, often the harshest criticism that we experience doesn't come from other people, but from *within*. Some of us are simply not comfortable with who we are, and as a result can harbour destructive and negative feelings towards ourselves. Quite often when we are struggling with an issue, the angst is compounded by the fact that we berate ourselves for actually having the issue! I have seen this happen a lot in practice. For instance, I regularly see individuals who suffer from fatigue, who are also annoyed at themselves for not having the energy to do the things they want to do in their lives. Also, individuals who want to lose weight are often intensely critical of how they look. Whatever the precise nature of your health issue, do you sometimes find that you give yourself a hard time about it?

The very act of focusing on what we perceive as our problem is what often causes it to perpetuate. As the saying goes: 'What you resist, *persists*'. One thing that is critical in enabling us to move forward in our lives is to accept ourselves as we are.

Accept yourself

You cannot get away from the fact that you are going to spend the rest of your life living with yourself. Now, you can choose to do this by judging and criticizing yourself, making each day an emotional battlefield. Or, you can choose to accept yourself for who you are. Self-acceptance can take the struggle out of life. Self-acceptance, however, is not the same as complacency. I am not for one moment suggesting that if we perceive there is an issue in our life we should merely accept it without question. Self-acceptance does not mean never endeavouring to improve ourselves or striving to attain our goals. It does, however, mean recognizing what it is we would like to change about ourselves and our life, *without judging or finding fault*. The drive for self-improvement is completely healthy as long as it comes from a place of self-love rather than a feeling of inadequacy.

Focus on what you do want, not on what you don't

If we want to create positive change in our lives then we need to focus on the positive changes we want. Essentially, change comes when we are moving towards something we *do* want rather than when we are running away from something we *don't*. So, whatever it is we want to transform, whether it is essentially physical or emotional in nature, it makes sense for us to put our focus and attention on the end result we desire.

See it

The first step in achieving change is to have a clear image in our mind of what it is we really *do* want. For instance, if you feel that shyness is 'holding you back' and not allowing you to live your life to the full, firstly visualize yourself acting with confidence. Imagine a situation in which you have felt self-conscious in the past, such as at a party. Put yourself in that situation in your mind's eye, this time seeing yourself acting in the way you would prefer. Maybe see yourself approaching someone with self-assurance, engaging them in easy conversation.

If your issue is of a more physical nature, then the trick is to see yourself as you would ideally like to be. If you are struggling to lose weight, for instance, imagine yourself the size and shape you aspire to. If you are troubled by fatigue, see yourself going about your daily life with abundant energy.

Feel it

Once you have this positive image in your mind, the next step is to engage with the emotion you may feel as the result of the change. For instance, how would you feel to have more confidence socially? Experience the excitement you might feel if you were to have lost the weight you want to lose. What would it feel like to have all the energy you want? Allow yourself to tap into the positive emotions that your positive image brings forth.

Be it

The final, and critical, step in actualizing change is to act! This means behaving in a way which is in accordance with this new image you see and feel. As much as possible, act in a manner which you would expect this transformed version of you to behave. If confidence in social situations is the issue, throw a party! If your weight is keeping you from joining a dance class, join anyway. If your fatigue is keeping you from your favourite hobby of walking, put on your gear, get outside and see how far you can get (you might be pleasantly surprised). By acting in the way you would prefer to be you are actually sending a very strong message to your unconscious. What you are telling yourself is that you can be whatever it is you want, and this can be a very powerful catalyst for positive change.

When Richard first came to see me, his major preoccupation seemed to be that he was soon to turn fifty. I couldn't help him with this! However, he did also have a number of physical symptoms (principally fatigue, poor mental concentration, athlete's foot, and a degree of excess weight) which I felt were relatively easily explained and treatable from a physical perspective: candida overgrowth, food sensitivities and blood sugar imbalance seemed to be the core issues.

However, his comment about the imminent chronological milestone made me feel that there were perhaps some other issues that could benefit from discussion. As the consultation unfolded, it was clear that Richard was far from happy. By his own admission, he had seemingly made a number of 'bad' choices in his life. In particular, he had chosen financial services as a career, which he was less than passionate about to say the least.

Richard told me his father had been a dominant character, and a strict disciplinarian. Richard confessed to feeling frightened of his father, and was an obedient child as a result. Richard also bought into the disciplined and controlling environment he was exposed to at school. He was a 'good' student, and worked hard to enable him to go to university. Soon after leaving college, Richard married a 'strong' woman, who he continually looked to for guidance. In his work, he had generally taken a back seat, and was unhappy that he was not able to exercise more control in his business dealings. In pretty much every area of his life Richard appeared to have denied his true self, choosing instead to satisfy the expectations of others. It was clear that his choices in life had been largely dictated by all sorts of influences other than his own.

On a conscious level, Richard felt that he needed to address his physical health through his diet. Clearly, though, there was more to it than that! I broached the subject of the need to honour oneself. In an effort to highlight what I saw as Richard's core issue, I simply asked him what he would really love to do in his life. He hesitated. When I pushed him, he said he didn't know. Richard appeared to have become so far adrift from his core self, he had even lost sight of what he wanted from life.

I encouraged him to use his imagination and not be bound by any beliefs about what is 'right and proper'. After a bit more prodding he told me that ever since he was a child he had always loved gardening. We explored this. Richard told me that when he was small, he often spent his pocket money on flower seeds. He would plant these in the central strip of grass on the driveway of the family home. He told me of the intense excitement he would feel as the seeds germinated and grew into flowers. As he recounted this story to me, tears of joy filled his eyes. Richard suddenly seemed to come alive for the first time in the consultation. Yet, even as Richard told me this story, I sensed some sadness. It seemed odd to me why he would plant the seeds in the driveway. Why not the garden? Even at a young age, Richard had not wanted to draw attention to his flower-growing hobby. Somehow, at this tender age, Richard had come to the conclusion that gardening was not a 'worthy' pastime.

Although Richard had a garden, he did no gardening. He said he just didn't have the time. Richard had suppressed his passion, and added that even the thought of gardening was now a painful and vivid reminder of how 'lost' he had become in his life. When I asked Richard what he was going to do about all this, he still seemed resigned to working in financial services. In Richard's eyes, gardening was not a 'proper job', and one that would not sustain him financially.

I felt this belief needed breaking down. I cited the example of musicians and artists who can appear very passionate about their work, but nonetheless earn a living from it. Richard then began to talk to me about his younger brother. According to Richard, his brother had always appeared to do 'exactly as he pleased'. He refused to bow to his father's rather patriarchal ways, and did not apply himself at school. Instead, he preferred to spend much of his time listening to music and playing the guitar. He left school and went on to become a respected session musician, playing with a string of successful and high-profile rock bands. Here, in Richard's own life, was a glaring example of how living in accordance with one's true self can be not only fun, but might also be sustaining and supportive. I suggested to Richard that his 'little' brother might have a lot to teach him about life!

I asked Richard to close his eyes and imagine himself tending a garden. As he did this, a smile came to his face. I encouraged Richard to experience the pleasure that this image conjured up to the full. Richard was able to do this with relative ease, and became more animated than he had been at any other point during the consultation. I then simply suggested Richard do something practical in the next day or two, however small, that was in keeping with this new vision of himself.

When I saw Richard two months later, he seemed like a different person. After our initial consultation he had visited a garden centre where he had bought a selection of books about gardening, and some gardening gloves. He was already spending a considerable part of his weekends tending his garden and was more than enthusiastic about this. He had reassessed his finances and come to the conclusion that he could afford to work part-time. He planned to continue working three days a week as a financial adviser, and spend the other two 'working' days in the garden. His wife was utterly supportive of Richard's plan, and his change of direction had even seemed to impact positively on their relationship. Along with some dietary change and the taking of supplements designed to combat his specific physical imbalances, Richard was feeling physically stronger and his original symptoms were considerably better.

Richard did indeed go on to realize his dream of part-time gardening. But it did not stop there. Within two years he and his wife had left London and bought a small farmhouse with some land in the south-west of England. This 'downsize' had freed up some money, which meant that he could resign from his job. The last I heard, Richard was in excellent health, and mixing his time giving independent financial advice a day or two each week along with tending a substantial garden and smallholding.

Richard's story exemplifies the kind of dramatic move forward in our circumstances and sense of fulfilment we can experience by simply honouring ourselves. How, though, do we know what is truly representative of who we are? What signposts can we use to tell us which path to take in life? While some of us may put our faith in the advice of a counsellor, tarot reader or clairvoyant, or seek guidance from horoscopes or the I Ching, the fact is all of the guidance we need is contained within us. The key to making the right choices in life is to *trust our intuition.*

Summary

- Each of us possesses a unique set of emotions and beliefs

- Honouring our innate selves is fundamental to our ability to live satisfying and fulfilling lives

- The effect of external influences such as our parents, teachers and the media can lead us to become detached from our true selves

- Believing that there is something better for us than what we truly desire for ourselves is often a key component in our failure to honour ourselves

- Accepting who we are and the innate needs we have is critical to the process of honouring ourselves

- Focusing on what it is we want to change can actually perpetuate the issue – what we resist, *persists*

- An important key for change is not to focus on what we *don't* want, but on what we *do* want

- It helps to see a vision of the positive change we desire

- Experiencing the positive emotions associated with this perceived change is also a powerful catalyst for change

- Acting as though change has already come further accelerates the process of transformation

8. Trust Your Intuition

One thing that all of us have in common is the need to make decisions. From day-to-day choices such as what clothes to put on in the morning and what to eat for lunch, to life's bigger questions such as which career to pursue and whether or not to start a family, there is no getting away from the fact that life is full of decisions. When considering our options a swift decision allows us to get on with the actual experience or at least frees us to move on to something else! The more quickly and confidently we make decisions, the richer our experience of life.

Yet, while decision making is of undoubted importance in our lives, it is an area where many of us can stall. Decisions over fundamental areas such as work, personal relationships and family may leave us hesitant and unsure. Wavering over which path to take in life and the choices open to us encourages stagnation, not flow. And while making decisions can be hard, making the *right* ones can be even harder. Even once we have made a decision, how often do we find ourselves wondering whether it's for the best? And how many of us have had occasion to look back at our lives and conclude that we have made some 'bad' choices along the way? The internal angst this can cause has the capacity to erode both enjoyment of life and our physical health.

So, what is it that hinders our ability to make decisions or causes us to make what appear to be the 'wrong' ones? There seems to be a common perception that problems with decision making stem from not giving them enough thought. However, my view is that problems with decision making are not the result of too little thought, but too *much*.

It's not the thought that counts

One approach to making a decision is to 'weigh things up' in our mind. Using some logic, going through the pros and cons, and giving a decision 'some serious thought' are all concepts we are familiar with. There is no doubt that engaging our brain before making decisions has some merit. If you are looking to buy a family car then your logical mind can be relied upon to do the job of telling you a two-seater sporty number is out of the question! However, have you ever found the mental dialogue you engage in when endeavouring to make a decision can tie you up in knots? Do you find yourself 'agonizing' over a decision, spending time and mental energy considering the choices, only to find that there is still no real clarity at the end?

While our culture and education system generally put a lot of emphasis on the need to use intellect and reason in one's daily life, these attributes do not necessarily assist us in our pursuit of happiness. While we may put a lot of store in things which 'logically' should bring us happiness, such as wealth, success, marriage and a family, we only need to look around to see that while this theory is one thing, reality is often another!

You may know, or at least know of, individuals who have wealth, or fame, or success or whatever, who nonetheless appear to have come up seriously short on the happiness stakes. There are plenty of people about who one might think *ought* to be happy, who nevertheless *aren't*. And, many of us know of people who have none of what are thought to be the external trappings of happiness, but who are nonetheless content and fulfilled.

Happiness is an emotion

Whatever achievements we may 'think' will bring us happiness in life, let us not lose sight of the fact that happiness is not an achievement, but an *emotion*. While deciding what will make us happy in our head may seem to be logical and correct, this approach may fail to satisfy us on a deep level. Because what we are truly striving for is *emotional* satisfaction, does it not make sense to live our lives based not so much on what we *think*, but how we *feel*? That's where our intuition comes in.

Intuition – a barometer for life

I like to think of our intuition as a sort of internal barometer. Intuition is a signal from our unconscious that reflects our true selves. These messages from the unconscious tell us much about our innate wishes and desires. We may not be consciously aware of these, but they are there. When making a decision or planning a course of action, our intuition points the way for us. The critical thing here is for us to tune into (and not ignore!) our intuition, because it tells us everything we need to know about what we really *feel* about the options and choices that present themselves in life.

When something 'feels right', that is a sign that it *is* right! On the other hand, if our gut says 'no', then we need not be in any doubt about the message here either. All we need to do is trust our intuition, and act on it.

In the last chapter we explored how our true wishes can get buried under beliefs and attitudes that are influenced and conditioned by factors such as our parents, teachers and the society 'norm'. Because our intuition comes from our subconscious, it reflects a part of us that has not been conditioned by these influences. The beauty of listening to our intuition is that it strips away what doesn't belong to us, revealing our true selves as it does this.

I have found trusting my intuition to be a powerful force in my own life:

In the last chapter I wrote about how I finally made my mind up to leave conventional medicine. There was certainly no 'logic' to this decision. Medicine, after all, is a relatively secure and well-paid job which many people believe still confers a degree of kudos and social status. Plus, in my final examinations I had won academic prizes which generally earmark young doctors for rapid progression in their chosen speciality.

All of this may be true, but the plain and simple fact of the matter was that I didn't feel comfortable about staying in medicine. Whatever my academic achievements were, and however long I had spent studying medicine, something in my gut was telling me that a career in conventional medicine was just not for me.

When I left conventional medicine, it took me a couple of years to 'find my feet'. I toyed with a number of different ideas including becoming an actor and retraining as a psychotherapist. Having left the secure environment of conventional medicine, I found myself with no career, no regular income and no real idea of what to do. I felt vulnerable and quite alone. Throughout this time, though, I clung to the idea that although I didn't know what I really wanted to do, at least I was not doing something I knew I didn't want to! I reasoned that at least by leaving medicine I had created the space for something else to come in.

While contemplating what was to become of me I took temporary jobs as a junior doctor in hospital medicine. On one such posting, I saw an elderly man who had come in for a hernia repair. Although he was in his seventies, he didn't look older than sixty. He was fit and robust, and, unusually for his age, had not been in hospital before. I was fascinated with how this man had managed to keep himself in such good health. When I asked him about this, he told me that he'd always eaten a simple but healthy diet, which now included organic vegetables grown on his allotment. Most days, he would cycle several times to and from this allotment, and worked hard tending it. He also confessed to taking nutritional supplements, in particular the mineral selenium which is known to have anti-ageing and disease-protective effects.

During my conversation with this man it dawned on me that perhaps the real secret to health was not so much a matter of luck, but more to do with how we live our lives. Maybe factors such as diet, exercise and our emotional health were the real determinants of health. This may seem obvious now, but to me at that time it was a major revelation. That very afternoon I bought a book on nutrition and began reading it that evening. I am not exaggerating when I tell you that from almost the first page, I was gripped.

For some months I read voraciously about natural medicine and nutrition. I was excited by the information I was discovering, and eager to learn more. I cannot express what a joy it was for me to be studying something not because I felt I had to, but because I wanted to. I was so enthralled by the whole subject that I decided to make natural medicine my career.

The problem was I knew nothing about the natural health industry, and what opportunities lay within it. My decision to embrace natural medicine was made without planning or much in the way of thought. However, I felt that this was the right move for me, and to this day, have had no regrets. I don't want to sound smug or self-satisfied, but my experience with natural medicine, both personally and professionally, has been an incredible journey. It has not always been 'easy', and there have been challenges along the way, but I have no doubt that I am doing the work I was born to do. I truly believe that I have come to this point not through some grand plan or logical scheme, but simply through following my intuition.

Excitement points the way

If I were to use one word to sum up how I felt about natural medicine when I became reacquainted with it, it would be excitement. Whatever it is we are contemplating, we can rest assured that if it's excitement we feel, then our intuition is shouting 'yes!'. All we need do then is act on it. Fundamental to living a truly fulfilling life is doing what excites us. As long as we keep doing precisely what sings to us on an emotional level, how can we fail to be emotionally fulfilled? The answer, of course, is that we can't.

The idea of acting on what excites us is clearly counter-intuitive in a culture that teaches us about concepts such as 'living up to our responsibilities' and 'planning for the future'. And I'm not saying there is anything 'wrong' with these and similar ideals. So long as they excite and resonate with us on some level, then why not utilize them in our lives? However, if how we live our lives is dictated more by duty and responsibility than excitement, then the danger is we can easily find ourselves short on happiness and contentment.

Sometimes it can take time to re-learn the art of listening to our intuition and following what excites us. If this is true for you, then it might help to keep in mind the following advice:

Take time

Some of us have become so far removed from our essential selves that we have simply forgotten what it is like to feel truly impassioned. I think that children have a lot to teach us in this respect. Have you noticed how children can get almost delirious with excitement about, say, the thought of a family holiday or a birthday party? The eager anticipation and delight with which a child unwraps a present is a joy in itself. Unfortunately, for many of us, such a sense of excitement can be a bit of a distant memory!

If this is true for you, then do allow yourself a little time. If you have spent years, even decades, doing a good job of ignoring your intuition, it can take just a wee while to get back in touch with it. Be kind on yourself and give yourself some time.

Practice makes perfect

When I speak to individuals who seem to be having real difficulty tuning in to their excitement, I suggest that they start by surveying all the options available to them. Even if none of these seems particularly exciting or appealing, the trick is to tune into the one which is even *slightly* more attractive than the other ones. This at least starts the process. Gradually, we can grow more accustomed to responding to our excitement, finally finding that following our heart becomes natural to us. As with most things, practice makes perfect.

What's the big idea?

One thing I have found that may hamper our ability to follow our heart is if we wait for that eureka! moment when we glimpse a grand vision so utterly exciting and compelling we are powerless to resist. Hanging out for 'the big idea' can mean that we spend our time waiting for an elusive explosion of inspiration. Of course this can happen and it's wonderful if it does, but it doesn't have to.

Excitement can come in different ways and to different degrees. While it may manifest as an explosion of enthusiasm and zest, it may also translate into a sense of peace and calm. For instance, while I was excited about the thought of working in natural medicine all those years ago, I wasn't jumping up and down about it. I did, however, have a certain 'knowing' that the direction I was taking was right for me. It's fine if you find yourself barely able to contain your enthusiasm and emotion, but remember a sense of inner knowing does just as well.

Everything is valid

Another thing that can derail us moving towards what excites is the belief that our dream is somehow unworthy. Remember Richard from the last chapter? Even though Richard's true passion was gardening, one of the main reasons he had not acted on that was because he did not view gardening as a 'worthy' occupation. Some of us may be tempted to believe that if our excitement is not attached to something 'significant' or 'proper', then it's simply not valid.

However, whatever it is that you want to do, the fact that it is a reflection of your true desires is justification enough to do it. If saving the world from ecological disaster is what truly excites you then of course that's fine. However, anything that excites you, however 'grand' or otherwise the vision appears, is as valid as anything else.

Make it easy on yourself

Another factor which can cause some hesitation and put a brake on our moving forward is when we seem to be faced with two or more concepts which seem equally exciting. My advice in this situation is to do the thing that you are most capable of acting on. Why not take the path of least resistance? For instance, if you find the idea of starting an organic vegetable patch in your garden equally as exciting as running an organic food company, start the vegetable patch and see where it leads you. Life does not need to be difficult, so don't make it!

What's stopping you?

Even when we are excited about the prospect of doing something with our lives, and have the means to act on this excitement, there is no assurance that we will actually *take action*. What, though, is it that stops us from acting on our excitement? Often, it's that head again!

Time and time again I have found that the reason why we fail to follow our joy is because we end up talking ourselves out of it. It's amazing how we can sometimes conjure up in our heads all sorts of reasons and unpleasant scenarios which may cause the excitement to fade and the dream to die. Is there anything we can do to protect our excitement from the mental processes that can sound the death knell for our excitement? I think so, but critical to this is to understand the nature of motivation.

To my mind, there are only two motivators in life. One is to get pleasure. The other is to avoid pain. Basically, if we are failing to act on our excitement, then we have come to the conclusion that doing so would either give us less pleasure or more pain. The belief that forms the basis for this conclusion needs shifting if your idea is going to be compelling enough for you to act.

Let's look at an example. In Richard's case, one of the beliefs was that gardening would not sustain him financially. In Richard's head, less money meant less pleasure (and perhaps more pain too). However, by changing this belief, and seeing downsizing as a viable proposition, Richard was able to remove the self-imposed obstacle which was a major factor in keeping him from living his dream. So, if you are hesitating, examine what negative beliefs you have about the outcome of your proposed action, and change them to beliefs that work for you.

Still teetering?

If you still find you're teetering on the brink, it will normally be because doubt has crept in. Maybe you feel that you simply cannot trust your intuition and follow your excitement. However, in these situations it can help to remember that there is no such thing as a lack of trust. Doubt is not a lack of trust. What doubt really is, however, is trust in a reality we simply don't prefer. You are always putting 100 per cent of your trust in something. The secret is to put your trust in a reality you *do* prefer. So, decide what it is you want, and trust that you can have it. If you still have any 'doubt' about taking the leap, I suggest the following approach:

Look to the future

Projecting into the future can sometimes be very useful for bringing about change. Let's assume that you have a vision of something that excites you, but still find it difficult to take action. As we have discussed, a fundamental belief here will be that acting will either bring you less pleasure or more pain. If you are having difficulty trusting the concept that the change will bring you more pleasure, another approach would be to trust in the idea that *not* changing would bring you *more* pain!

It won't come as any surprise to you to learn that I do not advocate people experiencing more pain than necessary, however I have found the following approach works well when all is needed is that final little push. The trick is to project some time into the future, say a year, and imagine how you might feel if you had still not acted on what excites you. Let's say, for instance, that you want to leave your job and set up on your own. Go a year into the future and imagine how you might feel if you have not made the break. Are you feeling any discomfort? Is emotional pain creeping in? If not, go further into the future, say five or ten years, and ask yourself the same question. Go as far into the future as you need to bring on enough pain and discomfort so that you are left in no doubt at all that acting on your excitement really will bring you more pleasure and less pain.

Trusting our intuition and acting on our excitement can take the doubt and hesitation from life, and transform it into a thrilling journey. However, as we proceed through life we can have our experience of it tainted by experiences we have had in the past, or by expectations we have of the future. Living our lives in the past or the future can take us away from the only time we have – *now*. A fundamental tool for experiencing life to the full is the ability to *live in the moment*.

Summary

- Life is full of decisions – the quicker and more confidently we make them the richer our experience of life

- Happiness is an emotion which is not inherently 'logical'

- Because of this it makes sense to live our lives not in accordance with how we *think*, but how we *feel*

- Our intuition gives us messages from our unconscious that are free from external influence

- Doing what excites us is the key to our enjoyment of life

- Getting back in touch with the emotion of excitement can take time

- Acting on what seems at least slightly more exciting to begin with, and seeing all visions as equally valid can help this process

- When faced with more than one option that seem equally exciting, it makes sense to choose the option that is easiest to act upon

- What stops us from taking action is the belief that doing so will give us less pleasure or more pain

- Projecting into the future can help motivate us to make a change and may be a powerful catalyst for transformation

9. Live in the Moment

Stop and think for a moment about how we experience life. We travel from one 'present' moment to the next. Behind us we leave our past; in front of us is our future. Yet, whatever has gone before, and whatever is to come, the plain and simple fact remains that the *only* time we have in which to experience life is *now*. A key to living abundantly is the ability to extract as much as possible from each and every 'now' moment in our lives. Well, that's the theory, anyway.

In *practice*, though, many of us find living in the present moment a real challenge. Some of us find that 'bad' experiences in our past continue to tie us in emotional knots and erode our sense of peace and contentment. Another common issue that can impact on our enjoyment of the present is the belief that happiness is for the future, and something that will only come once we have satisfied certain ambitions. Whether we are allowing our past to cast a shadow on our present, or we are putting our happiness off to the future, learning the art of living in the moment is a fundamental key to experiencing true happiness and fulfilment.

What happened to you?

Many of us can have our feelings of contentment and fulfilment dampened by past experience. Perhaps the traumatic break-up of a relationship is the reason why we find it difficult to trust new partners. A poor relationship with our parents can cause us to conclude that we are simply not 'good enough' as we are. Maybe a business failure has made us fearful of starting a new venture. It sometimes seems as though life has dealt us a 'bum deal', and that in some way we are suffering for this. The hurt and pain that we may have felt earlier in life, and which perpetuates to this day, can put a major brake on our emotional well-being. In practice, I have seen many individuals whose physical health issues seem to be related to their interpretation of painful events in the past. Transforming past experiences is often a key to regaining abundant health and well-being.

Healing the past

It is not uncommon for us to internalize and interpret past experiences in a way that simply does not serve us. Should this come as much of a surprise? After all, when we are young we do not necessarily have the emotional or intellectual maturity to find our own truth in the experience we have. As we discussed in chapter 7, we can end up taking on views and beliefs that are not innate to ourselves. The seeds for problems here are generally sown early in life, often through interaction with our parents. While the parent–child relationship is perhaps unlike any other, and offers unique potential for growth and fulfilment on both sides, it can be an emotional minefield too!

Some of the most common and destructive emotional issues I see in practice concern low self-esteem and insecurity. Very often, individuals say they spent their childhoods feeling unloved, and as a result, now feel *unlovable*. Whatever the precise cause of such an issue, it is clear it does nothing to enhance our experience of life. This may seem like I'm stating the obvious, but if we're not happy with ourselves, then it's virtually impossible to be happy, period! For many people, regaining a sense of self-esteem and learning to love themselves is a key to true happiness and fulfilment. The question is, how? The first step, is to take responsibility for how we feel.

Take responsibility

It's quite a commonly held belief that people outside of ourselves can *cause* us to have certain emotions. We might believe, for instance, that the way our parents raised us has made us feel insecure and inadequate. Or that our partner leaving us is the reason why we feel angry and resentful. However, other people do not implant emotions in us. Emotions are something we generate internally. While we may believe our parents or siblings or teachers or whoever are responsible for how we feel, the fact is *we* are.

Some of us do not immediately warm to the idea of being responsible for our emotions, because this suggests we are somehow to *blame*. I am keen to point out, however, that responsibility is not the same as blame. Break down the word responsibility and what we get is *response-ability* – the ability to respond. Through our ability to respond to life's experiences, past and present, we have the power to see all of life in a way which allows us to learn and develop as individuals.

My belief is that the events in our lives have no inherent meaning, only the meaning we give them. This concept will be discussed more fully in chapter 11, entitled 'See the Positive in Everything', and I'll save the ins and outs of this until then. However, what I want to say here is that there is nothing anywhere that says any experience *must* be 'good' or 'bad', it's up to *us* to decide. By giving past events positive meaning, we can integrate these into our lives in a productive way. When we see events that have occurred in our lives in a positive light, this effectively dissolves the emotional debris that is attached to them.

The present is the result of the present

Sometimes, it can be difficult to see how we can transform the effect past experiences have on our lives. Surely, what went before *must* impact on us somehow? Many of us believe that 'bad' experiences in the past inevitably lead to a 'bad' experience of the present. However, by changing our interpretation of past events, and therefore the emotions that go with them, we have the capacity to change their effect on us in the present. The present is not the result of the past, it's the result of the *present*. This concept is exemplified by the following story.

I was once consulted by a young actress called Sally. She came complaining of a range of symptoms, principally fatigue and digestive discomfort. It was my impression that Sally was suffering from poor digestion, principally related to low levels of stomach acid. I discussed the management of this with her, but also suggested she have a test for stomach acid secretion.

This indeed showed low acid secretion, and we went on to take steps to manage this naturally.

When Sally returned some weeks later, she had made some progress, but not as much as either of us would have liked. Plus, Sally mentioned that she had had a problem with anxiety for as long as she could remember, and wondered whether we could tackle that too. This seemed a good time to explore any emotional factors which might be playing a part in Sally's health.

On the outside, Sally was very engaging and outwardly content. However, she was very critical of her work and not at all accepting of her evident talent. She told me that even when she was complimented on a performance, she found it difficult not to focus on something that she felt she could have done better. Clearly, Sally was a perfectionist in her work, but self-criticism did seem to colour her experience of life and detract from her enjoyment of it.

Sally and I began to discuss the idea that nothing she did was ever really good enough. She was open to this idea, so I then asked her where or from whom she had learned this idea. Without any hesitation at all, Sally replied that she believed this idea had come from her mother. Sally proceeded to tell me how nothing she did seemed ever to satisfy or give real pleasure to her mother. I asked her to think back to the first time she felt like this. She told me that at the age of six, she had prepared a little play with her older sister to perform in front of her parents. She and her sister had spent much of the day rehearsing the play and getting their costumes ready. In the afternoon, they presented their self-written play excitedly to their parents. At the end, Sally remembers her father clapping and getting up to give her and her sister a big hug.

What had really stuck in Sally's memory, however, was her mother's comments. Apparently, she remarked that the girls had not learnt their lines properly, and what was needed was more rehearsal time! Sally remembers feeling upset and deflated at her mother's comments. Another event Sally recalled was coming home with a school report. Although her grades were good, Sally's mother had focused on her weakest subject, mathematics, suggesting that she must 'try harder' in this area. Sally told me that similar such episodes peppered her childhood.

It appeared that Sally had learned from these experiences that nothing she did was ever really good enough. Sally appeared to be playing out this belief in her own life, and this seemed to be manifesting as an extreme criticism of herself, particularly her work. I was keen to see if Sally might be able to change her sense of self-worth. I asked her to tell me more about her mother, and in particular, whether she was a critical person generally. Not surprisingly, it turned out that she was. Sally could clearly remember her mother's criticism of pretty much everyone including other family members and friends and acquaintances. Sally said her mother always seemed to be nit-picking about someone or something.

I suggested to Sally that it appeared no one was immune to this trait in her mother. While Sally had seemingly taken her mother's criticism personally, I suggested it was quite possible that the issue was not 'personal' at all. She could go on believing that her mother viewed her as never quite good enough and perpetuate this feeling in her life, or perhaps it would serve her better to see the issue as one coming from her mother's critical nature. Basically, it seemed quite possible that her mother's tendency to find fault had simply spilled into Sally's life.

Sally now had the choice about what she wanted to believe. More importantly, she now had the option of transforming her experience of the present by changing her interpretation of the past. As Sally contemplated the idea of viewing her childhood experiences in another light, I could almost see a weight lift from her shoulders. The next time I saw Sally was several months later. Purely by chance, between visits I had seen her on the television, and complimented her on her performance. She did not dismiss my praise, but thanked me for it. Most importantly, Sally seemed much more at ease with herself. The anxiety she had suffered from for years had gone, as had her stomach symptoms.

As Sally's story demonstrates, taking responsibility for our emotions and changing our beliefs about the past can have a positive effect on our experience of the present. 'Letting go' of pain from the past and resolving feelings of bitterness, anger or resentment can be very liberating for both body and mind. Another critical element in the letting go of past events is *forgiveness*.

Forgive, don't forget

When we have been 'wronged' by another, we sometimes get stuck on the idea that we are simply unable to forgive the person who has wronged us. This does nothing to resolve the pain associated with the experience, and only serves to perpetuate it. As we continue to feel the pain associated with past events, it's natural to do what we can to protect ourselves. One way we can do this is to 'bury' issues somewhere in our psyche so that we need not look at them. In short, we may feel it's better to forget than forgive.

Yet, experience shows that sweeping our emotions under the carpet usually just stores up problems for later on. While attempting to forget the past may appear to give us some respite from whatever it is that is causing us angst, in the long term the problems usually return to bite us on the ankle. Holding anger, bitterness or resentment in one's heart is a major drain on our emotional energy, and may well have unwanted repercussions for our physical health too. Anger, for instance, has been found to increase the risk of heart disease.

See it their way

For some of us, forgiveness is easier said than done. When we find forgiveness difficult, it helps to understand why someone has acted in the way that they have. Look, we all have issues. I do, you do, and everyone else does too. A lot of our issues, as we have been exploring, come as a result of our past experiences. Sometimes, people behave the way they do because often that's the way they've been *taught* to behave. We've all heard the statistics about how individuals who abuse their children were very often abused by their own parents. It's no one's fault, it's something that happens. Sometimes, seeking to understand the issues others have allows us to feel the compassion we need to extend true forgiveness. The concept of understanding and compassion as a route through to forgiveness is aptly demonstrated in the following story.

Bethan, by her own admission, did not have a good relationship with her father. The main issue seemed to revolve around the events which occurred more than ten years previously. Her parents had divorced when Bethan was twelve, and her father had subsequently remarried. When Bethan was twenty she learnt to drive, and her father offered to 'go halves' on a car. However, once she had bought a car, her father rescinded the original offer without explanation, finally giving only what Bethan viewed as a nominal sum. Bethan felt simply unable to forgive her father for this, and had not spoken to him since. She commented to me that if she never spoke to her father again, it would not bother her. However, while Bethan appeared to be giving off an emotionally detached attitude to her father, her body language and tone of voice told another story – one of hurt and resentment.

As we started to talk more about this issue, Bethan became very upset. A lot of suppressed emotion that had got buried along the way seemed to be bubbling to the surface. It seemed that Bethan would do well to heal the issue with her father, and I felt that forgiveness was critical to the healing process. Maybe, through understanding better why her father had behaved in the way he did, Bethan would be able to resolve the issue. I asked about whether similar issues had come up when she was very small. Did, for instance, Bethan's father promise her things when she was a girl but not deliver? Bethan did not recollect this, and believed that the issues she had with her father started after he left the family home and remarried.

In an effort to seek to understand Bethan's father's behaviour, I asked if she knew much about his own upbringing. This seemed to trigger a whole new stream of consciousness for Bethan. In particular, she remembered a conversation she had had with her father about his own father. Bethan's grandfather had himself divorced and remarried, after which he seemed to give Bethan's father very little support, either financially or emotionally. Bethan's father had never reconciled the feeling of resentment he had for his own father over this. I suggested to Bethan that her father was repeating a pattern from an unresolved issue which he himself had experienced. In the light of this better understanding of what perhaps lay behind the issue over the donation towards the car, Bethan could see that she at least had the ability to forgive her father.

Bethan wrote to her father expressing why she had been so upset, and asking him to 'give his side of the story'. In particular, she wanted to know why he had rescinded his financial offer. Bethan was very happy to get a letter back from her father. In it he explained that his second wife had persuaded him not to give the sum he had promised for the car, insisting that Bethan was no longer financially dependent on him. Bethan's father said he had bowed under pressure, and that he had felt guilty about this ever since. Try as he might, he just couldn't seem to make amends. Bethan's letter, however, had 'broken the ice', and he was keen to re-establish a relationship.

Bethan responded well to her father's letter. It helped her to understand much better her father's actions. This understanding is what allowed Bethan to forgive her father, and they went on to resume a close and loving relationship.

Everything is significant

One final point I'd like to make before we leave the issue of the past is this: every single experience we ever have has meaning and is valid. The reason I point this out is because I often find that when we are letting go of the past, we can fail to move forward because we judge our 'old' behaviour. When an age-old issue evaporates into the mist just by seeing an experience in a more productive light, some of us berate ourselves for not resolving the issue earlier. This is just getting rid of an issue, only to replace it with another one! Do remember that each and every experience we ever have in our lives has led us to where we are now. This basic fact allows us to see that all of life is both meaningful and valid.

Living in the future

While dwelling on the past can impair our ability to enjoy life to the full, so can living in the future. Many of us may feel dissatisfied with our lives, but cling to the idea that we will be happy when (and only when!) certain conditions are met. Perhaps we feel fulfilment will come with a job promotion and an increase in salary. Or that finding a 'soul-mate' is the key to our eternal bliss. Does the idea of having another child seem as though it will make everything all right?

Setting external conditions on our happiness in this way is basically putting happiness off for the future. Yet the future does not exist and never will exist. I know I've said it before, but I'm going to say it again – the only time we have is *now*.

Happiness is not something that we have to plan and strive for. It isn't something to be earned, or only goes to those who 'deserve' it. Happiness is an emotion. Like all emotions we have the power to create it. Either we choose to be happy, or we do not. We can choose to look at our life in a positive, abundant way, or we can choose to see it through a lens of negativity and scarcity. What is important to remember here is that our ability to be happy does not depend on us meeting some arbitrary criteria we have set for ourselves. The only conditions there may be on our happiness are the ones that we make. We can expend a lot of time and energy searching for a reason to be happy, when in reality there may be no reason *not* to be!

Count your blessings

In a world which can sometimes be so geared to consumerism, it comes as no surprise that we can tend to feel like we're lacking something. When we compare what we have to what we might have, it's easy to feel we've been short-changed somewhere. A good first step to embracing happiness in the moment is to appreciate what you *do* have in your life.

A useful trick here is to imagine how you might feel if you were suddenly stripped of all you have. You may feel you would like a larger home. Imagine, though, how you would feel if you had nowhere to live at all. Maybe you would like more friends. Think for a moment, however, what it would be like if the friends you have suddenly disappeared from your life, never to be seen or heard again? Perhaps you are feeling underpaid in your work. What if your salary was even lower or perhaps you had no job at all? The point of this is not to make you feel miserable! However, imagining life without what it is you have can be a useful way of getting in touch with the emotion of appreciation.

There's more to abundance than wealth

Another tool which can be used to allow happiness into the present is to change our definition of what it means to be 'abundant'. Many of us think that the word abundant refers to money and possessions. If we lack these things, how can we possibly be abundant? However, I would like to challenge this notion. The only reason we believe abundance is essentially about wealth is because we have been taught to believe that.

However, it often serves us better to view abundance as the ability to do what we want to do, when we want to do it. Money and possessions are simply not a prerequisite for this. The fact is, we don't actually need anything at all to be abundant. For instance, if what you really want to do is lie in a field and soak up the sun, is that being as abundant as lying on a beach in the Caribbean? Is a good heart-to-heart with a close friend over a cup of tea not every bit as abundant as an expensive restaurant meal with some business colleagues? Is not looking at a fabulous sky or some trees as fulfilling as having a priceless oil painting on the wall? Loosening up our definition of what abundance really means, and seeing it more as a state of being rather than a statement of ownership, can help us see how happiness is for us in the here and now, and not something to be put off to the future.

Living in the moment is critical to our ability to move ahead in our lives. As we do this, we must keep alive to the fact that what we want out of life can change. When we sense this, we may want to change our circumstances to match our new desires. However, what we see in our lives is really a reflection of ourselves. The secret to changing what appears to be on the outside is to change what's going on *inside*. Whatever it is we would like to transform in our lives, it helps to *see life as a mirror*.

Summary

- The only time we have to experience life is *now*

- Sometimes we may feel that 'bad' experiences from our past have cast a shadow over our present

- We may believe that other people or external events are responsible for how we feel, but the fact is *we* are

- Our emotions depend on the beliefs we have about events – changing our beliefs is what allows us to transform our emotions

- Forgiveness is often an important key to letting go of negative past experiences

- Seeking to understand the behaviour of others and extending compassion to them often helps the process of forgiveness

- Seeing all our past experiences as valid is important if we are to learn from them and move on in our lives

- Happiness is not something to be put off to the future – the only time we have to experience happiness is *now*

- Appreciation of what we have is key to experiencing happiness in the moment

- Seeing abundance as the ability to do what we want to do, when we want to do it, helps free us from the concept that wealth is a prerequisite for happiness

10. See Life as a Mirror

Sometimes, we can get the impression that the world is dishing us out more than our fair share of bad luck. When things go 'wrong' in our lives, it's easy to feel buffeted by fate and bad fortune. Often elements of our lives can seem completely beyond our control, somehow external to us and unpredictable. And even when we attempt to change our lives for the better, it can sometimes seem like our best efforts come to nothing. Many of us seek to improve our lives through changing circumstances such as our work, home and personal relationships, but often end up feeling no more fulfilled in the end.

It is my belief that we have the power to manifest the lives we truly desire. Sometimes, though, we just go at it all wrong. While life may appear to be external to us and essentially uncontrollable, I believe this is far from the truth. In this chapter we will be exploring the idea that life is like a mirror, and merely reflects back to us what we project into it. If we want to change our lives the secret is not to try and change the mirror, it's to change what we reflect into it.

All change

When we sense some dissatisfaction in our lives, it's natural to want to change things. Don't like our house? Build an extension. Better still, move somewhere else. Don't like our job? Ask for a pay rise. Or maybe get a new one. Not happy with our relationship? Tell our partner that things have got to change. Or maybe just chuck the whole thing in and get someone new. Despite the fact that we can strive to change the circumstances of our lives, it is amazing some-times just how the 'same' we can feel. Once the excitement of moving home, starting a new job, or embarking on a new relationship has faded, how often do we find we have the very same sense of dissatisfaction as we had before. The reason for this is because, as we shall explore, life is like a mirror. What we give out is what we get back.

Imagine you are in a car driving along the motorway. Say the speed limit is 70 m.p.h., but you and some other drivers are doing 80 in the fast lane. Quite suddenly, the cars in front of you slow to 70 m.p.h. At first it is not clear why they have, but then you notice a police car in the inside lane! Imagine for a moment how motorway driving must seem to the policeman driving the police car. For the most part, he sees other motorists on the motorway complying obediently with the speed limit. Imagine now the policeman comes to the end of his shift, and is driving home along the motorway in his civilian clothes in an unmarked car. What he experiences now is motorists charging along in the outside lane at 80! So, the reality the 'policeman' sees depends on whether he looks like a policeman or not. What reality the policeman has reflected back to him from the mirror of life depends on what he projects into it!

The mirror of life reflects our beliefs

We know that if we go around being kind and considerate to others we generally get a better reaction than if we are rude and aggressive. This sort of cause and effect is obvious in our lives. However, the mirror of life has other more subtle qualities. What the mirror also reflects back to us are beliefs we have we may be totally unaware of. Let me explain.

If we want to see a 'happy' reflection in our reality, we have to project happiness into it. As we discussed in the last chapter, happiness, like all emotions, comes from within. And like all emotions, happiness stems from belief. If we are feeling unhappy it is because we *believe* that we have something to be unhappy about.

Seeing isn't believing

You'll be familiar with the expression 'seeing is believing'. However, if we accept that what we see in our lives is a reflection of our emotions, and that emotions stem from beliefs, it becomes apparent that seeing isn't believing at all, it's the other way round!

Believing is seeing is the truth of the matter. Sometimes there may not seem to be any point to the 'bad' experiences we have in life. However, once we accept the idea that life is of our making, it means that we can see every single experience as an opportunity to learn more about what really makes us tick. Once we find out what beliefs we have that are creating any sense of pain or unhappiness, we can (if we choose) change those beliefs to ones we prefer. Changing our beliefs gives us the power to take control of our lives and make them what we want.

You don't get happiness by contorting the mirror

Looking for happiness by changing the external circumstances of our life is akin to attempting to contort the mirror. Many of us attempt to bend the mirror a little this way or that to improve the reflection we see. This may work, but not for long! Even if we do get a slightly different reflection in the mirror, the effect can be difficult to sustain. In terms of changing what reflection we get, contorting the mirror generally does not work! Quite frankly, the simplest, most effective way of changing what we see in the mirror of life is to change what we project into it. Changing our beliefs is the key to changing our reality.

Lose control

Another area where we might try to exert some control is with other people. Some people are desperate to manipulate and 'force' people into being a certain way or doing certain things. Commonly referred to as 'control freaks', these individuals can often spend enormous time and energy getting people to be who they want them to be in order to fulfil their own needs. It's exhausting work. And, try as they might, control freaks generally don't get the satisfaction they seek.

Here again, the real power to get what you want from your life, including other people, comes from the recognition of the fact that reality is a reflection. Whatever you want to change, remember it's you who has to. This is what puts real power in your hands. When you understand this, you will see how changing your reality need not be exhausting, and requires only the deftest touch.

One of the most profound experiences in my life concerns how changing our beliefs can be mirrored in our experience of life.

My father has what you might call 'a good mind'. I remember him helping me with my Latin homework when I was at school. Well into his fifties he still had good command of Latin, a subject he had not studied since his schooldays some forty years previously. In stark contrast, within a couple of years of leaving school, I had forgotten pretty much every bit of Latin I had ever learnt!

Another recollection I have from my schooldays concerns my learning of a Shakespearean speech for an English lesson. I asked my father to check me as I attempted to recite the piece from memory, and handed him the book opened at the relevant page. As I fumbled my way through the speech I became irritated when it was clear he wasn't even looking at the book. However, while I thought he was simply not paying attention, the fact was he could remember the speech from his own days at school. I challenged him to recite the speech from memory. Which he did. My memory, on the other hand, is so bad that I simply cannot remember which speech it was or even the play it came from!

You might think from these stories that I had a very close relationship with my father. This, however, was not the case, in fact it was what you might term 'strained'. While he had obvious powers of intellect, I wasn't really interested in that. The issue, from where I was standing, was that he didn't really seem to be very in touch with his emotions, and did not demonstrate his love to me in a way that I wanted.

After I moved from home to go to medical school, our relationship appeared only to become more distant. This did not seem to be helped by me failing my examinations at the end of the first year at college. We talked occasionally when I could be bothered to pick up the phone, but then only briefly. In the six years I spent at medical school, I remember my father called me once, and that was because of some crisis.

Some years after leaving medical school, I attended a lecture on feng shui. Feng shui is the oriental art and science behind how the physical nature of our environment can affect the energy flow around us. Feng shui teaches that the placement of objects and the design of the space around us can have a profound impact on every aspect of our lives. However, the lecture that I went to wasn't about which direction to face your desk in your office and where to put the rubber plant, it was about feng shui from the inside out. The concept here is that if we clear and order our internal 'emotional' space, then we do not need to worry so much about putting candles in the 'relationship area' and plumbing water fountains into our living rooms.

One of the areas covered in the lecture was that of elders or parents. The lecturer pointed out that one of the issues children have with their parents is that they often feel they are not loved by them. Sometimes children feel that their parents' love is 'conditional'; in other words it depends on them being a certain way. However, the lecturer pointed out that parents generally do love their children, but often they may have difficulty showing it! More than that, however, if we feel we cannot love our parents until they love us in a way we want, then we are being conditional. And if we are being conditional, bearing in mind life is a mirror, is it any surprise that we feel we are getting conditionality back?

These messages struck a real chord with me. I left the lecture theatre making a strong commitment to opening my heart to the concept that my father did indeed love me. And secondly, it dawned on me that for my relationship with my father to change, it was not he who had to change, but me. I knew in that instant that the secret to this was to extend unconditional love to my father.

The following day I was writing at my desk. The phone rang. It was my father. My immediate reaction was that there was a crisis. But, as it turned out, my father had just phoned for a 'chat'. He told me he had been in the newsagents that day and found an article of mine in a magazine. Apparently, he had shown it to a shop assistant and announced that he was my father. The shop assistant, he said, just looked at him as though he was mad.

The very next day after me making my internal adjustment, my father and I were communicating in a way I always hoped we would. For me, this was utter confirmation of the idea that we can transform our lives once we see them as a mirror of ourselves.

Don't wait for the reflection to change

While attempting to manipulate and mould our external reality is not the best way to transform it, neither is waiting for it to change spontaneously. Some of us, when confronted with a reality we don't prefer, sit back in the hope that our reality will finally give us something we can be happy about. This is akin to staring into the mirror with a frown, hoping that at some point we will see a smile coming back at us. I was doing this. Frowning into the mirror I was waiting for the reflection (my father in this case) to smile back at me. I don't need to tell you that this approach doesn't work! If we see something in our external reality that we don't like, the only person that has the real power to change it is *us*.

It's not about forcing a smile either

In the last chapter we touched on the importance of not burying our emotions, lest they may just fester in our consciousness and cause problems down the line. One way some of us can hide our emotions is simply to gloss over them, to ignore them, to pretend they're not there and that everything's fine. Sometimes, it seems the best thing to do is put a brave face on and move on regardless. However, this is like looking in the mirror and forcing a smile. It's not a real smile, and you can't fool yourself that it is. For things to really change, we have to change our beliefs. How, though, do we know when we really have changed?

What tells us that we really have changed, is when we have no expectation that our external reality will change. Once positive change has occurred on the inside, we need to detach from the idea of any change on the outside. If we are constantly on the look-out for signs of improvement, it is clear that we are simply not trusting that change will come. If we truly believe that change will come, and have 100 per cent trust that this is so, then we need not have any expectation about how our reality may change. We know that we have truly changed when we respond differently to our reality, even if it still looks the same.

When I walked out of the feng shui lecture I felt something had shifted. The moment I recognized my father's love and was willing to extend mine to him without condition I felt very different. I honestly had no expectations about what might happen. My commitment to change my beliefs and attitudes was without condition. It was this, I believe, that led to such an immediate shift in my external reality.

See yourself in others

Sometimes we can get angry, hurt or frustrated by the actions of others. Yet, if we see life as a mirror, it opens us up to the idea that often what we see and don't like about others may well be the very things we don't like about ourselves! The upside of this is that other people can alert us to aspects of ourselves that are not serving us. If you ever feel resentful of how someone else has behaved (we all do from time to time), then it often helps to pause for a moment, and ask yourself honestly whether that person is exhibiting traits you yourself have.

For instance, while I was feeling resentful of my father for offering what I thought was conditional love, there was I doing precisely the same thing! Once you recognize something about yourself that you would prefer not to exhibit, then you have the choice about whether to exhibit it or not! However critical you may be of someone at first sight, remember that you may end up thanking them for making you aware of something about yourself you now choose not to exhibit. The next story is a good example of this.

Robin was in his mid-fifties and came to see me complaining of low libido. He separated from his second wife some months previously, and was now with a new girlfriend. However, Robin's low libido was causing problems in the relationship. His girlfriend was taking his apparent uninterest in sex personally, and Robin was feeling under pressure to perform. Up until recently, Robin had always enjoyed a healthy sexual appetite, so what had gone wrong?

I enquired about his separation. After twenty-three years of marriage, his wife confessed that she was having an affair with a family friend. Robin was devastated and had immediately filed for divorce. However, according to Robin, his wife was keen for them to 'sort things out'. She suggested joint counselling. However, Robin could not see his way to forgiving his wife, and clearly still harboured a lot of bitterness and resentment toward her.

It seemed entirely possible that Robin's issues with low libido were related to the unresolved issues with his wife. He may have tried to patch his emotions up with a new relationship, but perhaps the wound was a little deeper than that. Because life is like a mirror, I thought I might dive in and ask him if he had ever been unfaithful in his marriage. Robin admitted that he had had three affairs during their marriage but quickly added: 'But they were different, they didn't mean anything.' As we delved a little deeper, it turned out that Robin's infidelities were really a reaction to what he felt were deficiencies in the relationship. Was it not possible, I suggested, that his wife's affair had also been a reaction to a certain dissatisfaction with the marriage? In this way, was not her own behaviour really just a mirror of his?

What had not been obvious to Robin suddenly was. Once he saw his wife's behaviour as nothing more than a reflection of his own, a lot of the 'bad' feeling he had towards her just evaporated. I asked him whether he loved his wife, which he did. So then I asked him what he was going to do about his situation. Quite voluntarily (and without prompting!) he said he was going to 'come clean' with his wife about his own infidelities. His plan was to tell all, and see if they could work on the real issues that had not yet been dealt with.

I didn't see Robin again, but I did get a letter from him some weeks later. He had spoken frankly to his wife, and she was very receptive to his honesty. They did indeed go on to have joint counselling which enabled them to look at issues that had been simmering for many years. Through more open communication they resumed their relationship, and were enjoying a healthy sex life once again.

★

While other people can exhibit 'undesirable' qualities that can alert us to our own issues, they can also reflect back to us aspects of ourselves that are welcome and positive. This is useful to remember because, quite frankly, many of us simply do not recognize our more attractive qualities. How often do you give yourself credit for your 'good' qualities? For that matter, are you even aware of them? If you see something you like in someone else, just stop for a moment and look within you for that same quality. You may be surprised at how often you find attributes you never even knew you had!

Seeing ourselves in other people is a useful aid to learning more about ourselves. When we see something we don't like, it allows us to explore those things about ourselves we would like to change. And when we see something we do like it can help us appreciate things about ourselves that we are not aware of or perhaps do not give ourselves enough credit for. In short, either way we win! In fact, all of life is like this. Whatever we experience in life, we always have the opportunity to learn and grow through it if we choose. Another fundamental tool to living abundantly is to *see the positive in everything*.

Summary

- Life can often appear external to us and uncontrollable

- Life is like a mirror – what we give out is what we get back

- Our external reality reflects our core beliefs

- The secret to changing our reality is not to attempt to change the circumstances of our lives, but to change our beliefs (without expectation)

- Other people can alert us to our own characteristics

- Seeing undesirable qualities in others can help make us aware of our own traits that we might like to change

- Seeing positive qualities in others can serve to remind us of our own attributes

11. See the Positive in Everything

Life is rich with experience, some good, and some bad. Generally, we don't mind the good stuff, it's the bad that causes the problems! But what is it about events that occur in our life that make them 'good' or 'bad'? We may view events such as having our car stolen or losing our job as bad, but is this always the case? If the insurance payout on our stolen car enables us to buy a brand-new one, what's so bad about that? If being made redundant leads us to find more fulfilling work elsewhere, are we going to grumble? This chapter explores the concept that nothing that happens in life has any inherent meaning – only the meaning we give to them. By being open to the idea that *you* are the one that gives your life meaning, you can choose to take something positive from any and every experience you have.

Often, the reason why we interpret an event as either 'good' or 'bad' is because we've been taught to. Through the sort of influences we explored in chapter 7 such as those coming from our parents and teachers, we *learn* to ascribe certain meanings to certain experiences. For example, winning the lottery is 'good', while being declared bankrupt is 'bad'. Yet, we've all heard stories about people who win the lottery and tell of the headaches this has caused. I personally know of someone who had a successful building company which went to the wall. He is now a yoga instructor and says he is happier than ever! The point here is that winning the lottery is not *always* good, and being declared bankrupt is not *necessarily* bad.

Reality is not 'fixed'

Nothing, and I mean *nothing*, in life is fixed. Even our experiences of life which seem completely indisputable are essentially a matter of opinion. Let's take the colour of grass as an example. We all know grass is green, right? However, for argument's sake, let's imagine an individual who is colour-blind and sees grass as blue. So, is the grass green or blue? You might argue that most people are not colour-blind, and will therefore *see* the grass as green, so therefore the grass *is* green. However, it is also true that if someone sees grass as blue, to them it *is* blue. And even if people with 'normal' sight have numbers on their side, does this invalidate the experience of the person who is colour-blind?

If for one moment we let go of our sometimes rigid perception of our world it becomes clear that grass is neither green nor blue – it's *both*. What colour we see it as depends on our perception. This is an important idea because it throws up the possibility that more than one reality can exist at the same time. Even something that appears fixed, such as the colour of grass, can vary depending on who is viewing it. Grass could, indeed, be any colour under the sun!

Even 'science' is open to interpretation

From my background in medicine, I know that there are plenty of people who believe that life is indeed fixed, and that science has the capacity to dissect the realities of the universe. Yet, when we look closely, we very often find that science does not give us the clear-cut answers we expect. I can think of countless examples in the scientific literature where two similar studies have produced quite different results. For example, recently I became aware of two studies which examined the effect of vitamin E on the heart. One study concluded that vitamin E was of benefit, the other did not. What is more, these studies came out within two days of each other. Talk about confusing! There are good arguments on both sides of the debate about vitamin E and its role in preventing heart disease. Which camp someone falls in is essentially down to *opinion*.

Even when the answers science gives us do appear to be clear-cut, even these are open to interpretation. Let me give you an example. Imagine a scientific study designed to establish the effectiveness of a new treatment for an incurable disease. One group of people is treated with the real treatment, and another group is treated with an inactive treatment or 'placebo'. At the end of the study it is found that the drug cured 50 per cent of people. Looks good so far, doesn't it? However, it turns out that the same study found that 50 per cent of people taking the placebo were also 'cured'. From a *scientific* perspective, the real treatment is viewed as ineffective. Yet, one might argue that because it cured 50 per cent of people with what was thought previously to be an incurable condition, the treatment does indeed have some merit. Some might argue that withholding a treatment shown to help 50 per cent of people is morally objectionable. Who says medical treatment needs to be 'scientific' anyway? Not everyone may agree that scientific evidence for the benefit of a treatment need be a prerequisite for its use in medicine.

I'm not making a case that any of these views is 'right' or 'wrong'. However, the point is that even the principles and practice of something as apparently 'correct' as scientific research are open to question, and demonstrates just how much the events around us are essentially a matter of opinion. If we accept that the nature of reality is not fixed, then it is certainly true that our interpretation of events around us is not either. This throws up the possibility that we may, if we choose, see all of life's events in a positive light. How though?

Let go of the negative

In the last chapter we explored the concept that life is like a mirror. The secret to seeing the positive in our experiences of life is to approach them from a positive point of view. The first step here is to let go of whatever attachment you may have to the idea that any event may be inherently negative. Whatever the event, we sometimes need to suspend our judgement about it for just a moment. Once we have, we can then start to look for the positive in the experience.

Look for the positive

Once we have suspended any negative judgement, we can start to look for the positive meaning in our experience. This is obviously a personal matter, and the positive you find in any experience will be individual to you. The principle of seeing the positive in our experience of life assumed great relevance in my own life when it helped to transform my relationship with my mother.

In the last chapter I wrote about how I had viewed my father as very much a 'head' person. My mother, on the other hand, is what I regard as a more 'heart-centred' person. My mother is a person who feels a lot. She has great intuition, and is very sensitive to the way others feel and the experiences they have. No doubt these skills were of great value to her when she was practising as a doctor, and I know that she still uses them in her daily life. Yet, while I now recognize the beauty of my mother's heart-centred approach to life, when I was younger it was a source of great irritation to me.

When I was at medical school, I developed this idea that my mother was not intellectual enough. Despite the fact that my mother was a doctor, I regarded her as not well-read enough, and intellectually inadequate (I cringe as I write this but it's the truth). Now, I realize this attitude was simply a reflection of my own insecurities (for much of the time I was studying medicine I believed that I was academically inferior to my peers). However, at the time this was not obvious to me, and I just thought that my mother was simply not 'brainy' enough. As with my father, communication with my mother was not great, and we had an 'at arm's length' relationship.

Relatively soon after embarking on my career in natural medicine I saw a patient who was a psychic and healer. I didn't know much about healing, but I was certainly interested in it. After talking about the concept of healing, he asked me if I would be interested in developing my own healing potential. I was excited by this but didn't know where to start.

Quite spontaneously, he suggested that I start by recognizing that I had inherited a lot of healing potential from my mother. He then went on to describe some of my mother's attributes, including her ability to sense a person's issues and offer advice and support. In this instant, I saw my mother in a whole different light. Whereas before I viewed her as intellectually inadequate, I could now see wonderful qualities which I had simply failed to recognize. In fact, I could even see that not being bound up in her intellect might be the very thing that allowed her to make best use of her more subtle qualities. In the space of just a few minutes, I experienced a complete sea change in how I felt about my mother, which came from having my eyes opened to the 'positive' in her.

This really was a turning point for me. There is no doubt in my mind that this change in perspective has greatly enhanced my relationship with my mother. Over the last few years I have learnt a lot from her approach to life. I now recognize her to be a very intuitive woman, who often seems to feel people's experiences without them having to tell her anything. She has a distinctly positive approach to life, and does not seem at all phased by the challenges that life can bring. Now I realize that her attributes have, in many ways, been an inspiration for the emotional and spiritual component of this book.

Likewise, I also understand my father's qualities as being an important influence on me too. While I used to see his 'intellectual' approach to life as an encumbrance, I now see this also as an immense gift. In my own life, I see that the ability to use a modicum of logic and rationale is what got me through medical school, and has afforded me the ability to understand better the way the body works, what can go wrong, and what can be done to put it right. This has clearly been invaluable in my work.

It is my belief that seeing the positive attributes in my parents, and drawing from these in my own life, has been invaluable in the writing of this book.

See the positive in your emotions

If we are open to seeing the positive in the events around us, we may also be able to see some positive in our emotions too. In my experience, one of the destructive – if not the most destructive – and paralysing emotions of all is fear. Fear is one of the major reasons why we choose not to do things in our lives and follow our heart's desire. Whether it is fear of failure, fear of feeling pain, fear of making the wrong decision, or even fear of success, fear can be a major block. However, it doesn't have to be this way. Remember, *everything* can be positive if we choose to view it from a positive perspective. So, what's so great about fear?

Transforming fear

The first step to transforming fear is to recognize that you have it. Quite often because we believe fear is something bad, we push our feelings down, and divert ourselves away from the issue, hoping that it will just go away. In chapter 9 we touched on the idea that glossing over our emotions and pretending they're not there does not work, and often makes things worse. Fear that is pushed down has not actually gone anywhere. If you still have the fear, then this may be reflected in your external reality.

Recognize the fear

Imagine an individual who has an unresolved fear of abandonment stemming from childhood and the time their father left the family home. Let's assume that this fear is now manifesting as an inability to feel trust in romantic relationships. In order to deal with the relationship issue, it makes sense to deal with the fear at its root. The first step is to recognize the fear is there in the first place.

What are you doing to protect yourself?

Once you acknowledge the fear, the next step is to ask yourself what you might be doing in your life to protect yourself from that fear. For instance, the person with a fear of abandonment may choose not to get involved in close relationships. No relationship, no chance of abandonment, right? The problem here, of course, is that the real issue, the *fear*, has not been dealt with. Protecting yourself from a fear just gives a false sense of security. Facing the fear by exposing yourself to it gives you the opportunity of resolving it for ever.

Find the beliefs that are at the root of the fear

As we discussed in the last chapter, emotions, including fear, stem from beliefs. If you don't have a belief about something, then you cannot have an emotional response to it. Whatever it is you may feel fearful about, there must be some belief that is driving that emotion. It is because of this that fear can actually be a very positive thing. Why? Because, quite simply, it alerts us to beliefs that we have that do not serve us. The next step, therefore, is to find what belief you have that has caused the fear. In the case of the individual who fears abandonment, the issue may revolve around a feeling of rejection from their father.

Change the belief to something you do prefer

The final step in transforming fear is to choose a belief that works better for you. As we explored in chapter 9, the present is not the result of the past, it's the result of the present. So, for an example, the individual fearing abandonment, whose fear is based on a fear of rejection by their father, might choose to recognize that what led to the father going were relationship problems with his wife, and not to do with rejection of his child. Seeing the event in a new light can help the feeling of abandonment, and the fear that goes with it, to evaporate.

Using fear as a tool to unearth and transform the beliefs that do not serve us is aptly demonstrated in the following story.

Patricia, a lady in her mid-fifties, came to see me complaining of arthritis in her hands and spine. These problems seemed related to a number of different underlying factors including food sensitivity and hormonal changes that had come with the menopause four years previously. I recommended dietary and lifestyle changes which, along with some nutritional supplementation, was designed to help her symptoms. I enquired about her domestic situation to gauge whether or not she had any help in the home.

At this point Patricia became very upset. Her husband to whom she had been married for twenty-eight years had left her only two months before.

He had, she told me, fallen in love with a lady from the United States whom he met on the Internet. Without warning, he suddenly announced to Patricia that he was leaving and left the very same day. Patricia was devastated. Not only had her husband leaving come as an incredible shock, she did not even know where he was. Her only means of contacting him was by e-mail. She had sent him a string of e-mails pleading for him to reconsider. However, she only had two replies; one to say he was safe, the other to say he was not coming home.

Patricia was upset and confessed that she had no idea what to do. It occurred to me that if her husband had run off to America to be with a woman he hadn't even met, then perhaps there were issues with the relationship. Sure enough, Patricia told me that there were, although she had thought that things weren't 'that bad'. I asked what issues they had. It turned out that their relationship had taken a distinct turn for the worse after the death of her father six years before. She felt that her husband had offered her little support at this time, and was very resentful of him for this.

Yet, despite this simmering bitterness towards her husband, Patricia never actually discussed how she felt with him. Their relationship had become quite functional. He went out to work while she looked after the home. She had previously worked as an office manager, but had given this up a few years ago after some pressure from her husband. Their sex-life had become very sporadic, and by her own admission, there was little in terms of companionship either. Yet, however unfulfilling the relationship was, Patricia seemed to have come to the conclusion that it was better than no relationship at all. Patricia was clearly fearful of life on her own, and believed that this would be somehow worse than continuing a relationship with her husband.

I challenged Patricia's beliefs about life without her husband, and also discussed with her the principle that no event or experience has any inherent meaning. I suggested that she might transform the situation by opening up to the potential of a positive outcome, and changing her beliefs about the after-effects of her husband's departure. Possibly, Patricia could see this event as a release. Plainly she was not fulfilled in her relationship; could its end therefore spell a whole new chapter in Patricia's life – one of liberation and adventure? I wondered also, whether her joint pain might be a physical metaphor for her sense of feeling 'stuck' in her relationship. Perhaps liberating herself from the relationship would also 'free up' her hands and spine.

Looking at her situation from a more positive perspective seemed to have an immediate impact on Patricia. Her mood changed from one of despondency to one of self-assurance. Clearly, Patricia had at least glimpsed the benefits that were evident in her husband's leaving. I was keen to learn how she got on.

She returned three months later saying that her attitude to her husband leaving had changed from one of sadness and desperation to relief. While Patricia had been fearful of life without her husband, she now was choosing to believe that life was infinitely better without him. The fear evaporated as a result, and this gave her the impetus to get on with her life. Immediately after the consultation she went home and e-mailed her husband saying that she wanted a divorce. She also vented her spleen regarding her resentment she had felt since her father's death. She told me her husband agreed to a divorce, and that she had sought the advice of a solicitor. Her joint pain was considerably better and for the first time in years she was feeling 'alive'. Her friends had been a tower of strength to her, and she was enjoying an active social life. Patricia was also intending to resume work, and in the meantime had taken a temping job as a secretary in an architect's office. She was, undoubtedly, optimistic about the future.

As Patricia's story demonstrates, personal relationships can be challenging. In a way, our interactions with other people possibly afford us the greatest potential for growth. Yet, as many of us know, they can also be the source of great heartache and pain. The following chapter explores ways in which we may enrich our relationship with ourselves, and how to use that as a basis for the love we extend to others. In short, this final chapter is about how to *be love*.

Summary

- Nothing in life has any inherent meaning, only the meaning we give it

- The first step to seeing the positive in any event is letting go of the concept that it is inherently 'bad'

- Once we have let go of the negative, we can seek what positive learning an event or experience has for us

- Even fear can be positive in that it alerts us to beliefs we would prefer not to have

- Recognizing fear and not protecting ourselves from it allows us to learn more about ourselves

- Changing the beliefs that are at the root of our fear is critical to transforming this emotion

12. Be Love

Our experience of life is not generally one of isolation. Living in today's world inevitably brings us into contact with other individuals, and from this contact many different kinds of relationship can be born which enrich our lives. It is through our interaction with others, whether they are family, friends, acquaintances or 'love interests', that we get to experience all facets of life. And while relationships can give us true pleasure, they can also be the source of intense pain. It is not uncommon for issues to spring up between family members, for instance. And most will know the challenges that romantic relationships bring. Friendships sometimes offer their own challenges.

In this chapter, we will be exploring some of the major reasons why relationships can falter. And we'll also be looking at ways of approaching relationships which can enhance our experience of them. A key element in truly fulfilling relationships is love. Love, like all emotions, is not something to be lost or found, it comes from *within*. The secret to having truly loving and fulfilling relationships with others is to first have a truly loving and fulfilling relationship with ourself.

You're always in a relationship with yourself

For most of us, the word 'relationship' is generally taken to refer to a connection between *two* people. Those of us who are not currently romantically engaged usually regard ourselves as being 'not in a relationship'. The fact is, though, we are *always* in a relationship – with *ourselves*. What is more, this is undeniably *the* most important relationship we will ever have. While relationships with others may come and go, we will *never* be out of a relationship with ourselves. What is more, the better the relationship we have with ourselves, the better our relationships with others.

In chapter 10 we explored the concept that life is like a mirror – what we give out is what we get back. The more love we experience internally, the more love we experience in our lives as a whole. But how many of us really do have true love in our hearts for ourselves? For instance, do you believe some aspect of your physical appearance is simply unacceptable? Or perhaps you find some aspect of your personality unpalatable? Maybe you have a feeling of low self-worth because of an issue with a feeling of being unloved as a child.

Love yourself

The bottom line is that many of us do not love ourselves, and as a result, have made the judgement that we are not 'worthy' of love. If we do indeed feel this way, is it likely that we'll find throngs of people falling over themselves to show us otherwise? Even if we do find ourselves in a relationship, if deep down we feel we do not 'deserve' true love, what are the chances that we are going to derive emotional satisfaction from that relationship and find that it endures?

Many of the concepts in the preceding chapters have explored ways of developing nurturing and loving relationships with ourselves. In chapter 7, we discussed the concept of honouring ourselves. Within the context of relationships, knowing who you are is important because if you don't, how do you really know who you're in a relationship with? Would you commit to a life-long relationship with someone you didn't know? Well, exactly. Another important lesson from chapter 7 is the idea of self-acceptance. Accepting yourself and allowing yourself to be who you are is critical to having a loving relationship with yourself, and others too.

Once you know who are and have accepted that whole-heartedly, the critical thing is to *be who you are*. This is essentially the theme of chapter 8. An important element here is not to compromise your true wishes and desires. When you do this you have sacrificed a part of yourself. Sacrifice is a sign that you believe you don't deserve what it is you want, including your heart's desire. When you honour yourself by being who you are, and act on that without compromise, the message you are sending out to the world is that you know what you want, you believe you can have it, and that nothing less will do. Once you love who you are, and honour your true wishes and beliefs, then your reality has no choice but to reflect that back to you. We may look to others to supply us with the love we feel we need, but we're really looking in the wrong place. Remember that everything you need is right inside you. If you are 'looking for love', you need look no further!

Transforming the past

Learning to love ourselves can sometimes mean transforming our experiences of the past. In chapter 9 we explored the idea that past events can leave a 'negative' imprint on us, and colour our experience of the present. Quite often, an individual's issues with relationships, romantic or otherwise, can stem from experiences in childhood. It is not uncommon for someone to feel unloved by one or both parents, and therefore essentially feel *unlovable*. Quite often, the root through to more fulfilling relationships involves the healing of a relationship with one or both parents.

As we discussed in chapter 9, the way to transform the emotions associated with the past is to change our *beliefs* about them. In particular, it can help to change the belief that our parents did not love us, to the belief that they *did*. As children, we can sometimes be very exacting about how we want the love of parents demonstrated to us. Our parents may indeed love us, but whether they express that in a way which we recognize and accept is another matter! It is by having the *belief* that our parents love us that we can begin to experience that love. I saw this work dramatically in my own life when I accepted my father's love and at the same time dropped the conditional nature of my love for him.

Another emotional sticking point for many of us can be our experience of past romantic relationships. Sometimes, we can feel emotionally bruised by one or more relationships which did not 'go our way'. Again, these experiences can often do with being transformed. I have found that one useful thing to bear in mind here is that nothing has any inherent meaning, only the meaning we give it. This theme was discussed in the last chapter. Because of this, we have the potential to look back at past relationships and see them in a more positive light.

What, for instance, did the experience of a 'bad' relationship help us learn about ourselves? Maybe looking back at a relationship we can see how the experience stemmed from an issue with our own insecurity. Perhaps the judgement and criticism we feel for an ex-partner can help alert us to the judgement and criticism we feel for ourselves. Whatever the precise experience of a relationship, it can always teach us more about ourselves, and help us become aware of things we'd like to change. Seeing all relationships in this positive light is often very effective in dissolving the negative emotions that go with them.

A relationship cannot 'fail'

Sometimes, our feelings about past romantic relationships can be based around a sense of failure. When a relationship comes to an end, we often say it has 'failed'. However, there is no such thing as a *failed* relationship. All relationships, however long and whatever the precise experiences they bring, are an opportunity to learn and grow. The success of a relationship is not determined by its longevity or how fulfilled we felt within it. It's determined by our willingness to take from it the learning it offers. By understanding that all relationships are equally valid, it can free us from the negativity that comes with the notion of failure.

There's no need for need!

There are essentially two ways to approach relationships: one is to believe we *need* to be in one, the other is to feel we *want* to. Neediness is a feeling that comes when we believe we are dependent on that relationship for our happiness. If our belief is that our sense of fulfil-ment and happiness comes from our relationship with another person, then the idea here is that they, not us, are in control of our happiness. This is not a particularly empowering place to be in! Let us not forget that the idea that someone else controls our happiness is an illusion. Everything we need we already have – *inside us*.

Once we see happiness as something that we choose and of our own making, then we can let go of the idea that a relationship is something we need. If we do not need relationships, what purpose do they serve? There are plenty of good reasons for being in a relationship. It is often through our relationships, romantic and other-wise, that we get to learn more about ourselves. All relationships are an opportunity to grow and develop emotionally and spiritually, and they can be a lot of fun too. There is not any reason why we should not engage in relationships, learn from our relationships, and above all *enjoy* our relationships. The important thing, though, is that we do not lose sight of the fact that while we may *want* to be in a relationship, it is not something we *need*.

Marriage

A lot of people express the desire to be in a 'committed' relationship, and commitment is generally regarded as a 'good' thing in a relation-ship. In modern-day society, the most common way couples declare their commitment to each other is through marriage. To this day, marriage retains a rather sacrosanct image; one of enduring love, monogamy and stability. A lot of people regard marriage as something which provides stability and security – the ideal environment in which to raise children. But for all its positive public image, is there any evidence that marriage lives up to its reputation?

In the UK, more than 40 per cent of marriages end in divorce. In the USA, more than half of all marriages 'fail'. Of the marriages that remain, we can only guess at how many of them are truly happy. Couples may state their eternal love for each other during the marriage ceremony, but for how many couples does this actually turn out to be true? The fact is, the way two people feel about each other can *change*. People fall in love, and they can fall out of love too. Individuals can want to be in a relationship with someone, but later find that they don't. Sometimes, relationships run their natural course.

And while marriage may seem to provide a suitable environment to raise children, it does not provide immunity from trouble. It won't be news to you to learn that there are some pretty unhappy families out there (you may have had experience of this yourself). And while some couples stay together 'for the children's sake', there is no assurance that this is for the best at all. For instance, I have a good friend whose parents separated and divorced when he was fourteen. He says, in all honesty, that after years of disharmony, he was genuinely relieved when his parents finally parted.

Despite our beliefs about marriage, it is true that many do not last the distance, and they can be the cause of considerable emotional distress. Why, though, can marriage turn out to be such a bitter disappointment for many? Why, one might ask, does marriage often fall short of expectation?

The illusion of security

If we find our expectations of a relationship are not met, it makes sense to look at what those expectations are. What is it that drives a desire to be married? Social convention is an obvious motivating force for many. But what other reasons are there for tying the knot? For many, marriage appears to give stability and *security*. Yet, as we have discussed, this is often far from true. Could it be that if we are looking for marriage to give us security, we are looking in the wrong place?

As we have discussed before, all emotions come from within. The only place we can find true security is inside ourselves. Remember, life is like a mirror. For many, getting married is simply contorting the mirror – a conscious or unconscious effort to create a *sense* of security. If there is a desire to create security, it perhaps suggests the real issue for many of us is insecurity? Could it be that being married and in a 'committed' relationship can in some way protect us from having to deal with this issue?

Challenging whatever insecurity we feel means examining the beliefs we have which are at the root of this emotion. Do you, for instance, believe that you can only be happy within the context of a life-long relationship? Have you come to the conclusion that only by being married are you socially acceptable? Whatever your belief, the fact remains that your sense of happiness and fulfilment is not dependent on *anything but you*. Once you are secure in this fact, then the need to seek security in relationships simply evaporates.

Marriage can sometimes tie people together through fear

Marriage can sometimes cause people to stay together not through love, but through *fear*. Some people view the financial, social, legal and emotional ramifications of divorce as a deterrent against one or both parties just walking away from a relationship. Let's face it, divorce does not appear to be a particularly attractive proposition to most people! Could it be that some people remain married, however bad it gets, because they are fearful of the implications of divorce? Can fear really be a healthy basis for a relationship?

Commitment can only really be for now

When we 'commit to' or marry someone, we are making a promise to them. The problem is, do we know this is a promise we are going to want to keep? Can we really predict with any certainty how we are going to feel in the future? Ask yourself honestly: do you feel the same about all elements of your life as you did ten years ago? Or even five years ago? The fact is, we simply do not know how we are truly going to feel in the future. Not in ten years, not in ten weeks, and not in ten minutes for that matter.

We cannot predict the future. Remember, all we have, and will ever have, is *now*. Because of this, the *only* time we can be absolutely sure about how we feel is *now*, and therefore if we are being truly honest, the *only* time we can truly commit to someone else in a knowing way is *in the moment*. This, I know, may seem like relationship heresy. I don't deny that this concept is challenging. While there is undoubtedly a certain 'logic' to marriage and long-term commitment, as we have said, we only need to look around to see that these concepts provide no immunity from relationship issues, and do not necessarily ensure security.

While our perception may be that marriage makes it more likely that our partner may stay put, marriage is no prerequisite for this. Two people don't need to be married to want to explore and resolve whatever issues come up. And marriage is not a prerequisite for a happy family life either. Is it not entirely possible for a couple who are not married to have children and bring them up in a loving and nurturing environment?

While I may sound like I'm rampantly anti-marriage, this is actually not the case. However, it does occur to me that sometimes our deepest motivations for being married can revolve around insecurity. Unearthing the root of the insecurity, and resolving this, is what will ultimately lead to enduring security. It is this which allows us to be truly empowered in a relationship (married or not!).

Communication is key

Have you ever found yourself in a relationship where so much seems to be *unsaid*? Maybe you have harboured the desire to marry someone but have been fearful of bringing the subject up. Perhaps you have felt real love for someone but not been able to express it. Have you ever harboured a grudge against a partner for something that they said or did, but did not communicate to them how you felt? Whatever our feelings (good or bad), communicating them is key to successful relationships.

One of the main reasons why problems perpetuate between two individuals is because of a breakdown in communication. For instance, Patricia (from the last chapter) was seething with resentment about her husband's lack of emotional support, and yet had not communicated her feelings to him. For six years, Patricia had endured a bubbling bitterness and resentment which she had said nothing about. This was probably affecting her health, both physically and emotionally, and did not seem to be doing much for the relationship either. As the relationship drew to a close, however, Patricia's expression of how she felt about her husband's lack of support appeared to be accompanied by a considerable physical and emotional release.

Expressing the issues we have is only half the story. It also helps to communicate to others what we like and love about them too. Yet, many of us can have real difficulty with this. Sometimes, we may feel uncomfortable about paying our partner a compliment. Perhaps we simply take for granted our partner's qualities. Some of us may *feel* love but have real difficulty uttering the words 'I love you'.

If any of this resonates with you, it can help to take some time to look at this. One useful question to ask yourself is whether the failure to express love and affection to others is a reflection of a failure to express love and affection to yourself? How often do you give *yourself* a pat on the back for who you are? How many of your attributes do you think you might be taking for granted? Be honest now, do you *ever* say 'I love you' to yourself? Again, because life is like a mirror, by recognizing your own positive qualities, you are likely to find it easier to articulate your love and appreciation to other people.

Tell the truth

Truthfulness is a fundamental component in successful relationships. But how many of us truly believe that honesty really is the best policy? Some of us will have had the experience of not being completely honest about our feelings towards someone. Perhaps we have sometimes kept our qualms about a relationship to ourselves. How many of us have not told someone else how much we love them? How often have we done things which we have deliberately kept from someone to whom we are close? If any of this is resonating with you, then it might help to look at what value honesty brings to relationships.

First of all, though, what is it that compels us to keep the truth from others? A desire to protect is often at the root of this. Sometimes, by not telling the truth we are seeking to protect *ourselves*. For instance, if we are being unfaithful to our partner, we may fear that being honest will cause us grief. Not telling the truth can protect us from the pain, but it doesn't get rid of the *fear*. In fact, it perpetuates it. We explored this concept in the last chapter. By not looking our fear square in the eye, and failing to confront what beliefs we have that are at the root of it, we are unlikely to take much from the experience.

While we may be keen to protect ourselves in a relationship, another motivation for not telling our truth is to protect the other party. After all, what they don't know can't hurt them, right? The assumption here is that learning the truth will have a 'bad' effect on them. This may turn out to be the case, but remember that precisely what effect it has is up to *them*. They can interpret the truth in any way they choose, including positively.

For instance, in chapter 10 I wrote about Robin, and how his wife had told him about an affair she was having. Initially, this did not get a good reaction from Robin. However, later on he chose to see it as an opportunity to be honest about his own infidelities, and explore with his wife deeper issues in their relationship. While we may feel that not telling the truth protects someone else, it is also robbing them of a valuable opportunity for personal growth.

Another problem with not being completely honest in a relationship is that it simply does not give the other person the opportunity to know *who* they are really in a relationship with. If you are not being your true self, then your partner is not really in a relationship with you, but someone else. Clearly, this is no basis for a 'real' relationship. Being who you are in every respect, and that means telling the truth, allows others to know who they are involved with!

Control games

Have you ever found yourself in a relationship where you have wanted to change your partner in some way? Maybe you have even sought to manipulate that person to fulfil your own needs. A common example of this is when people who feel insecure in a relationship attempt to feel more secure by undermining the other person. A comment about their appearance here, a jibe about their personality there. It can all go to erode another's sense of self-worth and self-love and create the illusion that they, in a way, depend on the relationship.

Attempting to manipulate another person is akin to contorting the mirror in an effort to see a different reflection. Within the context of our relationships we need to realize that whatever our needs, only *we* can fulfil them. Our experiences with others may facilitate that, but they can't do it for us. Once we have a complete relationship with ourselves, we can dispense with any need we have to control and manipulate others.

Give unconditional love

Once we drop the need to control other people, it can also open us up to the idea of unconditional love – love that is given without the other person needing to fulfil any criteria. In reality, though, we often offer our love only as long as our needs are fulfilled and our expectations of that person are met. Setting conditions about how you want another person to be does not make for truly fulfilling relationships. It perpetuates the illusion that our sense of happiness and peace comes from other people satisfying certain criteria. The fact remains, however, that the only person who can really meet your needs and expectations is *you*. It is by honouring yourself completely and having unconditional love for yourself, that you will be able to give and receive unconditional love within your relationships.

Summary

- The most important relationship we will ever have is with ourselves

- Knowing who we are, and honouring that is key to a good relationship with oneself

- All relationships are valuable learning experiences if we see them as such

- The idea that we may *need* another person for our happiness is an illusion and can often lead to disempowerment

- Insecurity is a common motivating factor in marriage and pledged commitment

- It is having internal security which allows us to be in relationships in a knowing, empowered way

- Because all we have is now, the only time we can be truly committed in a relationship is *now*

- Communication and truthfulness are key to loving, fulfilling relationships

- Unconditional love for oneself is what allows us to experience unconditional love within the context of relationships

Ultimate Health A–Z

The A–Z of health issues which follows includes scientific references where these are relevant. Often, studies known as 'placebo-controlled, double-blind studies' are referred to. These studies are designed to assess the effect of a treatment by comparing it to an inactive treatment or 'placebo'. 'Double-blind' means that neither the individuals administering the study nor the subjects receiving the treatment know whether active or placebo treatment is being used until after the study. Placebo-controlled, double-blind studies are designed to discriminate between the real effects of a treatment and any response that might be due to chance or spontaneous healing.

Abdominal Bloating Abdominal bloating can have several underlying causes, more than one of which can coincide in an individual. One of the most common causes of bloating is overgrowth of the organism Candida albicans. Information about how to go about diagnosing and treating this condition can be found in chapter 3 on pages 53–62. Food sensitivity is also a common factor in bloating. Wheat is often an offender here, but other foods, especially dairy products, can be implicated. Chapter 3, pages 34–43 contains information on how to diagnose and manage food sensitivity.

The failure to properly digest the milk sugar 'lactose' is another common cause of abdominal bloating (see *Lactose Intolerance*). Abdominal bloating can also be related to poor digestion, with inadequate chewing, and low levels of stomach acid (hypochlorhydria) and/or digestive enzymes common factors. See pages 44–8 for information on how to diagnose and treat poor digestion. Finally, a rarer but important cause of abdominal bloating is parasitic infection of the gut. Parasites can be hard to identify, though specialist laboratories that have expertise in this area do exist (see Useful Information at the back of the book). If parasites are found to be present, their successful elimination usually leads to a reduction in bloating and an improvement in general digestive function.

Acne vulgaris (see also *Rosacea*) Acne vulgaris is the most common form of acne, and is caused by blockages in the glands responsible for making a skin-waterproofing agent called 'sebum'. Acne is generally more common in adolescence, when hormonal changes may alter sebum secretion.

In natural medicine, acne is often viewed as a problem of excess toxicity within the body. For this reason, sufferers are often advised to eat as 'clean' a diet as possible. This means avoiding foods which contain significant quantities of fat (particularly what are known as 'partially hydrogenated' and 'trans fatty acid' found in many margarines and most fast, baked and processed foods). Other food components to avoid include artificial colourings, flavourings, preservatives and sweeteners. More information about how to identify and treat body toxicity can be found in chapter 3.

A common factor in acne is overgrowth of the yeast organism Candida albicans. Identification and successful treatment of this problem almost always leads to a significant improvement in skin condition. More information about the diagnosis and treatment of candida can be found on pages 53–62. For some women, their acne tends to flare up before a period (also known as 'pre-menstrual acne'). This sort of acne is often helped by taking 50 mg of vitamin B6 each day (*ref* 1). The herb agnus castus, probably through its hormone-balancing effects, has also been found to be of benefit here (*ref* 2).

Research has shown that a significant proportion of women with acne have high levels of 'male' hormones (androgens) such as testosterone in their systems. One study found that almost two-thirds of women with acne had raised levels of at least one type of male hormone (*ref* 3). This study suggests that elevated levels of androgens is a much more common factor in female acne than was previously thought.

High levels of androgens in women are often, but not always, associated with a condition known as 'polycystic ovarian syndrome' (PCOS). As its name suggests, PCOS is associated with multiple cysts in one or both ovaries. Common symptoms of this condition include breast pain, menstrual irregularities, and excess facial and/or body hair. More information about how to treat this condition can be found in the section entitled *Polycystic Ovarian Syndrome*.

Certain nutrients may be useful in controlling acne. The mineral zinc has been found to help acne sufferers (*ref* 4). One study found that zinc therapy worked as well as antibiotic medication (*ref* 5). I generally recommend acne sufferers take 30 mg of zinc, three times a day for three to four months, after which the dose can be reduced to once or twice daily. Studies show that zinc therapy takes time to work, with twelve weeks being the amount of time most people seem to need to get good results. My preference is to use a form of zinc which is readily absorbed by the body such as zinc citrate or zinc picolinate. Because zinc can induce copper deficiency, 1 mg of copper should be taken for every 15 mg of supplemental zinc.

Age Spots In the body, energy is generated through reactions in which food is 'burnt' with oxygen. These reactions result in the manufacture of waste products called 'free radicals' which have damaging and destructive effects on the body. The damage caused by free radicals forms a debris called 'lipofuscin'. Lipofuscin may accumulate in the skin, where it can give rise to brown spots (usually on the face and back of hands) which are commonly referred to as 'age spots'. The number and severity of age spots is thought to be an indication of the amount of free radical damage in the body as a whole.

Free radicals in the body are neutralized by substances known as 'antioxidants' which include the vitamins A, C, and E, and the mineral selenium. To help prevent age spots, it is therefore wise to take a good quality antioxidant supplement each day. In addition, it can be helpful to rub a cream containing vitamin C into the affected areas twice a day. The direct antioxidant effect this may have in the skin can help break down the lipofuscin in time.

Alcoholism Alcoholism, like other chemical addictions, is generally viewed as a psychological problem. However, addictions generally have a biochemical and physiological component as well, and addressing this usually makes overcoming any psychological component easier. As with perhaps all health issues, a holistic approach is usually the most successful.

From a biochemical standpoint, there is some thought that alcohol craving can be associated with fluctuations in blood sugar. When blood sugar levels drop, the body tends to crave foodstuffs that replenish sugar quickly in the body. For some people that might be chocolate or biscuits, but for others it is alcohol. I have seen many patients successfully reduce their alcohol consumption by taking steps to balance their blood sugar. More information about this can be found on pages 69–84. In particular, supplementation with the formulation Glucoguard (specifically designed to help stabilize blood sugar levels) can help.

Alcoholism may respond to supplementation with certain nutrients. Alcoholics are very often nutrient deficient, and studies in animals suggest that nutritional deficiency, particularly in the B vitamins, can increase the desire to drink alcohol (*refs* 1, 2, 3). More importantly, work with alcoholics has shown that nutrient supplementation has the ability to reduce alcohol consumption (*refs* 4, 5). Individuals wanting to stop or reduce their alcohol consumption might do well to take a good quality multivitamin and mineral supplement, combined with a B-complex supplement which provides 25 to 50 mg of vitamins B1, B2, B3, B5, and B6 each day.

Other nutrients which might be deficient with alcoholism are the essential fatty acids (EFAs). One of the final breakdown products of EFAs is a hormone-like molecule known as 'prostaglandin E1' (PGE1). PGE1 is believed to have mood enhancing and antidepressant action in the brain. Short-term alcohol consumption appears to increase PGE1 levels, while longer-term drinking appears to have the opposite effect. It has been theorized that alcohol craving is sometimes related to low PGE1 levels. Studies do suggest that supplementation with EFAs can be beneficial in terms of reducing alcohol intake and preventing symptoms of withdrawal (*refs* 6, 7). Because of its high EFA content, taking evening primrose oil (1 g, three times a day) might help to control drinking in the long term.

One other nutrient which appears to help reduce alcohol craving is the amino acid glutamine. In one study, nine out of ten alcoholics thought that glutamine at a dose of 1 g per day reduced their desire for alcohol. In this study, glutamine was also found to help reduce nervousness and improve sleep (*ref* 8).

Alzheimer's Disease Alzheimer's disease is caused by the gradual destruction of nerve cells in the brain, which ultimately leads to senility and dementia. The condition is characterized by a reduction in mental function, loss of short-term memory, and mood problems such as irritability or childish behaviour. Alzheimer's disease can occur at any age but is most common after the age of fifty.

What causes Alzheimer's disease is not known, but there is at least some evidence that a proportion of cases are linked to the toxic effects of the metal aluminium. More than one study has found accumulations of aluminium in the part of the brain affected by the disease (*refs* 1, 2). In one study, using aluminium-containing deodorants appeared to increase risk of Alzheimer's disease by 60 per cent (*ref* 3). However, some studies have not found a link between aluminium and Alzheimer's disease (*ref* 4). Clearly, this is a controversial area, but it does seem prudent for people to do what they can to avoid aluminium exposure. In general, aluminium-containing antacid medication, and food packaged in aluminium cartons or cooked in aluminium pans should be avoided. The use of aluminium-free deodorants is another wise precaution, and these can usually be found in health food stores.

There does seem to be some important links between diet and Alzheimer's disease. A high fat diet seems to increase the risk of the condition, while a diet rich in oily fish (e.g. salmon, trout, tuna, mackerel, herring) and other 'omega-3 fatty acids' such as flaxseed oil seems to protect against the disease. A high level of monounsaturated fats (e.g. extra virgin olive oil) has also been found to slow brain function decline. A diet rich in cereals and grain also appears to be protective (*ref* 5).

There has been a lot of recent interest in the role of damaging molecules called 'free radicals' in Alzheimer's disease. Interestingly, vitamin E (an important 'antioxidant' nutrient which can help reduce damage due to free radicals) at a dose of 2,000 IU (international units) per day has been shown to help protect against Alzheimer's disease (*ref* 6). High levels of the blood chemical 'homocysteine' have also been found in Alzheimer's disease sufferers, and there is potential for reducing this with vitamins B6 and B12 and folic acid. A raised homocysteine level (as ascertained by a blood test) can often be successfully treated with supplements of vitamin B6 (at least 10 mg per day), vitamin B12 (at least 50 mcg per day) and folic acid (at least 400 mcg per day) (*refs* 7, 8, 9).

There are a few natural treatment options for Alzheimer's disease, one of which is acetyl-L-carnitine. This substance can increase the production of the important brain chemical acetylcholine. Acetyl-L-carnitine has been shown to improve memory, and slow progression of the disease (*ref* 10). The normal recommended dose is 500 to 1,000 mg, three times a day.

Another natural substance that can be very effective in improving mental function is the herb ginkgo biloba. This can improve circulation to the brain, and appears to enhance memory and quality of life. Four double-blind studies have found ginkgo biloba to be of benefit in the early stages of Alzheimer's disease (*refs* 11, 12, 13, 14). The normal recommended dose is 40 to 80 mg of standardized extract, three times a day.

Anaemia – iron deficiency (see also *Anaemia – pernicious*) Oxygen is transported throughout the body by the red blood cells. The substance in the red blood cells responsible for carrying oxygen is called 'haemoglobin'. Iron is essential for the manufacture of haemoglobin, and any lack of iron (either through blood loss or inadequate intake) may lead to anaemia. Common symptoms of anaemia include physical fatigue, mental sluggishness and low mood. While anaemia is a relatively common cause of fatigue, it should be borne in mind that fatigue is not always caused by anaemia, and anaemia is not always caused by iron deficiency. See *Fatigue* for more information on the common causes of fatigue.

To complicate things further, it is possible that despite not being anaemic, individuals can be fatigued as a result of iron deficiency and may respond to iron supplementation. Other symptoms of iron deficiency include itching of the skin, 'spooning' (concavity) of the fingernails and, in women, diffuse thinning of the hair. Pregnant women and those who experience heavy periods are especially prone to iron deficiency. Other individuals at increased risk of this condition include vegetarians (their intake of iron is generally lower than that of meat-eaters), and those taking long term painkillers such as aspirin or non-steroidal anti-inflammatory drugs (these can induce bleeding in the gut).

While an individual's symptoms can point to low iron as a problem, iron does need to be handled with some care. Iron is what is known as an 'oxidizing agent', having quite the opposite effect of 'antioxidant' nutrients such as vitamin C and E which protect against disease. Some research suggests that high doses of iron induce changes which, at least theoretically, would increase the risk of heart disease. One study found that men with high levels of iron in their bodies have an increased risk of heart disease (*ref* 1). Also, a small percentage of the population suffer from a condition known as 'haemochromatosis' in which iron tends to accumulate in the body, depositing itself in various organs. More common in men than women, haemochromatosis can lead to problems with diabetes, cirrhosis of the liver, and heart rhythm abnormalities.

Probably the best way to determine iron levels in the body is with a blood test. The most commonly used test is known as the 'serum iron', which essentially measures the level of iron in the bloodstream. However, a better test for assessing the overall level of iron in the body is something called 'ferritin'. If a blood test shows a low ferritin level, then iron intake should be increased.

One way to do this is to increase consumption of iron-rich foods such as red meat, oysters, fish, dried fruit and green leafy vegetables. Coffee and tea should be avoided, as these can reduce the amount of iron absorbed from the diet. In addition, it usually helps to take iron in supplement form. A typical recommended dose is 100 mg of iron per day, though this may need to be adjusted according to changes in the ferritin level. Quite often, iron supplementation can cause gastrointestinal symptoms, the most common of which is constipation. It is well known that vitamin C enhances the absorption of iron, thereby reducing the amount of iron that needs to be taken in the long term. The less iron is taken, the less risk there is of side-effects such as constipation. A dose of 250 to 500 mg of vitamin C should be taken with each dose of iron. The most commonly prescribed form of iron is iron sulphate (ferrous sulphate), which is not very well absorbed and notorious for giving rise to gastrointestinal symptoms. Sometimes, it is a good idea to use a more absorbable and less irritating form such as iron fumarate.

Not uncommonly, individuals with iron deficiency fail to respond to supplementation. Despite using large doses of iron, the ferritin level may not increase much, and the individual may not feel much better. In this situation, it is important to consider the possibility of low stomach acid secretion (hypochlorhydria), as stomach acid is important for iron absorption. More information on the diagnosis and treatment of hypochlorhydria can be found in chapter 3, pages 44–8.

Anaemia – pernicious Pernicious anaemia is a particular form of anaemia caused by a chronic deficiency of vitamin B12. Classically, sufferers of this condition are said to lack the ability to make a molecule in the stomach called 'intrinsic factor' which is necessary for B12 to be absorbed by the body. As a result, dietary sources of B12, even in supplement form, are generally not well-absorbed. B12 deficiency can occur even when there are adequate levels of intrinsic factor, and the term pernicious anaemia is often used in these situations too. Common causes of low B12 absorption include Crohn's disease, coeliac disease and low stomach acid secretion (see pages 44–8 for more information about this).

Because the principal B12-containing foods are of animal origin (meat, fish, eggs and dairy products), vegans can sometimes become deficient in B12. Tempeh (a soybean product), spirulina and nutritional supplements are alternative sources.

Generally, only a small amount of vitamin B12 (say 3–4 mcg per day) is required to prevent a deficiency. However, if there is some problem with absorption, vitamin B12 injections (given into the muscle) may be recommended. After a course of injections, it may be possible to maintain B12 levels in the body by giving 1,000 to 2,000 mcg per day as an oral supplement (*refs* 1, 2).

Aneurysm – aortic The aorta is the main vessel which emerges from the heart to transport blood around the body. In some people, the wall of the aorta can balloon out, leading to a condition known as 'aortic aneurysm'. The concern with aortic aneurysms is that they may burst, a situation which often proves fatal. Because of this, some individuals are advised to have the aneurysm repaired by having a piece of synthetic tubing stitched inside the aorta.

There is some evidence to suggest that the development of aortic aneurysms is related to copper deficiency (*ref* 1). Much of the aorta is made up of elastic tissue, the normal production of which depends on copper. Also, one study found very low levels of copper in the bodies of aneurysm sufferers compared to normal subjects (*ref* 2). Although the effect of copper supplementation on the development of aortic aneurysms has not been studied, taking additional copper may help. While it is unlikely to reverse the aneurysm, it is possible that extra copper may slow or prevent further development of the problem. The normal recommended dose of copper is 3 mg per day.

Angina Angina is the result of reduced blood flow to the heart, and is normally felt as a dull, heavy sensation felt in the centre of the chest, neck or left arm, when the heart muscle is starved of oxygen. Angina is usually related to narrowing of the vessels that supply blood to the heart muscle itself known as the 'coronary arteries'. A common cause of coronary artery narrowing is a condition known as 'atherosclerosis' (see *Atherosclerosis*). Another cause of reduced blood supply to the heart muscle is spasm in the lining of one or more coronary artery. Usually, angina comes on during exercise but may also come on at rest.

Blood sugar balance is often important in the control of angina. When blood sugar levels fall, the body often attempts to correct this by secreting the hormone adrenaline which can help top up sugar levels by stimulating its release from the liver. Adrenaline may trigger angina, partly because it increases the oxygen demands of the heart muscle, but also because it may induce spasm in the coronary arteries. See pages 69–84 for more information about the diagnosis and treatment of blood sugar imbalance.

Certain nutrients may help to control angina symptoms. One of my personal favourites is the mineral magnesium. This is important for energy production in the body, enhancing muscle function (including the heart muscle), and reducing the risk of spasm in the coronary arteries. Magnesium injections appear to help control angina (*refs* 1, 2). One gram of magnesium sulphate might be given weekly for several weeks, with lower doses after this. I am not aware of any research that has looked at the effect of oral magnesium supplementation on angina, though it does seem sensible for individuals to consider this, especially when they do not have access to magnesium injections. I generally recommend 500 to 1,000 mg of magnesium per day.

Another natural substance which may help relieve angina is Coenzyme Q10 (CoQ10). This nutrient is essential for the production of ATP – the basic unit of energy in the body. One study showed that 150 mg of CoQ10 per day significantly lengthened the amount of time it took for angina to come on during exercise (*ref* 3). Benefits may also be obtained from supplementation with the compound L-carnitine. L-carnitine helps transport fat into parts of the body's cells called the 'mitochondria', where it can be burned for energy. Studies show that L-carnitine can increase exercise tolerance and reduce angina attacks (*refs* 4, 5). A typical dose would be 1 g of L-carnitine, once or twice a day.

One other 'natural' treatment to consider in angina is what is known as 'chelation therapy'. A chemical known as ethylenediaminetetraacetic acid (EDTA) appears to have the ability to open up clogged arteries when given intravenously. There is a wealth of anecdotal evidence to support the effectiveness of this treatment, and one review study concluded that it seems to help control symptoms in more than 80 per cent of individuals (*ref* 6). However, there still has not been any large double-blind studies on chelation therapy, and its use remains controversial. Nevertheless, it is my feeling that chelation therapy might be considered by anyone suffering from significant arterial disease because it does appear to help control and reverse artery blockage, and may prevent further disease.

Angular Stomatitis Angular stomatitis is a condition characterized by cracking at the corners of the mouth. It is often a painful condition that can make talking and eating quite uncomfortable. Occasionally, this condition is related to yeast infection (thrush) around the mouth. More often than not, however, angular stomatitis is related to a vitamin and/or mineral deficiency.

Sometimes angular stomatitis is associated with iron deficiency. The best test for iron deficiency is a blood test for a substance known as 'ferritin'. Because iron can have damaging effects in the body at high levels, it is advisable to have a ferritin test before supplementing with iron. Another factor which seems to be common in angular stomatitis is a deficiency in the B-group vitamins, particularly vitamins B2 and B6. In general, the diet should be rich in foods which contain vitamins B2 and B6 such as wholemeal bread, green leafy vegetables, eggs and fish. In addition, it can help to take a B-complex supplement each day containing 25–50 mg of the major B vitamins B1, B2, B3, B5 and B6. On this regime, angular stomatitis usually clears within a few weeks.

Anorexia Nervosa Anorexia nervosa is a form of eating disorder characterized by extreme weight loss, a morbid fear of becoming fat and an altered body image. Typically, anorexics are painfully thin, but actually 'see' themselves as overweight. Anorexia may be related to emotional issues such as problems with relationships in the family, feelings of deprivation and abuse. However, physiological and biochemical factors appear to play their part too.

It comes as no surprise that anorexia can lead to severe deficiencies of dietary elements such as protein, iron, calcium, B vitamins, folic acid and vitamin C. It is impossible to define the impact of such deficiencies on emotional and physical health, but it is likely that they will compound the health problems seen in anorexia. Taking a potent multivitamin and mineral supplement is one simple thing that sufferers can do to help themselves by reducing the risk of these deficiencies.

One nutrient which appears to have particular benefit in anorexia is the mineral zinc. Zinc has many important functions in the body, and one of these appears to be the normalization of brain function and perception. In one study, a daily dose of 45–90 mg of zinc led to weight gain in seventeen out of twenty anorexics after periods ranging between eight and fifty-six months (*ref* 1). In a double-blind study, 14 mg of zinc per day doubled the speed of weight increase in a group of anorexic women (*ref* 2). I generally recommend that in addition to a good quality multivitamin and mineral, anorexics also take 90 mg of zinc per day. Because zinc can induce copper deficiency, about 6 mg of copper should be taken with this dose of zinc. Once improvement is seen, the dose of zinc may be reduced, and more emphasis may be placed on a nutritious, varied diet.

Anxiety Occasional feelings of anxiety and tenseness are a normal response to some of the events and situations life can throw at us. However, in some people quite extreme feelings of unease can be experienced even when there does not appear to be any particular reason for this. From a natural health perspective, anxiety may be related to biochemical or physiological imbalance. One factor commonly seen in conjunction with anxiety is blood sugar imbalance. When blood sugar levels fall, the body often attempts to correct this by secreting the hormone adrenaline to help top up sugar levels by stimulating the release of sugar from stored forms of fuel. Adrenaline is well known to promote feelings of anxiety and sometimes panic. Blood sugar imbalance is discussed in depth in chapter 4. Weakness in the adrenal glands is also a common feature in anxiety and panic attacks (see pages 88–93).

A very important dietary factor that often features in anxiety is caffeine. Caffeine is a stimulant, and certainly has the ability to provoke nervousness. In one study, the severity of people's anxiety and depression correlated with the amount of caffeine they consumed. Interestingly, patients suffering from panic attacks were sensitive to the amount of caffeine found in just one cup of coffee. It seems, for those individuals who are prone to anxiety, the safest amount of caffeine to consume is none! (*ref* 1).

The conventional pharmacological treatments for anxiety revolve around beta blockers and tranquillizers. Beta blockers reduce the heart rate and the force of contraction of the heart, and may give rise to side-effects such as cold hands and feet, fatigue, dizziness and impotence as a result. Tranquillizers such as diazepam (Valium) and chlordiazepoxide (Librium) can help reduce anxiety, but may also induce unwanted symptoms such as dizziness, drowsiness and impaired coordination. Another downside to these drugs is that they can be addictive if taken for long periods.

A safe, natural alternative to these conventional medicines does exist in the form of a herb known as kava kava. Kava kava is rich in a group of compounds called the kavalactones, which appear to have a very calming effect on the mind. One double-blind study showed a significant reduction in anxiety compared with inactive medication (*ref* 2). The normal recommended dose is 50–75 mg of kavalactones, three times a day.

Please note: kava kava is not recommended for use by pregnant or lactating women and it should not be mixed with other sedative medications.

Asthma Asthma is a chronic lung condition characterized by recurrent attacks of breathlessness, often accompanied by wheezing. Asthma is due to inflammation in the air passages of the lungs, causing constriction of these passages (bronchospasm) which makes breathing difficult. Asthma can be classified into two main types: extrinsic, in which attacks are triggered by an allergy, and intrinsic, in which there is no obvious external cause for the attacks. Extrinsic or 'allergic' asthma tends to come on during childhood, while intrinsic asthma usually develops later in life. However, either condition can appear at any age.

Allergic asthma is often set off by an inhaled trigger such as animal fur, dust, feathers and air pollutants. However, there is also good evidence that asthma attacks can be linked to certain foods, especially in childhood asthma. One study showed that 90 per cent of children with asthma or allergic rhinitis (runny nose due to allergy) improved on a food elimination programme (*ref* 1). The most common offenders in this respect are dairy products, eggs, chocolate, wheat, corn, citrus fruits and fish. More information about the detection and elimination of problem foods can be found on pages 34–43.

It is well known that certain foodstuffs may promote inflammation in the body, which can then perhaps contribute to asthma and other allergic conditions such as eczema. Some of the foods which may do this are what are known as the omega-6 fatty acids. Omega-6 fats are generally found in quantity in margarine and vegetable oils such as sunflower, safflower and corn oil. Omega-6 fats can be converted into substances which tend to encourage inflammation in the body. On the other hand, fats of the omega-3 type, such as those found in oily fish, appear to reduce inflammation in the body.

There is an idea that an increased consumption of omega-6 fats (found in many margarines and vegetable oils), coupled with a decreased consumption of omega-3 fats, might increase the risk of asthma. One study in Australia reported that increased rates of asthma coincided with a five-fold increase in consumption of polyunsaturated fats, particularly of the omega-6 type (*ref* 2). This research also noted the increased consumption of these fats in New Zealand, the United States and the UK, all places where asthma rates are rising significantly. In contrast, countries where consumption of omega-3 fatty acids is high and omega-6 fats is low (such as Mediterranean and Scandinavian nations) have low rates of asthma. Research has also found that asthma symptoms appear to be better controlled in children who consume oily fish (*ref*3). Avoidance of margarine and vegetable oils, and the inclusion of oily fish such as salmon, trout, tuna, mackerel and herring in the diet may possibly help control asthma symptoms in time.

There is also some evidence linking salt consumption with asthma. Salt appears to heighten the response of the airways to histamine, causing increased constriction (*ref* 4). Asthmatics should therefore avoid adding salt to their food during cooking or at the table and minimize their consumption of processed foods which tend to have a lot of salt already added. Other substances that seem to provoke asthma include tartrazine (a yellow colouring found in some processed foods) and sulphites (used as a preservative in many alcoholic drinks and processed foods).

The mineral magnesium can be a useful supplement for asthmatics. Magnesium can help prevent the bronchi (airways in the lungs) going into spasm and might also help prevent histamine release (*ref* 5). I recommend that adult asthmatics take about 500 mg of magnesium a day, and for children adjusting the dose according to weight. Vitamin B6 is often deficient in asthmatics, and supplementation with this has been found to be beneficial in children (*ref*6) and adults (*ref* 7). The dose in the study in children was 200 mg per day. Because there is a slight risk of neurological symptoms at this dose, I recommend children on this regime be monitored by a medical practitioner. The dose used in the adult study was 50 mg, twice a day, which is a safe dose to take in the long term.

A herb which might help in cases of asthma is ginkgo biloba. Ginkgo appears to have the ability to block the action of a substance called 'platelet activating factor' (PAF), which is believed to be involved in the processes which trigger asthma. At least one study has found ginkgo to be effective in reducing asthma symptoms (*ref* 8). The normal recommended dose is 120–240 mg of standardized extract per day.

Atherosclerosis Atherosclerosis is a term used to describe the blockages that occur in the body's arteries as part of the ageing process. Ultimately, atherosclerosis can lead to heart disease (and heart attack), cerebrovascular disease (clogging of the arteries supplying blood to the brain, which may ultimately lead to stroke), and peripheral vascular disease (usually characterized by blockage in the arteries of the legs which may lead to gangrene and possibly the need for amputation).

The substance which causes blockage in the body's arteries is essentially composed of fat, so it makes sense to control fat consumption. However, there is good evidence to suggest that the type of fat we eat has an important bearing on the progression of atherosclerosis. The omega-3 fatty acids found in oily fish such as salmon, trout, mackerel, herring, tuna and swordfish have a number of beneficial effects on the cardiovascular system including protection from atherosclerosis. One study showed that supplementation with fish oil (6 g per day for 3 months followed by 3 g a day for 21 months) led to regression of atherosclerosis, and fewer complications (*ref* 1). Other dietary fats which appear to have a protective effect are those found in raw nuts and seeds, avocado and extra virgin olive oil.

While a lot of emphasis has been placed on the need to avoid saturated fat in the diet (red meat, dairy products, eggs), there is mounting evidence that the fats known as 'partially hydrogenated' and 'trans fatty acids' are also a cause for concern. These fats, found in many fast foods, baked goods, processed foods and margarine, have been found to cause atherosclerosis in animals (*ref* 2), and are associated with an increased risk of heart disease in humans (*ref* 3).

Studies show that consumption of homogenized milk correlates with heart disease, while butter and cheese consumption does not appear to increase risk (*ref* 4). The critical factor seems to be a substance called xanthine (pronounced zan-theen) oxidase. This enzyme appears to damage the lining of the arteries, predisposing them to atherosclerosis. Homogenized milk contains appreciable quantities of absorbable xanthine oxidase, while cheese and butter do not.

Sugar is another dietary element which might increase the risk of atherosclerosis. Sugar induces a variety of changes which might exacerbate this problem, such as a reduction in 'healthy' high density lipoprotein (HDL) cholesterol in the bloodstream and an increase in 'unhealthy' triglyceride levels (*ref* 5). What is more, sugar consumption has been shown to be closely related with an increased risk of heart disease (*ref* 6).

Atherosclerosis is also associated with high levels of a substance known as 'homocysteine'. Homocysteine is a break-down product of the amino acid methionine, and is normally converted in the body to a harmless substance called cystanthionine. However, this conversion is dependent on certain nutrients, namely vitamin B6, B12 and folic acid. A deficiency of one or more of these might cause homocysteine levels to rise. Anyone with a raised homocysteine level (as ascertained by a blood test) should take at least 10 mg of vitamin B6, 50 mcg of vitamin B12 and 400 mcg of folic acid per day. Studies show that supplementation with these nutrients can bring homocysteine levels down (*refs* 7, 8, 9).

In recent years, much attention has been focused on the need to control cholesterol levels in the bloodstream. However, studies suggest that cholesterol per se is not the problem. It is when cholesterol becomes damaged through a process known as 'oxidation' that it has the propensity to settle on the inside of the arteries. Vitamin E helps protect cholesterol from oxidation, thereby reducing its damaging effects. Studies show that men and women supplementing with 100 IU (international units) or more of vitamin E each day reduced their risk of suffering from a fatal or non-fatal heart attack by about a third (*refs* 10, 11). In another study, individuals with diagnosed heart disease were given either vitamin E (400 or 800 IU) or a placebo (*ref* 12). This study showed a massive 77 per cent reduction in risk of non-fatal heart attack in people taking vitamin E. However, the results of the study also indicated that there was no difference between the two groups in death rates. Further analysis found that of the fifty-nine deaths due to heart disease in this study, only six occurred in people actually taking vitamin E (*ref* 13).

Vitamin E may have side-effects such as digestive discomfort and reduced blood clotting, but the dose needed to produce significant problems is likely to be 1,500 IU or higher. However, because vitamin E can thin the blood at doses of 400 IU or more each day, individuals on an anti-clotting medication such as warfarin are advised to use vitamin E with some caution and under medical supervision. While vitamin E can be found in the diet in sunflower seeds, hazelnuts, almonds, avocado and vegetable oils such as olive oil and safflower oil, the average daily intake is probably only between 10 and 20 IU. For individuals wanting to reduce their risk of developing heart disease, I generally recommend that they supplement with 400 IU of vitamin E each day. For those with a history of heart disease, I usually advise higher doses be taken (about 800 IU per day). Vitamin E comes in two forms: d-alpha-tocopherol (natural) and dl-alpha-tocopherol (synthetic). The natural form of vitamin E appears to work better in the body and is therefore preferred.

Athlete's Foot Athlete's foot, also known as 'tinea pedis', is a fungal infection which normally causes cracking and itching of the skin between the toes. Some people experience a problem with persistent athlete's foot that often recurs and may be resistant to treatment. In this situation there is usually an underlying problem of yeast (fungus) overgrowth in the gut. My experience is that by controlling the overgrowth of the organism Candida albicans in the gastrointestinal tract, it is usually possible to get long term and even permanent relief from athlete's foot. Pages 53–62 contain details on how to diagnose and treat candida infection. Topical relief from athlete's foot can often be had from preparations containing tea tree oil (a natural anti-fungal agent).

Atrial Fibrillation The healthy heart beats in a consistent rhythmical fashion to pump blood around the body. In atrial fibrillation (AF) the heart goes out of sync and starts to beat irregularly. When this happens, the heart is temporarily unable to pump blood around the body as efficiently as normal. Commonly, AF is not continuous, but comes in fits and starts. This condition is called 'paroxysmal atrial fibrillation'. Common symptoms during an attack include palpitations, flutters in the chest, faintness or dizziness.

Caffeine has been linked to abnormal heart rhythm. Some individuals may be susceptible to as little as one cup of coffee (*ref* 1). A reduction in or complete elimination of caffeine from the diet may help to control heart rhythm. Deficiencies of both magnesium and potassium have been linked to an increased risk of heart rhythm disturbance such as atrial fibrillation (*ref* 2). Magnesium- and potassium-rich foods should be emphasized in the diet. Nuts, seafood, seeds, green leafy vegetables and whole grains such as wholemeal bread and wholewheat pasta are rich in magnesium, while potassium can be found in fresh fruits and vegetables, especially bananas. In addition, I generally recommend that people with arrhythmia take 500 mg of magnesium a day.

Another useful natural substance for the treatment of arrhythmia is the herb hawthorn (crataegus). One study showed hawthorn to be of value for treating arrhythmia in animals (*ref* 3), and I have often found it to be of benefit in practice. The normal recommended dose is 80–300 mg of herbal extract or 3–4 mls of tincture, three times a day.

Atrophic Vaginitis Vaginitis (inflammation of the vagina) can be caused by a number of factors including infections with Candida albicans or some other organism. After the time of the menopause, the reduction in oestrogen levels in the body can give rise to a particular form of vaginitis called 'atrophic vaginitis'. Here, the vaginal tissue can become thin and weakened, with a tendency to become inflamed. This condition often causes considerable discomfort, and can make intercourse difficult and painful. Taking natural steps to reduce the impact of menopause on the body (see *Menopause*) can help to control this condition. However, there is a natural remedy which does seem to be of particular value in atrophic vaginitis – panax ginseng. A dose of 100 mg of standardized extract should be taken three times a day until symptoms improve. After this, a once or twice daily dose is often enough to maintain health in this area.

b

Back Pain (disc degeneration) The spine is made up of a column of bones which are called the 'vertebrae'. Between the vertebrae lie discs of spongy material (known as 'intervertebral discs'), which act as shock absorbers and allow the spine to bend and twist more easily. Each intervertebral disc is composed of a hard outer layer with a soft jelly-like centre. As we age, one or more discs can start to break down, usually causing pain and a degree of immobility. If a disc becomes very damaged, surgery may be necessary.

Each disc in the spine contains a substance called 'collagen'. Collagen is largely responsible for the strength and resilience of the intervertebral discs. Vitamin C has a very important part to play in the formation of collagen, and taking this in supplement form does seem to help prevent further disc damage. It has been reported that vitamin C (1,500 to 2,500 mg per day) can often alleviate pain and spare the need for surgery (*ref* 1). Another useful agent in the treatment of disc problems is glucosamine sulphate. Glucosamine is the basic building block in the kind of tissue that intervertebral discs are made of. Taking 500 mg of glucosamine sulphate two or three times a day should also help to stimulate healing and repair in the damaged disc.

Bad Breath Bad breath is often believed to relate to a problem with oral hygiene. While this may be the case, the real cause of bad breath – also known as 'halitosis' – lies lower down in the digestive tract. Common causes of halitosis include problems with digestion and/or the elimination of waste from the bowel. Either of these factors can cause toxicity within the gut, and these toxins may come to be eliminated in the breath. More information on internal toxicity, and how to clear this, can be found in chapter 3.

Bed-wetting Bed-wetting, the medical term for which is 'enuresis', affects about one in ten five-year-olds. However, the problem is also known to persist after this age, even into a child's teens.

It is best to limit a child's fluid intake during the evening. The more a child drinks in those few hours before bedtime, the more likely he or she is to wet the bed. Caffeinated soft drinks should be avoided especially because caffeine is known to stimulate urine production, and is therefore likely to increase the risk of bed-wetting.

In my experience, a very common and frequently missed factor in bed-wetting is food sensitivity. While the mechanism for this is unclear, it does appear that unwanted reactions to certain foods and drinks in the diet can cause bed-wetting. Other symptoms to look out for that suggest food sensitivity include the presence of dark bags under the eyes (sometimes referred to as 'allergic shiners'), red ears, behavioural problems and frequent colds or other infections. Some of the most common problem foods are milk, cheese, wheat, eggs and citrus fruits. However, it is also worth bearing in mind that children tend to crave the foods to which they are most sensitive. More information on food sensitivity, and how to identify culprit foods, can be found on pages 34–43.

Benign Prostatic Hypertrophy The prostate is a walnut-sized gland that surrounds the first part of the tube that takes urine from the bladder to the outside (the urethra). As a man ages, the prostate gland may enlarge, and this can impede the flow of urine from the bladder. Prostate enlargement is normally due to a condition called 'benign prostatic hypertrophy' (BPH) which is a common condition after the age of fifty.

Like every gland in the body, the prostate has nutritional needs. Probably the most important nutrients in this respect are the mineral zinc and healthy fats known as essential fatty acids. Zinc can be found in fish, seafood (especially oysters) and seeds. Essential fats can be found in raw nuts and seeds, oily fish such as salmon, trout, mackerel and herring and extra virgin olive oil. Eating an abundance of these foods is likely to help maintain health in the prostate gland and may possibly reduce the risk of enlargement. Interestingly, essential fat consumption may help protect against prostate cancer. One study found that men consuming moderate or high amounts of oily fish had about a 70 per cent reduced risk of prostate cancer compared with men consuming no oily fish at all (*ref* 1).

Linseed oil is rich in essential fats, particularly the omega-3 variety, which seem to be important in maintaining prostate health. One study showed significant improvements in the symptoms and signs of prostatic enlargement (*ref* 2). One tablespoon of linseed oil should be taken daily for several months, after which the dose can be reduced to one to two teaspoons a day.

The mineral zinc is found in very high concentration in the prostate and supplementation with it (often in conjunction with linseed oil) seems to help reduce prostatic enlargement; 30–60 mg of zinc should be taken each day. Because zinc supplementation can induce copper deficiency, 1 mg of copper should be taken for each 15 mg of zinc taken.

The herb saw palmetto has been found to be effective in controlling prostate symptoms. A review of the available studies which looked at the effect of saw palmetto in BPH found that it is just as effective as the most commonly used drug for this condition (finasteride) (*ref* 3). The normal recommended dose is 160 mg twice a day, or 320 mg once a day. Another herb which may help in BPH is African pygeum. This herb contains a variety of compounds which appear to help combat BPH (*ref* 4). A dose of 50–100 mg of standardized extract should be taken twice a day.

Blepharitis Blepharitis is a condition characterized by inflammation of the eyelids. Typical symptoms include redness, irritation and scaliness around the margins of the lids. Sometimes the roots of one or more lashes may become infected or the surface of the eye may become inflamed. The conventional medical treatments for blepharitis are based around lid hygiene and eye-drops. Despite these measures, the condition often recurs.

A natural remedy that may well help to reduce symptoms is the herb Oregon grape (Mahonia aquifolium). This plant extract has traditionally been used to treat a variety of eye disorders including blepharitis and conjunctivitis. Oregon grape contains a substance called 'berberine' which has anti-microbial properties, and helps to combat the bacterial infection, which is often a feature in blepharitis. Oregon grape is also thought to strengthen delicate membranes around the body, including the eyelids.

Oregon grape should be applied topically and taken internally for best effect. To make a soothing eyewash, 10 g of the herb can be simmered in a pint of water for twenty minutes. The resulting fluid should be strained and allowed to cool. This mixture can then be applied with an eye bath or cotton-wool balls. The eyes can be bathed for ten minutes, twice a day. In addition, it usually helps to take a tincture (alcoholic extract) of Oregon grape internally. The normal recommended dose is 5 mls (1 tsp), three times a day.

Bone Spur Sometimes bones in the body may develop small pointed projections known as 'bone spurs'. This commonly occurs under the heel of the foot and can cause considerable discomfort; surgery may be deemed necessary. Supplementing the diet with calcium and magnesium can help to improve the symptoms caused by a spur. I generally use 1,000 to 1,500 mg of calcium along with 500 to 750 mg of magnesium. This treatment takes time, but benefits are often apparent after three to six months.

Breath-Holding Attacks Breath-holding attacks are most common between the ages of one and two, and are often accompanied by an expression of pain, anger or frustration. Often, a child will go red or blue in the face during an attack, and may even faint if it is very severe. Fortunately a reflex invariably restarts the breathing mechanism. Although breath-holding attacks are thought to be harmless, they can nonetheless be disturbing for parents and child. It is not clear what causes breath-holding attacks, but one theory is that children unconsciously bring on the attacks as an attention-seeking mechanism.

Some research casts doubt on the idea that children bring on breath-holding attacks themselves. There is now a theory that the condition may be associated with low levels of the mineral iron in the body. In one study, almost 90 per cent of children treated with iron suffered no more attacks or had the frequency of attacks cut by at least half (*ref* 1). In this study, ferrous sulphate, the most common form of iron, was used. The dose was 5 mg for each kg of weight, per day. While iron may be effective for controlling breath-holding attacks in many children, I would be cautious about using this approach until low iron levels have been shown in the child. The best way to assess levels of iron in the body is the 'serum ferritin' blood test.

Bronchitis Bronchitis is caused by inflammation in the airways of the lungs. There are principally two sorts of bronchitis; acute and chronic. Acute bronchitis is usually caused by a viral or bacterial infection, while chronic (long-term) bronchitis is usually related to prolonged exposure to an inhaled irritant such as cigarette smoke. Common symptoms of bronchitis include coughing (often with the production of phlegm), wheezing and shortness of breath.

For acute bronchitis, it is important to take steps to enhance immune system function. Three of the most important agents in this respect are vitamin A, vitamin C and the herb echinacea. Both vitamins A and C can boost immune function and vitamin A seems to be particularly beneficial in preventing lung infections. I generally recommend that individuals take 50,000 to 100,000 IU of vitamin A per day along with 1 g of vitamin C, several times a day during an acute attack. This large dose of vitamin A should not be taken in the long term because of the risk of toxicity. However, it is safe to take for a week or two. Echinacea, which has a widespread reputation as an immune-enhancer, may also be able to help control an infection. There are two main species of echinacea used therapeutically – purpurea and angustifolia. Because each form of echinacea has slightly different properties, it is probably a good idea to combine them for maximum effect.

For chronic bronchitis, it is important to avoid foods which tend to increase mucus formation in the airways. The classic offenders in this respect are dairy products, though other foods can cause problems too. For more information about food sensitivity, and how to identify problem foods, see pages 34–43. In addition, it may help to take certain nutrients. Of particular merit here is N-acetyl cysteine (NAC). This agent has the ability to break up and 'loosen' the secretions which commonly cause problems in chronic bronchitis. One study showed NAC had real benefit at a dose of 600 mg per day, three days a week (*ref* 1).

Bruising – Easy Bruises are caused by leakage of blood from the very smallest blood vessels in the skin known as 'capillaries'. The blood that collects in the skin appears purple or blue at first, but then turns yellow as it is broken down by the body. In some individuals, often young women, bruises can occur after the slightest bump or knock. Rarely, this problem may be due to some problem with the blood clotting system in the body. Despite the fact that such disorders are uncommon, it is nevertheless good practice for individuals with easy bruising to have appropriate blood tests.

Most commonly, individuals with easy bruising have weakness and fragility in the capillaries. Strengthening the capillaries is often effective in reducing bruising. Vitamin C and related nutrients known as 'bioflavonoids' found in many fruits can improve vessel strength and reduce the risk of bruising. Doses of 1,000 mg of vitamin C and 500 mg of mixed bioflavonoids, taken twice a day, normally control the problem within a few weeks. Half the initial dose is usually effective in the long term.

Bulimia Nervosa Bulimia, the full medical name for which is 'bulimia nervosa', is an eating disorder characterized by bouts of food bingeing, after which sufferers may make themselves sick or take excessive amounts of laxatives. There is good evidence that physiological and/or nutritional factors often underlie the condition, and that dietary management can be very effective in controlling symptoms.

Blood sugar imbalance seems to play an important role in the condition. In one study, a group of bulimic women were put on a diet designed to maintain a stable level of sugar in the bloodstream (*ref* 1). The diet excluded all alcohol, caffeine, refined sugar, white flour products, monosodium glutamate and flavour enhancers. All the women in the study stopped bingeing while they were on this regime, and were still binge-free two and a half years later. More information about the management of blood sugar instability can be found on pages 69–84.

Another factor which may be at play in bulimia is low levels of the brain chemical serotonin. Serotonin generally induces happy, feel-good emotions. It is manufactured in the brain from an amino acid called 'tryptophan' which itself is found in foods such as meat, tofu, almonds, peanuts, pumpkin seeds, sesame seeds and tahini (sesame seed paste). Tryptophan is absorbed into the brain more efficiently when there is carbohydrate present. This might explain why certain individuals gravitate towards sweet or starchy foods when upset or stressed. In one study, bulimic women were treated with tryptophan (3 g per day) or a placebo for about a month (*ref* 2). Those taking tryptophan were also given vitamin B6 (45 mg per day) as this is thought to help the conversion of tryptophan into serotonin. Those taking the tryptophan and B6 combination were found to have significantly improved measures of mood, eating behaviour and feeling about eating compared to those taking the placebo. Unfortunately, tryptophan is not available over-the-counter in many countries, including the UK and the US. However, 5-hydroxytryptophan (5-HTP) – the substance tryptophan is converted into before it is made into serotonin – is a good alternative. A supplement of 50 mg of 5-HTP should be taken, two or three times a day.

Burning Feet Syndrome Burning Feet Syndrome is a condition characterized by a burning sensation in the feet and sometimes the hands. It can often cause considerable discomfort and disturb sleep. There is no established medical treatment for this problem other than painkillers which may cause side-effects with extended use. Burning feet syndrome is related to a deficiency of vitamin B5 (pantothenic acid). Other potential symptoms of B5 deficiency include depression, fatigue, weakness and loss of appetite.

It is important to increase the consumption of foods that are rich in vitamin B5, including liver, kidney, eggs, nuts and whole grains such as wholemeal bread. In addition, 250 mg of vitamin B5 should be taken twice each day until the symptoms subside. After this, it is usually a good idea to take a B-complex supplement which contains 25–50 mg of the vitamins B1, B2, B3, B5 and B6 every day. This will help to prevent any deficiency in vitamin B5 in the future.

Burns The most important thing to do after a burn is to run cold water over it. This will take much of the heat out of the burn and is likely to help limit its severity. For maximum benefit, the burn should be kept under cold running water for several minutes and ice should be applied if possible. While minor burns can be treated at home, large or severe burns should be looked at by a doctor just in case there is a need for medical treatment.

A few natural agents can be beneficial for helping burns to heal and to reduce scarring. My favourites are pure essential oil of lavender, aloe vera gel, and vitamin E squeezed from a soft gelatine capsule. Applying one or more of these soothing and healing agents several times each day does seem to reduce discomfort and often seems to have a dramatic effect on the speed at which a burn heals.

Bursitis 'Bursae' are fluid-filled pockets which occur on or around the joints. Their function is to reduce friction. Sometimes a bursa may become inflamed, giving rise to a painful condition known as 'bursitis'. Physiotherapy, analgesics and steroid injections may all be tried in an attempt to control the pain of this condition. One study has showed that a useful natural treatment for bursitis is vitamin B12 injections given into the muscle. The typical dose was 1,000 mcg of B12 given daily for seven to ten days, followed by injections three times a week for two to three weeks, followed by once or twice weekly injections for another two to three weeks. The majority of patients experienced considerable relief with this treatment (*ref* 1).

C

Carpal Tunnel Syndrome Carpal tunnel syndrome (CTS) is a condition characterized by numbness, tingling or pain in the thumb and first three fingers of one or both hands. CTS is caused by the compression of one of the major nerves to the hand (the median nerve) as it runs through the wrist. Symptoms tend to be worse at night and can be especially bad on waking. Sometimes, CTS can be related to low thyroid function (hypothyroidism). If symptoms such as sensitivity to cold, cold hands and feet, dry skin and lethargy are also present, it may well be worth while considering this possibility. See chapter 5 for more details about the diagnosis and treatment of low thyroid function.

One nutrient apparently very effective in the treatment of CTS is vitamin B6. It reduces inflammatory reactions in soft tissues and some doctors believe that deficiency of this nutrient is a major factor in the development of CTS. There is good evidence that demonstrates significant relief for a large proportion of CTS sufferers with B6 supplementation (*refs* 1, 2). A dose of 100 mg of B6 should be taken three times a day for three months, followed by a good B-complex containing at least 25 mg of B6 daily.

Cataract Cataract (cloudiness in the lens of the eye) is a surprisingly common visual problem: almost everyone over the age of sixty-five has some degree of cataract formation, and most people over the age of seventy-five will experience some visual deterioration as a result of this condition. With an increasing ageing population, the incidence of cataracts is set to treble in the next fifty years. Fortunately, there is increasing evidence that cataracts can be prevented through dietary change and the use of nutritional supplements.

It is well established that cataract development is related to damage caused by destructive molecules in the body called 'free radicals'. The cloudiness induced in the lens by free radicals is similar to the change evident when an egg white is cooked. While a raw egg white is transparent, it becomes opaque when the protein within it is damaged during the cooking process. One lifestyle factor which is well known to increase free radical damage in the body is smoking. Stopping smoking cuts the risk of cataract by about 20–25 per cent in the long term (*ref* 1).

Free radicals are quenched in the body by 'antioxidant' nutrients such as beta-carotene, and vitamins C and E. Theoretically, increasing our intake of antioxidants should help protect our eyes from developing cataracts. Research has showed that individuals taking a multivitamin and mineral supplement containing vitamin C and/or E enjoyed a 60 per cent reduction in the risk of cataract (*ref* 2). However, because cataracts develop slowly over many years, supplementation does need to be long term to get real benefit. This particular study showed that the benefits of taking nutrients were only apparent after ten years of supplementation. Another study showed a 27 per cent reduced risk of cataracts through taking a multivitamin containing vitamin C and/or E for five years (*ref* 3). Yet another study found that taking vitamin C supplements for ten years or more reduced the risk of cataract development by 70 per cent (*ref* 4). On balance, this evidence suggests that taking 500 mg of vitamin C in addition to a multivitamin and mineral supplement each day is very likely to substantially reduce the risk of cataract formation in the long term.

While nutrient supplementation is of proven benefit in reducing cataract risk, making informed dietary choices also helps here. Research shows that eating foods rich in what are known as 'carotenoids' was associated with a reduced cataract risk (*refs* 5, 6). While beta-carotene is perhaps the best-known carotenoid, its less famous relatives lutein (pronounced loo-teen) and zeaxanthin (pronounced zee-ah-zanthin) appear to have significant antioxidant properties. Spinach, which is quite rich in beta-carotene, also contains significant quantities of lutein and zeaxanthin. Interestingly, of the range of food items that were studied, spinach was the one which seemed to be most consistently associated with a reduced cataract risk.

Cellulite Cellulite is the commonly used name for the dimpled, orange peel-like appearance which can affect skin at the back of the thighs. It seems to be an exclusively female problem. Cellulite is often related to toxicity in the body. See chapter 3 for more details about toxicity, and what to do about it. I have found that skin brushing (described on page 30) is often of particular value in clearing cellulite.

Cerebrovascular Insufficiency (see also *Atherosclerosis*) The brain is supplied with blood via two main vessels known as the 'carotid arteries'. As we age, these arteries may become gradually clogged with a fatty substance in a process known as 'atherosclerosis'. If this is so severe that the brain is starved of blood, symptoms such as short-term memory loss, dizziness and ringing in the ears (tinnitus) may arise. The medical term for this condition is 'cerebrovascular insufficiency'.

Eating a diet low in saturated fat should help reduce further clogging of the carotid arteries. For this reason, consumption of red meat, dairy products and processed foods should be limited. In addition, certain natural agents may help. By protecting it from damage due to oxidation, vitamin E reduces the risk of cholesterol depositing itself on the inside of the artery wall, and also has natural blood-thinning effects. A dose of 400 to 800 IU should be taken each day.

Another useful natural substance for cerebrovascular insufficiency is ginkgo biloba. This herb can improve circulation, including that to the brain, and may therefore help relieve the symptoms such as poor memory, dizziness or tinnitus. The recommended dose is a total of 120 to 240 mg of standardized extract per day.

Cervical Dysplasia The term 'cervical dysplasia' is used to describe potentially cancerous changes in the cells of the cervix (the neck of the womb) in women. Another term used to describe changes in the cervical cells is 'cervical intraepithelial neoplasia' (CIN). CIN is classified according to severity. CIN1, CIN2 and CIN3 denote mild, moderate and severe dysplasia respectively. If CIN is allowed to progress unchecked it will ultimately develop into early localized cancer (called 'carcinoma *in situ*') and then finally full-blown cervical cancer. Any woman found to have cervical dysplasia will normally be advised to have a repeat smear or an examination of the cervix with a viewing instrument (colposcopy). During colposcopy, samples of tissue are sometimes removed (biopsy) or the affected area is treated with laser or electro-coagulation (both of which use heat to destroy abnormal tissue) or cryosurgery (freezing of abnormal tissue).

The development of abnormal cervical cells is related to the number of sexual partners a woman has had; the greater the number, the greater her risk. However, some women develop abnormal cervical cells despite only having one or a small number of sexual partners. Risk is also increased if there has been contact with the virus that causes genital warts (the human papilloma virus). Using condoms during intercourse may reduce risk. Smoking also increases the risk of cervical dysplasia.

Studies show that cervical dysplasia is associated with low dietary or body levels of the antioxidant nutrients beta-carotene, vitamins A, C and E and the mineral selenium (*refs* 1, 2, 3, 4, 5). Eating a diet rich in these (fresh fruits and vegetables, avocado, and Brazil nuts) may help to prevent cervical dysplasia or keep it in check. One study suggests a diet high in lycopene (found in tomatoes) might help protect against cervical dysplasia (*ref* 6). Taking an antioxidant supplement each day that includes some lycopene (say 10 mg) might also help to prevent or control cervical dysplasia. A good example of such a supplement is NutriGuard Forte, which is available from VitaTech (see Useful Information at the back of the book).

Chilblains Chilblains are itchy, purple-red swellings which usually occur on the toes and are related to problems with circulation. Chilblains are caused by excessive narrowing and constriction of blood vessels, usually as a result of exposure to cold. Chilblains occur mostly in the young and the elderly, and are more common in women than in men.

There are several natural agents which may reduce the tendency to suffer from chilblains. I generally recommend that chilblain sufferers take 400 to 800 IU of vitamin E each day. Vitamin E helps to reduce the stickiness of blood components called platelets, effectively thinning the blood and thereby improving circulation. A supplement of the mineral magnesium may also help because it has a relaxant effect on blood vessels. A good dose is 250 to 500 mg per day. Finally, the herb ginkgo biloba is also likely to provide some relief, as it is well known to enhance circulation. The normal recommended dose is 40 to 80 mg of standardized extract, three times a day.

Chocolate Craving Chocolate is full of mind- and mood-altering substances, including caffeine, phenylethylamine (an amphetamine) and a marijuana-like compound. My experience is that the main addictive component in chocolate is usually sugar. Many individuals who experience episodes of low blood sugar (see pages 69–100) will crave foods which release sugar quickly into the bloodstream such as chocolate. Glucoguard, a supplement designed specifically to help blood sugar stability, is often very helpful here. This can be obtained from VitaTech (see Useful Information at the back of the book).

Cholecystitis (gallbladder pain) (see also *Gallstones*) The gallbladder sits underneath the liver and acts as a reservoir for bile, a substance made in the liver. Bile is then passed into the digestive tract. Its function is to dissolve fat, a bit like washing-up liquid, so that it can be properly digested in the gut. Gallstones are common in Western society. Mostly, they are symptomless, although some seem to give rise to recurrent bouts of pain and discomfort (cholecystitis), usually felt in the upper right-hand side of the abdomen. Some individuals who have their gallbladder removed (with an operation known as cholecystectomy) continue to have problems with abdominal symptoms. The presence of this condition, known as 'post-cholecystectomy syndrome', suggests that factors other than the gallstones themselves might be at play.

A frequent underlying factor in gallbladder pain is food sensitivity. In one study, sixty-nine individuals with symptomatic gallstones or post-cholecystectomy syndrome were put on a diet which consisted of only beef, rye, soy, rice, cherry, peach, apricot, beet and spinach for a week (*ref* 1). All of the sixty-nine subjects in this study became symptom free. Then foods were added one at a time back into the diet, to identify which ones appeared to provoke symptoms. The worst offenders were egg, pork and onion, though it is probably a good idea for sufferers to assess their food sensitivities on an individual basis. More details about this can be found on pages 34–43.

Another factor associated with gallbladder pain is low stomach acid (hypochlorhydria). In one study, more than half of individuals with gallstones were found to be suffering from this condition (*ref* 2). Hypochlorhydria can give rise to symptoms such as bloating, belching and digestive discomfort, which can be similar to those associated with gallbladder disease. Sometimes, 'gallbladder' symptoms will resolve once hypochlorhydria has been identified and treated. More details about the diagnosis and treatment of hypochlorhydria can be found on pages 44–8.

Chondromalacia Patellae Chondromalacia patellae is a knee condition that most commonly affects adolescents and young adults. The condition is caused by a degeneration of the cartilage that covers the back of the kneecap, causing pain in the front of the knee, often after running or when walking down stairs. Some sufferers of chondromalacia patellae may eventually have an operation that involves either scraping the inside of the kneecap and/or realignment of the kneecap so that it is less prone to damage.

One nutrient that may help heal this is glucosamine sulphate. This is an essential building block for cartilage formation and speeds up cartilage regeneration. A dose of 500 mg should be taken three times a day. Once symptoms have improved this may be reduced to 500 mg once or twice a day. Two other nutrients that experience shows may be very useful in combating chondromalacia patellae are selenium and vitamin E. Amounts of 200 to 300 mcg of selenium and 400 to 800 IU of vitamin E should be taken each day until a month after the symptoms are under control.

Cluster Headaches Cluster headaches are intense, migraine-like headaches, often manifesting as severe stabbing pains on one side of the head. Cluster headaches tend to last for a few hours at a time, and often come daily for several days or even weeks. The headaches may then disappear for months or even years, before they return again. Blood levels of the brain chemical melatonin have been found to be low in sufferers of cluster headaches, especially during an attack. In one double-blind study, the effectiveness of a daily dose of 10 mg of melatonin was compared with a placebo (*ref* 1). The individuals receiving melatonin experienced cessation of their headaches after three to five days of treatment, whereas the placebo group experienced no improvement in their symptoms. While the long-term effects of melatonin supplementation are not known, it is likely that its use for limited periods of time (such as in the treatment of cluster headaches) is safe.

Cold and Flu Both cold and flu are caused by viruses. Our susceptibility to these infections is essentially dictated by the efficiency of our immune system – the part of the body responsible for repelling unwanted organisms. The strength of the immune system is intimately related to lifestyle factors, including what we eat. An important dietary component in this respect is sugar. There is evidence that sugar has the capacity to disable the immune system (*refs* 1, 2). Sugar should therefore be limited in the diet, especially at the first sign of an infection.

Several natural agents have been found to be effective in treating the common cold, probably the best known of which is vitamin C. Vitamin C has several immune strengthening and anti-viral actions in the body. Most studies suggest that 1.5–4 g of vitamin C taken in divided doses during the day at the first sign of a cold reduce the number of ill days by about 30 per cent (*ref* 3). In accordance with the work of the late Linus Pauling, an ardent proponent of vitamin C, many people find larger doses more effective. Taking 1–2 g of vitamin C every two waking hours until a day or two after the symptoms disappear often seems to stop a cold or flu in its tracks. This large dose of vitamin C can sometimes cause some loosening of the bowels, though this side-effect resolves once the dose is reduced.

Another useful nutrient for combating the common cold is zinc. Zinc inhibits the virus responsible for the cold infections (rhinovirus). Sucking a zinc lozenge every two waking hours has been shown to reduce the average duration of colds by seven days compared to a placebo (inactive medication) (*ref* 4). The precise form of the zinc in the lozenge is important – it should be zinc *gluconate*. Other forms of zinc may not actually liberate sufficient quantities of zinc to exert a significant effect. The lozenge should not contain citric acid, tartaric acid, mannitol, or sorbitol either, as these can inactivate the zinc. Zinc lozenges taste awful! However, in my experience, most individuals will put up with the taste because the benefits of this treatment are usually so clear.

The herb echinacea has gained quite a reputation over the last few years as a potent infection fighter. Echinacea has proven immune system stimulating ability, and a review concluded that there was good evidence to support its use in the treatment of the common cold (*ref* 5). There are two main species of echinacea used therapeutically; purpurea and angustifolia. Purpurea is the type most commonly used, though angustifolia certainly has merit and contains anti-viral agents called echinacosides which are not found in the purpurea plant. Because of this, it is probably best to use a combination of both types of echinacea during a viral infection.

Another useful agent in the treatment of viral infections is Sambucol. This product contains a blend of black elderberries (*Sambucus nigra L.*) and rasp-berries (*Rubus idaeus L.*) which have the ability to inhibit the flu virus. One study found that if Sambucol was started within twenty-four hours of the onset of symptoms, 90 per cent of subjects became symptom-free in two to three days (*ref* 6). In contrast, individuals taking inactive medication did not recover for at least six days.

Cold Sores Cold sores are caused by the herpes simplex virus (HSV). Once it has infected the body, the virus lies dormant, but may reactivate and cause a cold sore at any time, especially when the immune system is weak or run-down. Cold sores typically last for seven to ten days, are unsightly, and can cause considerable discomfort.

The HSV virus needs an amino acid called arginine to multiply in the body. Arginine is found in high concentration in nuts, especially peanuts and cashews, chocolate and grains, and many people report that eating these foods can bring on symptoms. Avoiding these foods, especially at the first sign of an attack, is likely to help prevent problems.

While arginine encourages growth of the HSV, another amino acid – lysine – actually inhibits it. Most studies which have looked into this association show that lysine can reduce the frequency and severity of cold sore attacks (*ref* 1). A dose of 500 mg should be taken per day, increasing to 1 g, two to three times a day during an acute attack. To this regime it can help to add vitamin C and bioflavonoids, a combination of which has been found to reduce the duration of symptoms by more than half (*ref* 2). At the first sign of an attack 200 mg of vitamin C and 200 mg of bioflavonoids should be taken three to five times each day. Another nutrient which might help to reduce attacks is selenium. Selenium has the ability to inhibit several viruses, including the herpes virus. As a preventive 300 to 400 mcg should be taken per day. This dose should be doubled during an attack.

For topical relief I recommend vitamin E from a soft gelatine capsule. Soak a small piece of tissue in the contents of a capsule and apply to the cold sore. If this is done for fifteen minutes, twice a day, the cold sore will often resolve in a day or two (*refs* 3, 4).

Colic Colic is a common problem in infants which usually causes sharp, gripey abdominal pains, abdominal bloating, drawing up of the legs and crying. Colic seems to be more common in bottle-fed rather than breast-fed infants. There is good evidence to suggest that colic is related to a reaction to cow's milk-based infant formulas (*refs* 1, 2). Some children are simply unable to digest the large protein molecules in milk, and this is often at the root of the bowel symptoms typical of colic. Switching a child to a formula based on goat's milk or cow's milk specially treated to break down the protein molecules within it (known as 'hydrolysates') can often be very effective in reducing the symptoms of colic.

Studies also show that milk in the mother's diet may cause colic in breast-fed infants too. Breast-fed infants with colic often improve when cow's milk is eliminated from the mother's diet. Rice milk, oat milk and calcium-enriched soya milk make good alternatives. While cow's milk is commonly implicated in colic, it's not the only offender. One study showed that other foods in the mother's diet which commonly upset breast-fed children include cabbage, broccoli, cauliflower, onion and chocolate. Breast-feeding mothers with colicky children should consider eliminating these foods from their diet (*ref 3*).

Another useful strategy in combating colic is feeding on demand. There is a theory that if too long is left between a child's feeds, discomfort may result. This problem may be related to falls in the child's blood sugar level. One study showed that demand-based feeding dramatically reduced the incidence of colic (*ref 4*).

Constipation – see chapter 3, pages 27–8

Cough Coughing can be related to many different health issues including cold and flu (see pages 221–2), bronchitis (see page 214) and asthma (see pages 206–8). Dealing with the underlying nature of a cough is usually the best way to get rid of the symptom. However, it may also help to use a natural agent to help soothe the throat. A commonly used herb is thyme (*Thymus vulgaris*). This herb has a long history of use in Europe for dry cough. Around 1–2 g of thyme can be made into a tea with boiling water. This should be drunk several times a day.

Cradle Cap Cradle cap is an infantile form of skin condition known as 'seborrhoeic dermatitis'. It is characterized by the presence of thick yellow scales on the skin of the scalp. Other sites for this condition include the face, neck, and the nappy region. The condition is not related to poor hygiene or lack of cleanliness and is harmless. There is some evidence that cradle cap is related to a deficiency in the nutrient biotin which is one of the B-group vitamins (*ref 1*). An increase in the child's consumption of biotin may help to control the condition. If the child is being breast-fed, the mother herself can take the biotin as this will be conferred to the child in the breast milk. The mother should take 500 to 1,000 mcg per day. For bottle-fed children, 50 to 100 mcg of biotin can be added to the feed each day.

The application of starflower (borage) oil to the child's seborrhoeic dermatitis in the nappy region often leads to considerable improvement in the condition. This approach is also certainly worth trying in cradle cap too. Ten drops of starflower oil should be rubbed into the affected region, twice a day for two weeks. This can be repeated as necessary.

Cramp Cramp is a painful spasm in a muscle caused by excessive or prolonged contraction of muscle fibres, often in the calves, feet or back of the thighs. Cramps usually last for a few moments, but can quite commonly occur at night, which may disrupt sleep. It is usually related to a deficiency of magnesium, calcium or potassium. On a dietary level it is important to increase consumption of foods that are rich in these. Sesame seeds, tahini (sesame seed paste), and tinned fish are good sources of calcium. Magnesium can be found in nuts, seafood, whole grains and green leafy vegetables, while bananas and other fruits are rich in potassium. Eating more of these foods can sometimes be all it takes to stop recurrent cramp attacks.

Supplementing with magnesium is often very effective in relieving cramp. In a double-blind study performed in pregnant women with leg cramps, 365 mg of magnesium each day was found to reduce the severity of the cramps by more than 70 per cent (*ref* 1). I normally recommend 500 mg of magnesium per day, reducing the dose to about half this once symptoms have improved.

Crohn's Disease Crohn's disease is caused by inflammation in the wall of the bowel and is characterized by bouts of pain and diarrhoea that can be bloody. The condition can affect any part of the gut, but classically causes inflammation in the last part of the small intestine.

There are two approaches to Crohn's disease which I have found to be quite effective. One of these is to eliminate refined carbohydrates, and in particular sugars known as 'disaccharides' (e.g. sucrose and fructose). The concept here is that these foods feed organisms within the gut that might trigger or worsen Crohn's disease. This approach has been popularized by Elaine Gottschall, an American nutritionist who was introduced to this treatment through her work with the gastroenterologist Dr Sidney Haas. More details about the specifics of this diet can be found in Elaine Gottschall's book entitled *Breaking the Vicious Cycle*. There is at least some experimental evidence suggesting that a low carbohydrate diet can be effective in controlling Crohn's disease. In one study, a low-sugar, high-fibre diet led to a 70 per cent reduction in hospitalizations compared with individuals who did not change their diet (*ref* 1).

The other major approach I tend to use in Crohn's disease centres around the identification and treatment of food sensitivities. There is some evidence that food intolerance can be a factor in Crohn's disease. In one study, the most common food triggers were found to be cereals, dairy products and yeast (*ref* 2). For more information about food sensitivity, see pages 32–43.

Crohn's sufferers can have multiple nutritional deficiencies because they tend not to absorb nutrients very effectively. It is a good idea for them to take a potent, high-quality multivitamin and mineral preparation every day. Of particular importance are zinc, vitamin B12 and folic acid, as they can help in the repair of the cells lining the intestinal tract. Useful daily doses of these are 30–45 mg of zinc (balanced with 2–3 mg of copper), 800 mcg of vitamin B12 and 800 mcg of folic acid.

Fish oils such as eicosapentaenoic acid (EPA) and docosahexaenoic acid (DHA) might also help to control Crohn's and this may be related to their anti-inflammatory effect. One two-year study showed that a diet high in fish substantially reduced the relapse rate in sufferers (*ref* 3). The fish richest in EPA and DHA are the 'oily' fish such as salmon, trout, tuna, mackerel, herring and swordfish.

d

Depression Depression can have specific physiological and/or biochemical triggers. Common problems which I encounter in practice include low thyroid function (see chapter 5), anaemia and/or iron deficiency (see pages 201–2), seasonal affective disorder (see pages 278–9), food sensitivity (see pages 34–43), and blood sugar imbalance (see pages 69–84).

On a dietary level, it can often help to eliminate certain foodstuffs which tend to upset brain chemistry. The major offenders here are sugar, caffeine, alcohol and artificial sweeteners. Just getting these elements out of the diet often leads to a significant improvement in mood. In addition, further support may be had from natural substances.

The herb St John's Wort (*Hypericum perforatum*) has been shown to be effective in the treatment of depression. In one study, two thirds of individuals with mild to moderate depression improved on St John's Wort, compared to only about a quarter of individuals who were taking inactive medication (placebo) (*ref* 1). Although St John's Wort's antidepressant activity has often been ascribed to a constituent known as hypericin, more recent attention has focused on other elements including hyperforin, xanthones and flavonoids. There is some evidence that the overall effect of St John's Wort is to increase the levels of 'feel-good' brain chemicals such as serotonin, noradrenaline and dopamine (*ref* 2). The normal recommended dose is 300 mg of herb extract, three times a day.

Diabetes Diabetes, a condition characterized by abnormally high levels of sugar in the bloodstream, is a common problem and the third leading cause of death in the West after cardiovascular disease and cancer. In the long term, diabetes can lead to a variety of health problems including eye disease and blindness, kidney disease, heart disease, leg ulcers, gangrene and impotence. There are essentially two forms of diabetes: Type I and Type II. Type I diabetes (also known as 'juvenile onset' or 'insulin-dependent' diabetes) generally comes on early in life and is caused by a failure of the pancreas to secrete insulin. Sufferers of this form of diabetes must take insulin by injection to keep blood sugar levels from rising uncontrollably. There is some evidence to suggest that Type I diabetes is related to the consumption of cow's milk (*refs* 1, 2, 3). Some scientists have theorized that certain proteins in milk might trigger an immune reaction, which also leads to the destruction of cells in the pancreas responsible for making insulin.

In Type II diabetes (also known as 'non-insulin dependent' diabetes) the problem is often not that there is insufficient insulin, but the body is resistant to its effects. Type II diabetes is very often related to excess weight and inactivity. Fortunately, sufferers of this form of diabetes may be able to control their diabetes through changing their diet and taking more exercise. If this fails, oral medication may be prescribed. A proportion of Type II diabetics may need insulin to control their condition. Until recently, Type II diabetes was found almost exclusively in middle and old age, and was sometimes referred to as 'mature-onset' diabetes for this reason. However, in many industrialized countries the condition is being diagnosed in children as young as ten years old, which is why the term 'mature-onset' is generally no longer used.

Diabetics are normally advised to limit their consumption of sweet, sugary foods, and to keep their diet based around starchy carbohydrates such as bread, potatoes, rice and pasta. The basis for this is that unlike sugar, starches need to be digested before they can be absorbed, slowing their release into the bloodstream. However, in contrast to conventional wisdom, research suggests that many starchy foods can upset blood sugar control because they actually release sugar very quickly into the bloodstream. Foods which fall into this category include diabetic staples such as potatoes, white bread, white rice and pasta. More information on dietary approaches to stabilizing blood sugar levels can be found on pages 69–84. This chapter also includes information on herbs and nutrients which might help improve blood sugar, and therefore diabetic, control. Some of the most important agents in this respect include chromium, vitamin B3 (in the form of niacin), magnesium and the herb Gymnema sylvestre (400 mg per day).

Many of the complications of diabetes are caused by a process called 'glyco-sylation'. Here, sugar binds to protein molecules in the body, thereby damaging them. Vitamins C, E and B6 are all known to inhibit glycosylation, and may therefore help prevent diabetic complications in the long term. For this reason, diabetics may benefit from taking vitamin C (1 g, two to three times a day), vitamin E (400 to 800 IU per day) and vitamin B6 (50 to 100 mg per day).

Diarrhoea Short-lived diarrhoea is often related to infection with an unhealthy organism such as a virus (e.g. gastroenteritis) or bacterium (e.g. salmonella). These infections will very often resolve of their own accord. Having said this, one approach that I generally recommend during a diarrhoeal illness is to take probiotics (supplements of healthy gut bacteria). Probiotics may well help to speed up the resolution of symptoms by 'crowding out' the unhealthy organism(s), and may exert some anti-microbial effect. Using probiotics may also reduce the likelihood of persistent problems with long-term disruption of the gut ecology.

In long-standing diarrhoea, other underlying factors may be at work. The factors commonly seen include food sensitivity (see pages 34–43), lactose intolerance (see *Lactose Intolerance*), poor digestion and impaired absorption (see pages 44–8), diverticular disease (see *Diverticular Disease*), and Candida albicans infection (see pages 53–62). Working with and resolving these factors, if they seem to be present, often leads to an improvement in symptoms. Whatever the cause of diarrhoea, probiotics tend to be very useful in the majority of cases. Because healthy gut organisms have so many different roles in the intestinal tract, they are about as close to a 'cure-all' for diarrhoea as you can get. Details of two very good quality healthy gut bacteria supplements can be found on pages 63–4.

Diverticular Disease Diverticular disease is characterized by the presence of small out-pocketings in the wall of the large bowel. The condition is common in the Western world, and is usually symptomless. However, if one or more of the pockets becomes inflamed or infected, symptoms such as diarrhoea, pain, abdominal bloating and the passing of blood in the stool can occur.

Diverticular disease is almost always related to long-standing constipation. The key to controlling it is to ensure a healthy, regular bowel habit. It is important to eat a diet rich in high-fibre foods such as fresh fruits and vegetables, beans, pulses, oats and well-cooked brown rice. It is also a good idea to add a fibre supplement to the diet based on psyllium husks or ground linseeds (see pages 27–8 for more information on how to prevent and treat constipation). In addition to fibre, the other essential for bowel regularity is water; 1.5–2 litres of filtered or still mineral water should be drunk each day.

In my experience, the most useful supplements in diverticular disease are probiotics – preparations of healthy gut bacteria. A lack of these organisms, which itself may be related to the use of antibiotics, often seems to aggravate diverticulitis. A supplement which contains the organism bifidobacterium (thought to be the most important organism in the large bowel) should be taken for at least two or three months. A good example is the supplement Acidophilus Forte which is available from VitaTech (see Useful Information at the back of the book). A maintenance dose of this or a similar supplement (e.g. every other day), is often useful in the long term too.

Down's Syndrome Almost all cells in the body contain genetic information in the form of structures called chromosomes. Normally the cells contain 46 chromosomes each (23 pairs of chromosomes). However, in Down's syndrome, individuals have one extra chromosome. Instead of there being two copies of chromosome number 21, there are three. Down's syndrome is also known as 'Trisomy 21' for this reason. This extra chromosome has been shown to increase the work-rate of certain enzymes that increase free radical production and enhance what is known as 'oxidative stress' on the body. What this essentially means is that the body ages more quickly, and is more likely to run into problems with degenerative conditions earlier in life.

Scientists at Nutri-Chem Pharmacies in Ottawa in Canada offer a multivitamin and mineral supplement which contains antioxidants (to reduce oxidative stress) and has been specifically formulated for people with Down's syndrome (see Useful Information at the back of the book).

Dry Eyes (Sicca Syndrome) The surface of the eye is kept moist by tears secreted by what are known as the 'lachrymal glands'. Sicca syndrome is characterized by dry eyes caused by insufficient tear production, and is usually associated with a dry mouth. Wearing contact lenses will tend to worsen dry eyes, and sicca syndrome sufferers are generally recommended to wear spectacles instead for this reason.

On a dietary level, it is important to avoid salt in the diet. Salt in the body tends to draw moisture out of the surface of the eye, and can therefore worsen a dry eye condition. Alcohol and caffeinated drinks should also be avoided because of their tendency to dehydrate the body by stimulating the production of urine. Foods to emphasize in the diet include those rich in healthy fats known as the essential fatty acids (EFAs). EFAs have a very important role in the maintenance of moisture in the eye.

Healthy fats come in two main forms; omega-3 and omega-6. Omega-3 oils can be found in oily fish such as salmon, trout, herring and mackerel and linseed (flaxseed) oil. Omega-6 fats can be found in evening primrose, safflower and soya oils. Plenty of foods rich in beneficial fats including extra virgin olive oil, avocado, oily fish and raw nuts and seeds should be eaten. In addition, it can help to take an essential fat supplement, such as flaxseed oil. A tablespoon should be taken each day.

Dry Skin Dry skin is a common symptom of low thyroid function. If other symptoms of this condition such as sensitivity to cold, cold hands and feet, fatigue and weight gain are present, then this is likely to be an underlying factor. More information about low thyroid function can be found in chapter 5.

In general, dry skin is usually associated with a deficiency of healthy fats known as essential fatty acids (EFAs). In this respect, the condition has a similar cause to dry eyes and these two symptoms very often coincide. Increasing consumption of EFA-rich foods (see under *Dry Eyes*) is often effective in moistening the skin. In addition, it can help to take flaxseed oil at a dose of 1 tablespoon per day.

e

Ear Infections Ear infections (also called 'otitis media' by the medical profession) are common in childhood and a frequent cause of earache. Such infections are quite often related to colds. Here the viral infection may lead to the build-up of fluid and congestion, which then makes infection with a bacterial agent more likely. Bacterial infections are usually treated with antibiotics.

In natural medicine it is often found that recurrent ear infections in children are related to food sensitivity. In one study in children with recurrent ear infection, 78 per cent tested positive to food sensitivity. Elimination of offending foods led to a significant improvement in 86 per cent of children (*ref* 1). Some foods are renowned for their ability to stimulate mucus formation in and around the ears, with dairy products being by far the most common culprits. It is usually beneficial to remove cow's milk and dairy products made from cow's milk such as cheese and yoghurt from a child's diet. These can be substituted for rice and soya milk (available from good health and food stores), and cheeses made from goat's and sheep's milk. If a child does not improve on this regime, it might be worth eliminating other commonly implicated foods such as wheat, eggs and chocolate. More information on how to identify food sensitivities and appropriate substitute foods can be found on pages 34–43. Sugar should also be avoided as this suppresses the function of the immune system, which can make ear infection more likely.

Certain nutrients may help to maintain healthy immune function. For this reason, it is a good idea for children who are prone to ear infections to take a multivitamin and mineral supplement each day. Another useful approach is for the child to take a course of probiotics (healthy gut bacteria) for a month or two. Children who have ear infection will normally be given antibiotics. While these may help fight bacterial infection in the ear itself, they can also kill many of the beneficial bacteria in the gut leading to imbalance in the organisms here. In the long term this can lead to problems with irritable bowel syndrome, yeast over-growth and food sensitivity. Such supplements can be found in powder form or as capsules which can be opened into water and drunk.

Eczema Eczema is often a red, itchy rash which may cause the skin to become cracked and sore. Typical body sites include the face, hands, insides of the elbows and the backs of the knees. Eczema is caused by inflammation in the outer layers of the skin. Although such inflammation can sometimes be caused by some external irritant such as cleaning fluid or wool, a common trigger in eczema is actually food (*refs* 1, 2). More information about the diagnosis and treatment of food sensitivity can be found in chapter 3, pages 34–43.

Perhaps the most useful dietary supplements for eczema are the essential fatty acids (EFAs). These help to maintain moisture in the skin, and therefore combat dry skin which is a common feature in eczema. Some research suggests that many eczema sufferers have a defect in the way that they process EFAs in the body, leading to a deficiency in gamma-linolenic acid (GLA) (*ref* 3). Some studies suggest that supplementing with GLA can help individuals with eczema (*refs* 4, 5). Typically, twelve 500 mg capsules of evening primrose oil (each one of which contains about 45 mg of GLA) have been used to good effect.

Emphysema Emphysema is a chronic lung disease characterized by over-inflation of the lungs and a destruction of the alveoli, the tiny sacs where gaseous exchange occurs. Emphysema is usually, but not always, related to long-standing smoking. Over time it can give rise to shortness of breath, and ultimately lead to death due to respiratory and/or heart failure. Emphysema can occur on its own, but it is also quite commonly associated with chronic bronchitis (see pages 000–0). Both emphysema and chronic bronchitis are what are known as chronic obstructive airway diseases (COADs).

Nutritional supplementation can often help people with emphysema. Two of the most useful agents in this respect are Coenzyme Q10 (CoQ10) and L-carnitine. CoQ10 is essential for the production of ATP – the basic unit of energy in the body. One study showed that 90 mg of CoQ10 per day for eight weeks significantly lengthened the time COAD sufferers could exercise on a treadmill (*ref* 1). L-carnitine has the ability to help transport fat into parts of the body's cells called the mitochondria, where it can be burned for energy. One study showed that at a dose of 2 g, three times a day, of L-carnitine increased exercise tolerance in individuals with chronic lung disease (*ref* 2).

Endometriosis During each menstrual cycle, the lining of the womb builds up and then is shed if pregnancy does not take place. In endometriosis, womb tissue is found outside the womb itself. Common sites for the endometrial tissue include the ovaries, fallopian tubes, and ligaments that support the uterus, and the area between the vagina and rectum. This misplaced tissue develops into growths or lesions which respond to the menstrual cycle in the same way that the womb lining does, and this can cause considerable pain and discomfort. Some of the most common symptoms of endometriosis include menstrual pain, pain during sex, and painful urination and/or bowel movements during periods. The condition is also associated with some cases of infertility.

It is not clear what causes endometriosis. One theory is that it is related to exposure to environmental toxins called 'dioxins'. One study in rhesus monkeys found a clear correlation between dioxin exposure and endometriosis (*ref* 1). Many sanitary towels and tampons are contaminated with dioxins, and it seems prudent that women should use chemical-free sanitary wear. Suitable products are often to be found in health food stores.

There is good evidence that endometriosis is perpetuated by the female hormone oestrogen (*ref* 2). In fact, oestrogen therapy has been shown to worsen gynaecological conditions such as fibroids and endometriosis (*ref* 3). This opens up a couple of options for natural treatments for endometriosis. One is to reduce oestrogen levels through manipulation of the hormone balance in the body. Agnus castus (40 drops each morning) may help with this. Another approach is to improve liver function, which can help to reduce oestrogen levels by enhancing its breakdown. More details about enhancing liver function can be found on pages 31–2.

Epilepsy The classic symptoms of epilepsy are fits. Epilepsy can be a serious condition and may not respond to medication. Even when it does, the side-effects of the medication can be persistent and troublesome. Not unusually, though, epilepsy does seem to respond to a natural and/or nutritional approach. Sometimes an effective strategy is to ensure that the level of sugar in the bloodstream is maintained. Low blood sugar (hypoglycaemia) seems to be a common trigger factor. Frequent meals and snacks based on foods which release sugar slowly into the bloodstream should be taken. Certain supplements can also help stabilize blood sugar levels, including chromium, magnesium and vitamin B3. More about the regulation of blood sugar can be found in chapter 4.

Food sensitivity seems to be a common factor, at least in children. One study found that 80 per cent of epileptic children who also had other symptoms of food sensitivity (e.g. migraine, hyperactivity, abdominal symptoms) improved on a diet which excluded the foods to which people tend to be sensitive. More than half of the children became completely seizure-free (*ref* 1). More information about the diagnosis and treatment of food sensitivity can be found in chapter 3, pages 34–43.

There is some evidence that epilepsy is related to nutritional deficiencies. One study showed that more than half of epileptic patients had a deficiency of vitamin B6, and that about half of these responded to vitamin B6 therapy at a dose of 160 mg per day (*ref* 2). In another study, vitamin E was found to help a significant proportion of epileptic children. Ten out of twelve children (83 per cent) who were resistant to drug therapy had a reduction in seizure frequency of at least 60 per cent when given a dose of 400 IU of vitamin E per day (*ref* 3). Epilepsy is a potentially serious condition, and it is advisable to work with a practitioner experienced in its management.

f

Fatigue Fatigue can have a bewildering array of underlying nutritional, physiological or biochemical mechanisms. Some of the most common that are seen in practice include blood sugar imbalance (see pages 69–84), low adrenal gland function (see pages 88–93), food sensitivity (see pages 34–43), Candida albicans overgrowth (see pages 53–62), anaemia and/or deficiency of iron (see *Anaemia – iron deficiency*) or vitamin B12 (see *Anaemia – pernicious*), and low thyroid function (see chapter 5).

Identifying the true underlying cause(s) of the fatigue is key to overcoming the problem. However, sometimes, it can help to use a natural agent to boost energy and speed general healing. Panax (Korean) ginseng has been shown to improve the ability to think and work (*refs* 1, 2). It is these qualities which have led to its immense popularity as a general tonic. The normal dose is 100 to 200 mg of standardized extract containing 4 to 7 per cent ginsenosides per day. The dose for non-standardized preparations is 1–2 g per day or 2–3 mls of herbal tincture. It is generally recommended that Panax ginseng be used on a cyclical basis with treatment periods of two to three weeks interspersed with supplement-free periods of one to two weeks. While Panax ginseng is generally regarded as safe at the recommended dosage, it may cause insomnia if taken close to bedtime. It should not be used by those suffering from high blood pressure. Panax ginseng is known to cause breast tenderness and menstrual abnormalities in some women and is not recommended for pregnant or lactating women.

The other commonly used form of ginseng is Siberian ginseng. Like Panax ginseng, Siberian ginseng has been used in Chinese medicine for over 2,000 years, both as an energy booster and immune system enhancer. The active ingredients are thought to support the function of the adrenal glands (*ref* 3) and sharpen the mind as well as improve physical energy (*refs* 4, 5). A dose of 300 to 400 mg of concentrated solid standardized extract should be taken each day. The normal dosage for dried powder is 2–3 g per day. It is generally recommended that Siberian ginseng be used on a cyclical basis with treatment periods of six to eight weeks interspersed with breaks lasting one to two weeks. It may cause mild, transient diarrhoea and, as with Panax ginseng, insomnia if taken too close to bedtime. It should not be used by those suffering from high blood pressure and is not recommended for pregnant or lactating women.

Fibrocystic Breast Disease In fibrocystic breast disease (FBD) the breasts develop multiple cysts (fluid-filled pockets). The condition is thought to affect about 30 per cent of pre-menopausal women, with sufferers usually complaining of painful, lumpy breasts, which are generally worse just before a period. FBD is related to raised levels of the hormone oestrogen in the body, which is why it usually subsides after the time of the menopause (when oestrogen levels fall). Occasionally, FBD can be associated with low thyroid gland function. This association is more likely if the sufferer also has symptoms such as sensitivity to cold, cold hands and/or feet, fatigue, weight gain and dry skin (see chapter 5 for more details about this). Although the cysts that cause the lumpiness in FBD are benign (non-cancerous), any woman with a lump or lumps in her breast should have this assessed by a doctor.

It is well known that the symptoms of FBD are made worse by the consumption of caffeine and caffeine-like substances found in coffee, tea, caffeinated soft drinks and chocolate (*refs* 1, 2). Studies show that complete abstinence from these foodstuffs can be very helpful in controlling the symptoms. A high-fibre diet should be eaten, as this may help to reduce oestrogen levels in the body. Excess oestrogen is eliminated via the bowel, and the more rapidly food and waste passes through the intestine, the less opportunity there is for oestrogen to be reabsorbed back into the body. A low-fat diet can also reduce oestrogen levels in the blood, and a couple of studies have shown that this can lead to a reduction in symptoms after three to six months (*refs* 3, 4).

Studies show that vitamin E can be very effective in relieving the symptoms of FBD (*refs* 5, 6), though how it does this is not understood at present. A dose of 400 to 600 IU of vitamin E should be taken each day for several months. Evening primrose oil, which has anti-inflammatory and hormone-balancing effects, can also help relieve the symptoms (*refs* 7, 8). The normal recommended dose is 1 g three times a day.

Another natural remedy for the treatment of FBD is the herb agnus castus. This herb seems to increase progesterone production. Progesterone balances the effects of oestrogen in the body, and in so doing can help to alleviate the symptoms of FBD. A dose of 40 drops of concentrated agnus castus liquid (either fluid extract or tincture) should be taken each morning.

Fibromyalgia Fibromyalgia is characterized by generalized aches, pains and tender points in the muscles, fatigue, and sleep disruption. The sleep problems associated with the condition seem to be caused by the pain and discomfort which comes from lying on tender muscle areas. Fibromyalgia is a poorly understood condition and the underlying causes are complex. It often seems to be connected with either low thyroid function and/or adrenal weakness. More details about other signs and symptoms of these conditions, and how to go about treating them can be found in chapters 4 (pages 88–93) and 5.

There is some evidence that some individuals with fibromyalgia are deficient in the mineral magnesium (*ref* 1). Also, magnesium in combination with malic acid is thought to help relieve the symptoms of fibromyalgia (*ref* 2). In combination, magnesium (300 to 600 mg per day) and malic acid (1,200 to 2,400 mg per day) help in the production of ATP – the basic fuel source in the body's cells.

Fungal Infections Because yeast organisms thrive in warm, moist environments, fungal infections commonly affect the feet (see *Athlete's Foot*), scalp (see *Scalp – itchy*), groin, and toenails. Many people with persistent fungal infections seem to have an overgrowth of the organism Candida albicans in the digestive tract. Generally, only once this infection has been successfully dealt with (see chapter 3, pages 53–62 for more details about this) will the more superficial infections normally clear up for good. In the meantime, topical preparations containing the natural anti-fungal agent tea tree oil can help to control symptoms.

g

Gallstones (see also Cholecystitis) Gallstones form in the gallbladder, which sits underneath the liver. Gallstones can cause pain in the upper-right side of the abdomen, and this may be associated with nausea and vomiting. Gallstones come in different forms, with the most common being made of cholesterol. Because of this it is a good idea to reduce the amount of fatty food in the diet, including red meat, dairy products, fried and processed foods. Excess weight is often a factor in gallstone formation. The diet should be based on whole, unprocessed foods such as wholemeal bread, brown rice, beans, fruits and vegetables. High-fibre diets, such as this one, can often help with weight loss and are also associated with a reduced risk of gallstones.

A common underlying factor in gallstone formation appears to be hypo-chlorhydria (low stomach acid secretion). More information about this condition can be found on pages 44–8. Some individuals with gallstones may benefit from taking a South American herb called quebra pedra (which literally trans-lated means 'stone breaker'). Quebra pedra has been used by the indigenous people of the Amazon to treat both kidney stones and gallstones for hundreds of years. In the UK, quebra pedra is available as a powder that can be made into a tea. Two heaped teaspoons are boiled in about half a litre of water. This mixture can be drunk over the course of the day, either hot or cold. Quebra pedra is available from Rio Trading (see Useful Information at the back of the book).

Gilbert's Disease Each red blood cell lives for about 120 days. When it dies, its chief ingredient, haemoglobin, is broken down in the liver. The main breakdown product of this process is a substance called 'bilirubin'. Most of the bilirubin formed by the liver passes into the gut in the bile, and goes on to be excreted from the body in the stool. In Gilbert's disease, the ability of the liver to process bilirubin is faulty, causing bilirubin levels in the blood to rise. Once thought to be very rare, Gilbert's disease is now thought to affect as much as 5 per cent of the population. Usually, the condition does not give rise to symptoms, though a proportion of sufferers may experience problems with loss of appetite, general malaise and fatigue.

Nutritionally, it is a good idea for people with Gilbert's disease to avoid anything which tends to put stress on the liver such as alcohol and caffeine. In addition, 1½–2 litres of filtered or mineral water should be drunk each day to help detoxification and liver health. One natural substance which may help to protect the liver and minimize the effect of Gilbert's disease is the herb milk thistle (*Silybum marianum*). Milk thistle contains a substance called silymarin which enhances liver function and helps in the regeneration of liver cells. A dose of 70 to 100 mg of silymarin should be taken, three times a day.

Gingivitis The usual symptoms of gingivitis are red, swollen, often tender gums which tend to bleed easily. The condition can be caused by a bacterial infection where the gum and tooth meet, and is often related to a build-up of plaque in this area. The inflammation typical of gingivitis can be difficult to treat, and sufferers often have persistent problems. Adequate intake of vitamin C and substances called bioflavonoids (found in fruits and vegetables) are essential for gum health. One study showed that in combination (300 mg of each per day) these nutrients improved the health of the gum tissue (*ref* 1).

Another nutrient which has been shown to help resolve gingivitis is Coenzyme Q10 (CoQ10). This vitamin-like substance participates in the processes which generate energy within the body's cells, and has also been shown to improve the health and condition of the gums (*ref* 2). Anyone suffering from gingivitis should take at least 25 mg of CoQ10, twice a day. Piercing an oil-filled CoQ10 capsule and rubbing its contents into the gums from time to time might also help.

Glaucoma Each eye is filled with fluid that is essential for maintaining its normal shape. Sometimes the pressure in one or both eyes can increase giving rise to a condition known as 'glaucoma'. Ninety per cent of glaucoma cases are known as 'chronic glaucoma'. In this condition, there are usually no symptoms until significant elevations in eye pressure are present. When the pressure of fluids in the eye reaches high levels, a gradual loss of peripheral vision – sometimes called 'tunnel vision' – is experienced. Chronic glaucoma can lead to damage to the major nerve in the eye, causing gradual loss of vision over time.

Like many conditions, glaucoma may have one or more underlying physiological mechanisms. The imbalances that seem most relevant are low thyroid function (see chapter 5), food sensitivity (*refs* 1, 2) (see pages 34–43) and low adrenal function (see pages 44–8). Identifying which, if any, of these factors are present and successfully treating them can help to control pressure within the eye.

Some natural substances seem to have the ability to reduce eye pressure. Eskimos who eat a diet rich in oily fish (high in essential fatty acids of the omega-3 type) have been found to be at reduced risk of glaucoma. I am not aware of any studies which have looked at the effect of healthy fats on eye pressure in humans, although cod liver oil (also rich in omega-3 fatty acids) has been shown to be effective in animals (*ref* 3). Including plenty of omega-3 rich foods in the diet and taking a supplement of these oils (either as fish oil or linseed oil) might help to control eye pressure in the long term.

Another useful natural substance for glaucoma appears to be the bioflavonoid compound rutin. Just 20 mg, three times a day, was found in one study to help seventeen out of twenty-six eyes affected by glaucoma in individuals already taking conventional medication for this condition (*ref* 4).

Glue Ear Glue ear is a condition caused by the accumulation of fluid within the ear. Many children with this condition are recommended to have grommets (small plastic tubes) inserted into the eardrum. Grommets allow air into the ear cavity, which can help fluid drain from this area. Interestingly, studies suggest that glue ear does not impair intellectual development; but it is possible that the insertion of grommets may lead to some degree of hearing loss for several years after the procedure.

It is not uncommon for children with glue ear to have problems with their adenoids. The adenoids are glands (similar to tonsils) situated at the back of the nose. In some children, the adenoids enlarge, restricting breathing through the nose (sufferers often have a characteristic nasal voice), snoring and an increased risk of glue ear and ear infections. The usual medical management of enlarged adenoids is something called 'adenoidectomy', where the glands are removed surgically.

In practice, glue ear is often caused by food sensitivity. By far the most common food triggers are cow's milk, ice cream and cheese, with yoghurt often being a problem too. Butter is very rarely a problem. Other symptoms of dairy sensitivity include frequent colds and a blocked and/or runny nose. Often, children crave the foods which they are most sensitive to. If a child is especially keen on one or more dairy product, then this strongly suggests that he or she has a problem with this type of food. While dairy product sensitivity is quite likely to be a factor in glue ear, other foods may contribute to the problem. It can therefore be useful for a child to have his or her food sensitivities individually assessed. For more details about this, see pages 34–43.

Goitre A goitre is the medical term used to describe an enlarged thyroid gland. The condition can be related to a variety of underlying factors including iodine deficiency, low thyroid function, thyroid over-activity, inflammation of the thyroid (thyroiditis), benign (non-cancerous) lumps and cancer (rare). The thyroid can also enlarge due to hormonal changes induced by puberty, pregnancy and the taking of hormone-based medications such as the oral contraceptive pill. Thyroid enlargement should be investigated by a doctor to help ensure that potentially serious conditions are not missed. For more information about low thyroid function, and how to treat it, see chapter 5.

Gout Gout is a type of arthritis that is caused by the accumulation of uric acid in the body. Crystals of uric acid can form in a joint and this can lead to intense pain and inflammation. While gout is classically thought of as a condition which affects the big toe, in fact crystals of uric acid can deposit anywhere in the body. In some individuals, widespread deposition of uric acid in the joints and tendons can give rise to a condition known as 'gouty arthritis'. Commonly affected joints include the knee, ankle, wrist, feet and hands.

Uric acid is actually a breakdown product of a class of substances known as 'purines'. Anyone with a history of gout should avoid foods that are rich in purines including meat (especially organ meats such as liver and kidney), seafood, beans, peas and lentils. Sugar should also be avoided as this can increase the level of uric acid in the blood (*ref* 1).

Plenty of fresh fruits and vegetables should be eaten as this will help to increase the alkalinity in the body. This, in turn, can help to neutralize the effect of the uric acid. At least 1½ litres of filtered or still mineral water should be drunk each day to help dilute and speed the elimination of uric acid.

Cherries should be eaten when they are in season because they are rich in substances called proanthocyanidins which will help neutralize uric acid and reduce the inflammation which is characteristic in gout. In a study of twelve gout sufferers, consuming half a pound of cherries or the equivalent in cherry juice each day stopped gout attacks (*ref* 2).

Growing Pains Growing pains are vague aches and pains that occur in the limbs of children. The pains usually occur at night and generally affect the calves of children between six and twelve years of age. Although distressing, growing pains are usually of no medical significance. Occasionally, however, they may be related to juvenile arthritis. For this reason, children who have joint pain and swelling should be seen by a doctor.

While the precise cause of growing pains is unclear, it will often respond to a nutritional approach. A common and frequently overlooked cause of growing pains is food sensitivity. Advice about identifying culprit foods can be found on pages 34–43.

Magnesium, which is essential for muscle health, can often help relieve growing pains, especially when combined with vitamin E which improves blood flow to muscle tissues. A quantity of 100 mg of magnesium and 100 IU of vitamin E, given twice a day, is often effective. Manganese may also help relieve growing pains; it has an important role to play in maintaining the health of tendons which can become strained during periods of growth. A good dose is 5–10 mg of manganese, twice a day.

Gum Disease – see *Gingivitis*

Haemorrhoids (piles) Haemorrhoids or 'piles' are enlarged veins found around the anus. Sometimes haemorrhoids can be internal (not visible from the outside), but they may also protrude from the anus giving rise to what are known as 'external' piles. Haemorrhoids are very often related to constipation, and resolving this issue can help them to heal (see pages 27–8 for more information about overcoming constipation). In addition, certain natural supplements may help. Of particular importance here are substances known as flavonoids which have the ability to strengthen the walls of veins, including those around the anus. The herb horse chestnut contains a compound known as aescin which can strengthen blood vessel walls, and is therefore useful for haemorrhoid sufferers (*ref* 1). It is normally recommended that 50–75 mg of aescin be taken twice a day.

Hair Loss (women) Hair loss in women can be related to one or more of a number of physiological factors. Common underlying health issues include low thyroid function (see chapter 5), and low stomach acid secretion (see pages 44–8). Low stomach acid secretion quite often leads to poor absorption of minerals which are important for the manufacture of hair (and nails). Of particular importance here is the mineral iron (see *Anaemia – iron deficiency*). Occasionally, hair loss can be associated with high levels of the 'male' hormone testosterone, just as it is in men. Raised levels of testosterone are often associated with a condition known as polycystic ovarian syndrome (see *Polycystic Ovarian Syndrome*).

Hair – dull and lifeless The condition of the hair, skin and nails can give important clues to the nutritional state and internal health of the body. Hair that has lost its lustre and sheen is generally a sign of a deficiency in a class of nutrients known as the essential fatty acids (EFAs). Dry skin is another common manifestation of essential fat deficiency, so if this is also present then this points quite firmly to this particular problem.

Healthy fats come in two main forms; omega-3 and omega-6. Omega-3 oils can be found in oily fish such as salmon, trout, herring and mackerel and linseed (flaxseed) oil. Omega-6 fats can be found in evening primrose, safflower and soy oils. Dry hair is often helped by eating foods rich in beneficial fats including extra virgin olive oil, avocado, oily fish and raw nuts and seeds. Additional benefit may be had from taking an EFA supplement such as flaxseed (linseed) oil, at a dose of one tablespoon per day.

Hay Fever Hay fever is caused by an allergic reaction to pollen, causing the release of histamine around the nose and eyes. Characteristic symptoms include red, itchy eyes, and a runny or congested nose. The conventional medical approach to hay fever generally consists of three types of medication: antihistamines which block the release of histamine which is responsible for the swelling and congestion; steroid-based nasal sprays; and decongestants such as ephedrine. However, dietary changes and natural supplements may significantly reduce or even eliminate the need for conventional medication.

I often find that individuals with hay fever have food sensitivities too. When these foods are successfully identified and eliminated, the hay fever very often gets much better. It is thought that the reactions to food 'sensitize' the tissues in the eye and/or nose, making it more likely that pollen will trigger any allergic reaction there. More details about the identification of individual food sensitivities can be found on pages 34–43.

Vitamin C is a natural antihistamine and there is some evidence that it can help control hay fever symptoms (*refs* 1, 2). A dose of 1 g of vitamin C should be taken three or four times a day while symptoms persist. Another useful natural agent for the treatment of hay fever is quercetin. This 'bioflavonoid' compound appears to reduce the quantity of histamine released from immune system cells known as 'mast cells'. In practice, quercetin does seem to help a proportion of hay fever sufferers. The normal recommended dose is 400 mg, two or three times a day. The herb nettle (*Urtica dioica*) has anti-allergy properties, and may therefore be useful in treating hay fever symptoms. The normal recommended dose is 450 mg of leaf powder, two or three times a day.

Headache – see also *Migraine* and *Cluster Headaches* Many of the underlying features of common headaches are dealt with in the section on migraine. Factors which seem to crop up commonly are low blood sugar (see pages 69–84), food sensitivity (see pages 34–43) and toxicity (see pages 23–31). Stress is another common feature in many headaches. Stress-induced headaches are often referred to as 'tension headaches'. These are characterized by a steady, constant, dull pain that starts at the back of the head or the forehead, eventually spreading over the entire head. Tension headaches are caused by a tightening in the muscles of the face, neck or scalp as a result of stress or poor posture. Relaxation techniques, the Alexander Technique (a therapy which encourages correct posture), chiropractic manipulation and osteopathy may benefit anyone suffering from chronic tension headaches.

Another common and often overlooked cause of headache is dehydration. The tissues which surround the brain are mostly composed of water. When these tissues lose fluid, they shrink, giving rise to pain and irritation. Low levels of fluid in the body may also encourage the accumulation of toxins which have been implicated in headaches. Many people find that just drinking 1½–2 litres of water a day can lead to a substantial reduction in the frequency and/or severity of their headaches.

Another lifestyle factor which is often related to headaches is caffeine. It is often between times of caffeine consumption (caffeine withdrawal) that the headache tends to strike. Regular caffeine takers normally find that stopping caffeine cold-turkey leads to substantial headaches for a day or two, after which they are very much reduced or stop altogether. For the best results, all forms of caffeine-containing foodstuffs including coffee, tea, chocolate, cocoa and caffeinated soft drinks should be eliminated from the diet. Naturally caffeine-free beverages such as herb and fruit teas and coffee substitutes based on barley or chicory make good alternatives.

Hearing Loss Hearing, just like any other body function, is dependent on the supply of certain nutrients. Research has linked hearing loss to low levels of both vitamin B12 and folic acid (*ref* 1). Vitamin B12 and folic acid depend on good digestion for proper absorption, and it is quite possible that hearing problems might be related, at least in part, to reduced digestive function (see pages 45–6). To help preserve hearing, it may be wise to take a good quality multivitamin and mineral supplement each day with additional B12 (1,000 mcg per day) and folic acid (500 mcg per day).

There is some evidence that magnesium may help protect hearing. In one study in military recruits exposed to high noise levels, hearing loss was less common and less severe in individuals taking magnesium compared with those on inactive medication (*ref* 2). An amount of 250 to 300 mg should be taken each day.

Heart Disease (see *Atherosclerosis*)

Heart Failure The chief function of the heart is to take blood which has absorbed oxygen in the lungs and pump this to the rest of the body. If the heart should become weak – a condition known as 'heart failure' – fluid can accumulate in various parts of the body including the lungs (often causing shortness of breath) and the legs (causing swelling in the feet and ankles). Because a weakened heart does not pump blood efficiently to the body, including organs such as the brain and muscles, fatigue and weakness are also common symptoms of this condition.

The heart muscle has a wide range of nutritional needs. By supplying the body with nutrients that contribute to healthy heart function it is possible to improve heart function and improve the symptoms of heart failure. One of the most important nutrients for good heart function is the mineral magnesium. Individuals with heart failure tend to have lower than normal levels of magnesium in their bloodstreams and, in practice, many individuals with this condition seem to improve with magnesium supplementation. In particular, magnesium seems to protect against heart rhythm irregularities which quite often occur in cases of heart failure and can themselves lead to potentially serious complications (*ref* 1). A dose of 350 to 500 mg of magnesium should be taken each day.

Another nutrient that has been shown to improve heart function is Coenzyme Q10 (CoQ10). This is essential for the production of ATP, the basic unit of energy in the body. There is evidence that CoQ10 relieves the symptoms of heart failure (*ref* 2), and may increase general energy levels as well. CoQ10 is best absorbed into the body when dissolved in oil (as found in soft gelatine capsules). A quantity of 30–50 mg should be taken, three times a day.

The herb hawthorn (*Crataegus oxyacantha*) may also help people with heart failure (*refs* 3, 4). Hawthorn may increase blood flow to the heart and increase the strength of contraction of the heart. The normal recommended dose is 80 to 300 mg of standardized extract, two or three times a day.

Hepatitis Hepatitis actually means inflammation of the liver. This condition can be caused by a number of factors, including drugs, chemicals and poisons. However, by far the most common cause of hepatitis is infection with the hepatitis virus. There are several strains of hepatitis virus which are identified using letters of the alphabet. The most important strains are hepatitis A, B and C. Hepatitis A is passed through contact with infected water, food or faeces, while B and C are usually contracted through sex or via contact with infected blood.

Initial infection with the hepatitis virus often triggers a condition known as 'acute hepatitis'. This may start as a flu-like illness, after which jaundice (yellowing of the skin) may develop. In the case of hepatitis A, the illness is usually self-limiting, though a proportion of sufferers may complain of vague symptoms for weeks or months after the original infection. Individuals infected with hepatitis B or C are at risk of the infection persisting in the long term, a condition known as 'chronic hepatitis'.

In the acute phase, anyone recovering from a hepatitis infection should generally avoid anything which tends to put stress on the liver such as caffeine and alcohol. Fatty foods can also tax the liver by stimulating the production of bile. Plenty of water should be drunk (about 2 litres per day), as this helps to reduce the toxic load on the body. In addition, certain natural substances may help. The herb milk thistle (silymarin) has been shown to have beneficial effects on liver function, and may help restore health to the liver. A dose of 70 mg of silymarin should be taken three times a day.

Another nutrient that is likely to help is vitamin C. In addition to stimulating the immune system and its anti-viral properties, it is also known to promote tissue healing, and may therefore help to reduce the risk of damage to the liver over time. A dose of 2 g of vitamin C should be taken three times a day while symptoms persist, though this dose can be reduced as the condition resolves. There is also evidence that the mineral selenium inhibits the hepatitis virus; 600 mcg should be taken each day when there are symptoms.

In cases of chronic hepatitis, natural approaches often help to strengthen the liver and improve the sufferer's condition. Some of the most important nutrients include vitamin C (1–2 g, three times a day), selenium (200 mcg per day) and silymarin (70 mg, three times a day). Another useful natural agent for chronic hepatitis is licorice. Licorice root contains a substance called 'glycyrrhizin' which, like vitamin C, helps to protect the liver and also has anti-viral properties. A dose of 500 mg of licorice root should be taken, three times a day.

Herpes – Genital Genital herpes is caused by a virus very similar to the one responsible for cold sores. While cold sores are usually caused by what is known as the herpes 'simplex I' virus, genital herpes is generally caused by the herpes 'simplex II' virus. Once contracted, the virus lies dormant in the body but is normally kept in check by the body's immune system. However, the virus can reactivate and cause problems from time to time, especially if we are run down and the immune system is weakened. Normally, a herpes outbreak will start with numbness, tingling or pain in the affected area. The prevention and treatment of herpes simplex II is the same as that for herpes simplex I (see *Cold Sores*).

Hiatus Hernia Food enters the stomach via a tube called the oesophagus (gullet). The oesophagus passes through a sheet of muscle called the 'diaphragm', which forms part of a valve mechanism which is designed to keep the acidic contents of the stomach from leaking into the oesophagus. In a hiatus hernia, part of the stomach is pulled up through the diaphragm, allowing the escape of food into the oesophagus (acid reflux). Typical symptoms of a hiatus hernia include heart-burn and digestive discomfort.

While a hiatus hernia is often believed to be related to an over-production of stomach acid, quite the opposite problem – low stomach acid – is often an underlying feature. If the stomach fails to secrete enough acid, digestion can be impaired, causing food to linger in the stomach. This food may be prone to fermentation which increases the risk of it bubbling up into the oesophagus. Also, stomach acid is an important stimulus for the closure of the valve between the oesophagus and the stomach (the gastro-oesophageal valve). Low stomach acid levels can cause the gastro-oesophageal valve to remain open, predisposing to reflux and heartburn. A fuller account of the problems associated with low stomach acid and how to remedy this problem can be found in chapter 3, pages 44–8.

Taking steps to improve digestion is often very effective in controlling the symptoms of a hiatus hernia. In particular, chewing food very thoroughly, avoiding drinking with meals, avoiding late and large meals, and food combining (separat-ing protein and starch at meal times) can help. More information about these approaches can be found on pages 45–7.

High Blood Pressure (see *Hypertension*)

High Cholesterol Cholesterol is a waxy, fat-like substance that is transported around the body in the bloodstream. Cholesterol can build up on the inside of our arteries and increase the risk of cardiovascular diseases such as heart disease and stroke. The deposition of cholesterol in artery walls is known as 'atherosclerosis' (see *Atherosclerosis*). Generally speaking, it is thought that higher levels of cholesterol in the bloodstream predisposes to clogging of the arteries. While too much cholesterol is undoubtedly a bad thing, we do need some – cholesterol is an essential constituent of every cell in the body, as well as being an important ingredient in the manufacture of vital body substances including hormones and bile.

When we eat fat it is digested in the gut and then passed through the gut wall into the bloodstream. Cholesterol in the bloodstream is found in two main forms; low density lipoprotein (LDL) and high density lipoprotein (HDL). Raised levels of LDL are associated with an increased risk of atherosclerosis and for this reason LDL has been dubbed 'bad cholesterol'. HDL, on the other hand, is associated with a reduced risk of atherosclerosis and is therefore often referred to as 'good cholesterol'. If the cholesterol level is up, then knowing the relative proportions of 'good' to 'bad' cholesterol in the bloodstream is important. To do this, the total cholesterol level can be divided by the HDL level. A ratio of five or less is desirable, and the lower the ratio, the better.

If the total cholesterol level is raised, it can help to modify both the amount and type of fat in the diet. More information about this can be found in the section on atherosclerosis. In addition, it can help to increase the consumption of foods which appear to have a cholesterol-lowering effect such as soya milk and tofu, oat bran, 'live' yoghurt, walnuts, garlic and onions.

As well as reducing the level of LDL in the body, it can help to increase the level of HDL. Exercise has been shown to do this (*ref* 1). This is likely to be one of the reasons why regular exercise reduces the risk of cardiovascular conditions such as heart disease and stroke.

Niacin (a form of vitamin B3) and chromium are two nutrients which seem to have the property of reducing cholesterol. Large doses (3 g a day) of niacin have been shown to substantially reduce total cholesterol levels and increase HDL levels (*ref* 2). As a result, niacin is gaining increasing popularity as a cholesterol treatment even with conventional doctors. However, such large doses of niacin can be toxic to the body, particularly the liver, and may induce problems such as flushing, nausea and queasiness. Because of this, large doses of niacin should really only be taken under the supervision of a doctor.

Chromium can also reduce cholesterol levels (*refs* 3, 4), and increase HDL levels (*refs* 5, 6). It is believed that niacin and chromium work particularly well in combination, perhaps because they are the two main constituents of a molecule known as glucose tolerance factor chromium (GTF-chromium), which appears to have an important role in the regulation of insulin and blood sugar levels. One report suggests that just 100 mg of niacin combined with 200 mcg of chromium per day may be effective in reducing cholesterol levels for some people (*ref* 7). Magnesium is also useful for treating raised cholesterol. In one study, magnesium was shown to reduce cholesterol levels and increase HDL levels at a dose of 430 mg per day (*ref* 8).

The Indian herb guggul (*Commiphora mukul*) contains compounds called guggulsterones which have the ability to reduce LDL levels. Studies in humans have consistently confirmed that guggul reduces cholesterol levels (*ref* 9). The normal recommended dose is 25 mg of guggulsterones, three times a day.

High Triglycerides Fat is transported around the body in essentially two forms: cholesterol and triglycerides. Triglycerides are actually the major form of fat found in food and the body. While the precise impact of triglycerides on health is unclear, there is some evidence linking high levels of triglycerides in the blood with an increased risk of heart disease. They can be made in the liver in response to insulin. Because insulin itself is secreted in response to high levels of blood sugar, avoiding foods which tend to release sugar rapidly in the bloodstream is important (see page 76 for more information on this). Eating refined sugar has been shown to increase triglyceride levels (*refs* 1, 2). Alcohol, in excess, is an important cause of raised triglycerides (*ref* 3), and moderation of drinking is therefore important if levels of triglycerides are to be properly regulated.

Garlic has been shown to be an effective triglyceride-lowering agent (*refs* 4, 5). The effective dose seems to be 600 to 900 mg per day. One raw clove consumed each day, or a supplement containing about 5,000 mcg of allicin (thought to be garlic's main active ingredient) may be effective in reducing triglyceride levels.

The Indian herb guggul (*Commiphora mukul*) contains compounds called guggulsterones which reduce triglyceride levels (*ref* 6). In one study, triglyceride levels fell by almost one third (*ref* 7). The normal recommended dose is 25 mg of guggulsterones, three times a day.

Hives (urticaria) Urticaria, also known as 'nettle rash' or 'hives', is characterized by red, raised, itchy weals on the skin surface. The rash usually affects the trunk or limbs, tends to come and go, and normally lasts for a few hours at a time. Urticaria is known to be triggered by a variety of factors including prescription drugs, extremes of temperature, and sunlight. However, there is some evidence that many cases of urticaria are caused by reactions to food (*ref* 1) or food additives, particularly colourings, flavourings (salicylates), aspartame, and preservatives (*refs* 2, 3, 4). For more details about how to identify specific food sensitivities, see pages 00–00. Chronic urticaria has also been associated with low stomach acid secretion (*ref* 5). More details about the diagnosis and treatment of this condition can be found on pages 44–8.

Because urticaria seems to be related to the release of histamine, natural approaches which have an antihistamine effect may help. See the section entitled *Hay Fever* for more details about these.

Hyperactivity (attention deficit hyperactivity disorder) Some children exhibit extreme mood and behaviour disruption indicative of a condition known as attention deficit hyperactivity disorder (ADHD). More and more children are being diagnosed with ADHD, which is characterized by hyperactivity, mood swings and lack of focus and concentration. Sleep disturbance, bed-wetting and excessive thirst are other common symptoms. The diagnosis of ADHD is usually made by an educational psychologist, and treatment revolves around behavioural therapy and drugs such as Ritalin (methylphenidate hydrochloride). Even though Ritalin is an amphetamine (a form of 'speed'), it can have the paradoxical effect of calming the nervous system in some children. However, Ritalin does not work for a significant proportion of hyperactive children, and is also linked with a variety of side-effects such as insomnia and restlessness.

ADHD is very often amenable to a nutritional approach. Certain foods seem to be associated with an increased risk of mood and behaviour disturbance.

Eliminating caffeine, sugar and all food additives (artificial flavourings, colourings and preservatives) from the diet often helps to control symptoms. Not uncommonly, ADHD is related to food sensitivity. Here, one or more foods may provoke an unwanted reaction in the body, giving rise to symptoms typical of ADHD. Children suffering from food intolerance often have dark circles or bags under their eyes, and may exhibit very red cheeks and/or ears during fits of uncontrollable behaviour or screaming. While any food may produce unwanted reactions, the most common problems are wheat, milk, cheese, ice-cream, chocolate, citrus fruits and eggs. Children quite often crave the foods they are sensitive to, so it is wise to be especially suspicious of a child's favourite foods. Information about the identification of individual food sensitivities can be found on pages 34–43.

Another quite common feature in children with ADHD is fluctuations in the level of sugar in the bloodstream. The body generally keeps blood sugar levels within relatively narrow parameters, and this is especially important for normal brain function. The brain tissue uses a large proportion of the sugar in the bloodstream, and if fuel supply stalls, it can provoke significant problems with mood. Many children suffer from episodes of low blood sugar throughout the day which may manifest as mood swings, tantrums and uncontrolled behaviour. This problem is quite likely if the child craves sweet foods, or gets very irritable if he or she does not eat regularly and on time. These children will often respond to a diet designed to stabilize blood sugar levels. More details about this can be found on pages 69–84. Foods and drinks containing artificial sweeteners such as aspartame are also best avoided. At least one study has shown that aspartame can provoke mood disturbance in adults, and there is no reason to assume that this problem is any different in children.

Children with ADHD are often found to have nutrient deficiencies, especially in healthy fats known as essential fatty acids (EFAs) (*refs* 1, 2). Common symptoms of EFA deficiency include dry, flaky skin and excessive thirst. EFAs play an important role in the development and function of the brain. Possibly the most important nutrient in this respect is docosahexaenoic acid (DHA) which is normally found in fish oils. In practice, about 1 g of DHA per day may be effective.

Magnesium is another nutrient which may help in ADHD. Some children with ADHD have low levels of magnesium in their bodies and supplementation with this mineral has been shown to help reduce hyperactive behaviour (*ref* 3). The dose of magnesium should be adjusted according to age, but an average ten-year-old should be given between 100 to 200 mg per day.

Hypertension (high blood pressure) High blood pressure, also known as hypertension, affects about 1 in 7 adults in this country. A lot of people imagine that hypertension gives rise to headaches. Actually, the condition is usually symptomless, and its real danger lies in the fact that it increases the risk of major killers such as heart disease and stroke.

Not surprisingly, high blood pressure is often related to lifestyle factors. Smoking and excess weight should be avoided because they increase the risk of hypertension. Exercise, on the other hand, can help to reduce blood pressure. Individuals with high blood pressure should take some form of sustained exercise (brisk walking, aerobics, cycling and light jogging are ideal) for half an hour, on most days.

With regard to the diet, salt (sodium chloride) appears to raise blood pressure in a significant number of people (*ref* 1). If possible, salt should not be added to food during cooking or at the table. Also, processed and packaged foods should be avoided as these tend to contain a lot of salt. While the sodium in salt tends to put the blood pressure up, another nutrient – potassium – tends to lower it (*ref* 2). Eating a potassium-rich diet containing plenty of fresh fruits and vegetables (especially bananas) may help to bring blood pressure down. Another useful food is garlic: studies have shown that this can significantly reduce blood pressure (*ref* 3).

Calcium has been reported to help reduce blood pressure, and although the degree of blood pressure drop appears to be small (*ref* 4), some individuals (seemingly those sensitive to salt) may get significant benefit (*ref* 5). A twelve-week trial of 1,000 mg of calcium per day is certainly worth trying. A magnesium supplement may also lower blood pressure (*ref* 6). A good dose is between 350 to 500 mg per day. One other nutritional agent which may help is Coenzyme Q10 at a dose of 50 mg, twice a day (*refs* 7, 8).

Hypotension (low blood pressure) Doctors' opinions vary widely in their attitude to low blood pressure. Some believe that it is of no significance and often remark that it is desirable as it reduces the risk of high blood pressure later on. Others believe that it is often the sign of some imbalance or weakness in the body. I take the latter view. In practice, low blood pressure is often associated with a weakness in the adrenal glands. The adrenal glands manufacture a hormone called 'aldosterone' which helps the body to maintain blood pressure levels by retaining sodium. Weakened adrenal glands may under-produce aldosterone, causing sodium loss in the body and a lowered blood pressure. Adding salt to the diet can help by reducing the body's need to secret aldosterone from the adrenal glands. Taking steps to restore adrenal health as outlined in pages 88–93 usually brings long-term improvement in blood pressure, and often leads to a significant enhancement in well-being too.

Hypothyroidism – see chapter 5

i

Impotence A man's ability to attain and maintain an erection is to a certain degree dependent on the blood supply to the penis. The herb ginkgo biloba has a long history of use as a circulatory stimulant, and has been shown to help improve blood supply to the penis. One study showed that after nine months of treatment with ginkgo extract, there was significant improvement in 78 per cent of men with impotence. The dose used in this study was 80 mg of ginkgo extract, three times a day (*ref* 1).

Other herbs which have traditionally been used to treat impotence include catuaba (from the Amazon rainforest) at a dose of 1,000 mg, twice a day, and muira puama (also from South America) at a dose of 1,000 to 1,500 mg of 4:1 extract per day.

Incontinence – urinary Incontinence can be related to weakness in what is known as the 'detrusor' muscle, a proportion of which makes up the outer muscular coat of the bladder. In a condition known as 'detrusor instability', it is thought that this muscle does not function normally, giving rise to certain symptoms which may include incontinence, and frequent urination with the need to pass water at night. One nutritional factor which seems to have a significant effect in many cases of detrusor instability is caffeine. One study found that women older than fifty-five years of age who drank more than four cups of coffee per day had twice the risk of developing weakened bladder muscles (*ref* 1). While women older than fifty-five are especially vulnerable to this condition, researchers reported caffeine consumption increased risk regardless of age. Women who consumed an average of 484 mg of caffeine a day were more likely to have detrusor instability compared to women drinking an average of 194 mg of caffeine per day. It may therefore be important to keep caffeine consumption to a minimum, and certainly to less than 200 mg per day. Per cup, brewed coffee, instant coffee and tea contain about 130 mg, 70 mg and 40 mg of caffeine respectively.

Another useful approach to treating detrusor instability is to take a supplement of the mineral magnesium. In one study, it was found that symptoms of detrusor instability improved in more than half of the women taking magnesium. In contrast, only 20 per cent of women taking a placebo (inactive) medication reported any improvement (*ref* 2). Magnesium probably works by helping to relax and improve coordination in the detrusor muscle. A dose of 250 to 350 mg of magnesium should be taken two to four times a day, though this dose can usually be reduced as symptoms improve.

In practice, incontinence can often be very effectively treated using what is known as 'Kegel' exercises. These involve voluntary contraction of the muscles in the pelvic floor, which in turn can increase the strength and tone of the muscles here. Women practising this exercise focus on contracting the same muscles they would normally use to stop their urinary flow mid-stream. With frequent and systematic practice, and maybe the use of vaginal weights, it is often possible to get very good control of the symptoms of incontinence.

Indigestion (see also *Hiatus Hernia*) Indigestion, the feeling of pain, discomfort, or bloating after eating, is very often related to poor digestion. Inadequate chewing, low stomach acid secretion and/or low levels of digestive enzymes are frequent factors here. See pages 44–8 for more information about poor digestion and how to manage it.

Indigestion may also be related to infection with the organism *Helicobacter pylori*. This infection may respond to treatment with mastic gum, which is prepared from the resin of a tree which grows on an island in the Aegean Sea. Mastic gum has been found to kill *Helicobacter pylori* in the test-tube. Experimentally, mastic gum has been shown to reduce symptoms in 80 per cent of sufferers, and heal 70 per cent of duodenal ulcers (*ref* 1). A dose of 1 g of mastic gum should be taken each day for two weeks.

Infertility – female Infertility in women can have many different underlying causes, some of which may be amenable to a natural approach. Smoking (*ref* 1), caffeine and alcohol (*ref* 2) seem to be related to infertility. Low thyroid function (see chapter 00) can sometimes be a factor.

Infertility may be related to nutritional deficiency, and one double-blind study found that taking a multivitamin and mineral supplement helped (*ref* 3). Vitamin E taken at a dose of 200 IU per day for women and 100 IU per day for men has been shown to increase fertility (*ref* 4). The herb *Agnus castus* has been shown to enhance fertility, perhaps through its ability to normalize levels of progesterone, a hormone necessary for the maintenance of a pregnancy (*ref* 5).

Infertility – male Scientific studies suggest that male infertility is reaching epidemic proportions. One study which reviewed a mass of data from sixty-one research papers found a 50 per cent fall in the average sperm count between 1938 and 1990 (*ref* 1). One study showed that while 5 per cent of European sperm donors were found to have reduced fertility in 1980, by 1990 this figure had risen almost tenfold to 46 per cent (*ref* 2). The precise reason for this dramatic decline in sperm counts is unknown, though many scientists believe it is likely to be related to the ingestion of chemicals in the environment, which may mimic hormones such as pesticides (e.g. DDT and dieldren), and plastic residues.

Healthy sperm production is dependent on a number of different factors which can often be modified to improve fertility. Sperm production is better if the testes are kept cool. It is advisable for men to avoid tight-fitting trousers and underwear, as these tend to raise the temperature of the testes which can impair sperm production. For the same reason, showers are preferable to baths.

In addition, certain natural substances may help to enhance fertility. One nutrient which has been shown to improve sperm production is vitamin C. This seems to help prevent sperm from sticking together (something known as 'agglutination'), and also increases the percentage of normal sperm (*ref* 3). A sensible dose of vitamin C is 500 mg, twice a day. Zinc is also important for male fertility. In one study, men with low concentrations of zinc in their semen experienced increases in sperm count and motility (movement) by taking 55 mg of zinc per day (*ref* 4).

Another natural agent which may help fertility is the vitamin-like compound L-carnitine. In one study, 3 g of L-carnitine per day increased the proportion of sperm showing normal motility (*ref* 5).

Inflammatory Bowel Disease – see *Ulcerative Colitis* and *Crohn's Disease*

Insomnia Sleep disturbance can broadly be divided into two categories: difficulty in getting to sleep, and problems with waking in the night. If getting off to sleep is a problem, then it often helps to engage in relaxing activities such as reading, listening to music and taking a bath in the evening. Dietary factors also play an important part in determining our ability to get to sleep. For instance, one common cause of sleeplessness is caffeine, which has stimulant effects in the body. Studies have shown that coffee and tea drinkers are more likely to suffer from sleep disruption. The effects of caffeine can linger for up to twenty hours (*ref* 1), so cutting out caffeine from the diet, or at least avoiding it after breakfast, may be necessary for sleep patterns to regularize. Camomile tea, drunk in the evening, is a good alternative and is found by many to be an effective sleep aid.

Valerian (*Valeriana officinalis*) has been widely used in folk medicine as a sedative. The root of the valerian plant contains a number of constituents including essential oils which have calming and sleep-inducing properties. Valerian, unlike many of the conventional sleeping medications, does not seem to be addictive. The normal recommended dose is 300 to 500 mg of root extract or 5 mls of tincture, taken one hour before bedtime.

Sleep is induced by the production of certain brain chemicals including a substance called 'serotonin'. Serotonin is manufactured from the amino acid tryptophan. An intermediary in this process is the substance 5-hydroxytryptophan.

Many people find that supplementing with this substance can help induce and maintain sleep. The normal recommended dose is 50 mg, taken an hour before bedtime.

Some people find that while dropping off to sleep is not a problem, they tend to wake in the middle of the night, often finding it difficult to get back to sleep again. This problem is quite often related to a drop in the level of sugar in the bloodstream during the night. Normally, the body likes to keep an adequate and stable blood sugar level while we sleep. Should the blood sugar level drop, the body secretes certain hormones, notably adrenaline, to correct this. Peak adrenaline secretion is often at around three or four o'clock in the morning, which is perhaps why many individuals wake at this time. The secret to ensuring a good night's sleep is to maintain a stable level of blood sugar throughout the night. More details about this can be found on pages 69–84.

Intermittent Claudication Each muscle in the body is dependent on an adequate blood supply for its function. In some individuals, the arteries which supply blood to the muscles in the legs can become narrowed, essentially starving the muscle of oxygen and other nutrients. As a result, it is not uncommon for individuals with this condition to experience pain in their legs when they walk any distance, particularly on an uphill incline. Typically, the pain will be felt in one or both calf muscles and is relieved by resting.

Regular walks should be taken, and it can help to exercise through the pain if at all possible. It is thought that doing so helps to stimulate the development of other channels of blood flow into the legs. On a dietary level, animal fat and what are known as 'partially hydrogenated' or 'trans fatty acids' (found in most processed foods, fried foods, fast food and baked goods) should be avoided. Oily fish, extra virgin olive oil and garlic, all of which have a beneficial effect on diseased arteries, should be emphasized in the diet.

Vitamin E may help the symptoms of intermittent claudication. Vitamin E has blood-thinning properties and may also help to prevent further fatty build-up in the arteries. From 800 to 1,000 IU should be taken each day. Another useful natural remedy for intermittent claudication is a blend of Tibetan herbs called Padma 28. This supplement (760 mg, twice a day) has been shown to double the walking distance in individuals with intermittent claudication (*ref* 1). Treatment should continue for at least twelve weeks. This supplement can be obtained from Cedar Health/Padma UK (see Useful Information at the back of the book).

Irritable Bowel Syndrome – see also *Abdominal Bloating* Irritable bowel syndrome (IBS) is a common digestive problem, typical symptoms of which are bloating, excessive flatulence, abdominal discomfort and constipation and/or loose bowels. Very often IBS can be effectively dealt with by tackling one or both of two main underlying problems: food sensitivity and an imbalance in the organisms which normally inhabit the gut (especially yeast overgrowth). Chapter 3 contains details on how to go about diagnosing and treating these conditions.

IBS can also be related to insufficient digestion. Chapter 3, pages 44–8, contains information about the diagnosis and treatment of this problem.

k

Kidney Stones Stones that form in the kidney or bladder come in several different forms, the most common of which are made of calcium and a substance called 'oxalate'. It is thought that high levels of oxalate in the diet may predispose to the formation of these stones (*ref* 1). For this reason, anyone with a history of calcium oxalate kidney stones should cut down on consumption of oxalate-rich foods such as beans, cocoa, instant coffee, tea, parsley, rhubarb, spinach and chocolate.

Individuals who suffer from recurrent kidney stones are often advised to cut down on their consumption of calcium. Interestingly, calcium can bind to oxalate in the digestive tract, preventing its absorption into the body. There is some evidence that a calcium-rich diet can actually reduce the risk of developing calcium-based stones (*refs* 2, 3). Calcium supplements may promote kidney stones, but this only appears to be the case if they are taken away from mealtimes (*ref* 3). Calcium supplements should be taken with food for this reason.

Two nutrients which may help to reduce the risk of kidney stone formation are magnesium and vitamin B6. Both of these are used by the body to convert oxalate into other substances. One study showed that taking supplements with magnesium along with vitamin B6 reduced the rate of stone recurrence by about 90 per cent (*ref* 4). Good doses would be 300 mg of magnesium and 50 mg of vitamin B6 per day.

A natural remedy which can help to dissolve kidney stones is the herb quebra pedra (which literally translated means 'stone breaker'). Quebra pedra is usually available as a powder that can be made into a tea. Two heaped teaspoons should be boiled in about half a litre of water. This mixture can be drunk over the course of the day, either hot or cold. Anecdotally, the many individuals who try this remedy find that the kidney stone dissolves within about two weeks of starting treatment.

Lactose Intolerance Milk contains a sugar called lactose, which is made up of two other sugars – glucose and galactose. Lactose is normally broken down into its constituents prior to absorption. However, some individuals lack the enzyme in the gut responsible for digesting lactose, a problem which can give rise to diarrhoea, bloating and wind. This condition is called 'lactose intolerance', and is especially common in individuals of Asian, African and Middle Eastern descent.

In the gut, certain bacterial species have the ability to metabolize lactose. One of the most important in this respect is *lactobacillus acidophilus* – the name of which gives a clue to its lactose-digesting ability. Taking a good quality acidophilus supplement for two to three months, perhaps followed by a maintenance dose of this organism, seems to enhance lactose-digesting ability.

Another option is to treat milk with the enzyme responsible for digesting lactose called 'lactase'. Lactase can often be found in liquid form which can be added to milk twenty-four hours before it is consumed. Lactase may also be available in tablet form, to be taken when consuming milk or milk products such as ice cream. One final approach is to choose naturally lactose-free milks such as soya, oat and rice milk in preference to dairy-based milk.

Leg Ulcer – see *Ulcer – skin*

Leukoplakia Leukoplakia is a condition characterized by white 'plaques' in the mouth. The condition is itself quite harmless, but there is a chance it may turn cancerous in time. One study showed that 300 mcg of selenium taken each day for twelve weeks improved 7 out of 12 (72 per cent) individuals (*ref* 1). Other nutrients which also seem to help this condition include vitamin A and beta-carotene. A supplement of 10,000 IU of vitamin A and 25,000 to 50,000 IU of beta-carotene per day are likely to add to the beneficial effects of selenium.

Low Blood Pressure – see *Hypotension*

Macular Degeneration Light from the outside world is focused on to a structure at the back of the eye called the 'retina'. The central part of the retina – known as the 'macula' – is crucial for vision. In some individuals, the macula gradually deteriorates leading to visual problems. This problem is associated with the growth of tiny blood vessels called capillaries just behind the retina which may bleed, often causing the vision to deteriorate further. Macular degeneration is more common as we age, and a quarter of individuals over the age of sixty-five have at least the beginnings of this disease.

Macular degeneration is triggered by damaging, destructive molecules called 'free radicals'. In the body, free radicals are neutralized by substances called antioxidants such as beta-carotene. One study showed that eating beta-carotene rich foods such as red and orange peppers, apricots, cantaloupe melon, kale and spinach helped reduce the risk of macular degeneration (*ref* 1). Other nutrients that have been found to protect against macular degeneration include lutein and zeaxanthin (*ref* 2). These relatives of beta-carotene can be found in foods such as spinach, collard greens and kale. They can also be taken in supplement form – 6 mg of each would be a good dose, along with 15,000 to 25,000 IU of beta-carotene. Another natural agent which may help in the treatment of macular degeneration is the herb ginkgo biloba. Some research exists to suggest there may be a benefit from this herb in the early stages of the disease (*ref* 3). The normal recommended dose is 120 to 240 mg of standardized extract per day.

Memory and Concentration – poor (see also *Alzheimer's Disease*) Declining memory and mental function is common as we age and is sometimes referred to as age-associated memory impairment. This problem often seems to be connected with reduced blood supply to the brain and/or a failure of the brain cells to coordinate or communicate properly. While poor memory is sometimes regarded as an inevitable consequence of the ageing process, it is usually possible to improve brain function using natural means.

Generally speaking, the diet should be rich in whole, unrefined foods as this will help to provide the brain with the nutrients it needs for optimal function. Oily fish such as mackerel, salmon, trout or tuna should be eaten, as they are rich in the omega-3 fatty acids which play an important part in maintaining the structure and function of nerve cells in the brain. In addition, fresh fruits and vegetables should be emphasized, as they contain vitamin C and beta-carotene which have been associated with better memory in elderly individuals (*ref* 1).

The herb ginkgo biloba has been shown to enhance mental function (*refs* 2, 3), possibly through its ability to enhance blood supply to the brain. Another useful natural agent is acetyl-L-carnitine. This has been shown to improve memory in elderly individuals with mild brain function impairment (*refs* 4, 5). The normal recommended dose is 500 to 1,000 mg, three times a day.

Ménière's Disease Ménière's disease is a disorder which affects the part of the body responsible for maintaining balance – the inner ear. The condition is characterized by episodes of dizziness and vertigo. These symptoms can be very severe and can cause extreme disorientation and collapse. Ménière's disease can also be associated with other symptoms such as deafness and tinnitus (ringing in the ears). Although the precise cause is unknown, one theory is that restricted blood supply to the inner ear is a factor.

On a dietary level, it is important to avoid sugar and other foods that release sugar quickly into the bloodstream, such as white bread, white rice, and potatoes. These foods can upset the balance of sugar in the bloodstream, which seems to bring on symptoms in many sufferers. For more details about blood sugar control, see pages 69–84. In addition, salt should be limited, so should saturated fat (red meat and dairy products), coffee and tea. Plenty of fresh fruits and vegetables, nuts, seeds, extra virgin olive oil, and plain filtered or bottled water should be included in the diet. One study showed very significant improvement in the symptoms of Ménière's disease in sufferers who had followed this regime for a year (*ref* 1).

One very useful natural substance for the treatment of Ménière's disease is ginkgo biloba. A double-blind study has confirmed its value in treating vertigo, a common symptom in Ménière's disease (*ref* 2). The normal recommended dose is 120 to 240 mg of standardized extract per day.

Menopause During her reproductive years a woman's cycle is regulated by a variety of hormones, the most important of which are oestrogen and progesterone. At about the age of fifty, the production of these hormones by the ovaries declines sharply, which leads to an end to menstruation – commonly referred to as the 'menopause'. At this time, many women will complain of potentially troublesome symptoms such as hot flushes, low libido, depression, insomnia and vaginal dryness. The post-menopausal period is associated with an increased risk of certain conditions including osteoporosis and heart disease.

The conventional medical approach to treating menopause is centred around the use of hormone replacement therapy (HRT) which comes in pill, patch and implant forms. HRT appears to control menopausal symptoms in some women, and it has been claimed that it may also reduce the risk of osteoporosis and heart disease. With regard to osteoporosis, the best HRT can do is to slow down the rate of bone loss. However, this effect is lost once HRT is stopped, which means that women must continue treatment indefinitely if they want long-term protection. Also, there are plenty of natural approaches to osteoporosis that do not require the use of synthetic hormones (see *Osteoporosis*). The evidence for HRT's benefits for the heart are even more scanty. A study which looked at the collective results from twenty-two pieces of research found that HRT did not reduce the risk of heart disease at all (*ref* 1). More recent work has confirmed this finding (*ref* 2). HRT is also associated with significant health risks. In research which combined the data from fifty-one studies, taking HRT for five years or more (average duration of treatment in this group being eleven years) increased the risk of breast cancer by 35 per cent (*ref* 3).

There is no doubt that diet and appropriate nutritional supplements can help protect women from the negative effects of the menopause. It is interesting to note that in some cultures women tend to have relatively few problems with the menopause. In Japan, for instance, only a small percentage of women suffer significant menopausal symptoms, and there is no Japanese equivalent to the term 'hot flush'. The low rate of menopausal symptoms in Japan appears to be related to the consumption of significant quantities of soya-based foods including tofu and soya milk. Soya contains substances called isoflavones (also known as phytoestrogens), which can mimic the effect of oestrogen in the body. Including these in the diet may help to control some of the symptoms associated with a lack of oestrogen including hot flushes.

To help combat osteoporosis it is important to eat a diet rich in calcium. However, what is less well known is that calcium seems to have most effect when in combination with another bone-building mineral – magnesium. For this reason it is a good idea to include in the diet foods which are rich in both these nutrients – green leafy vegetables, sardines, mackerel, seafood and sesame seeds.

Another important concept that may help reduce the negative effects of menopause is blood sugar control. Fluctuating levels of sugar in the bloodstream tend to stimulate adrenaline secretion in the body, and this hormone is well known to promote bone loss. More details about how to stabilize blood sugar levels can be found in chapter 4.

To ensure that blood sugar levels remain stable, the diet should be based around foods which release sugar relatively slowly, such as wholemeal bread, brown rice, wholewheat pasta, vegetables, beans, pulses and fish. Fast-releasing foods such as sugar, potatoes, white bread and white rice should be avoided or eaten in moderation.

Vitamins, minerals and herbs will often provide relief from many of the symptoms and adverse effects associated with the menopause. Several studies show that vitamin E can be very effective in relieving hot flushes in menopausal women (*refs* 4, 5, 6, 7, 8). An effective dose seems to be 800 to 1,000 IU per day. Vitamin E may also substantially reduce the risk of heart disease (see *Atherosclerosis*).

Another natural substance that seems to have a beneficial effect on menopausal symptoms is the herb black cohosh (*Cimicifuga racemosa*). This has been shown to reduce hot flushes along with other menopausal symptoms in a significant number of women (*ref* 9). The normal recommended dose is 2–4 mls of tincture (alcoholic extract), three times a day.

Other herbs which may often be useful in relieving menopausal symptoms include agnus castus (40 drops of concentrated liquid herbal extract taken in the morning) and dong quai (3–4 g of the herb per day).

Menorrhagia (heavy periods) Heavy menstrual bleeding – referred to as 'menorrhagia' (pronounced men-or-ray-jah) by the medical profession – affects a significant proportion of women. While it is important for women with heavy periods to consult their doctor to exclude any potentially serious condition, usually no specific reason can be found for the problem. Often treatment options for menorrhagia involve hormonal medications or hysterectomy (removal of the womb). Fortunately, natural alternatives do exist.

Menorrhagia can have several potential causes including fibroids (non-cancerous growths in the womb) and hormonal imbalance. Another quite common cause of menorrhagia is hypothyroidism (see chapter 5 for more details on this). One nutrient that seems to be very effective in treating menorrhagia is vitamin A. One study showed that 25,000 IU of vitamin A taken twice a day for fifteen days brought about a significant reduction of menstrual flow in more than 90 per cent of women (*ref* 1). Vitamin A should not be taken in doses exceeding 10,000 IU per day by women who are pregnant or are planning pregnancy.

It is well known that iron deficiency is a common consequence of menorrhagia. However, what is less well known is that iron can also be used to treat menorrhagia. Iron appears to help blood vessels contract, which is important if the body is to bring an end to the bleeding from the womb. The 'ferritin' blood test is the best way to check the level of iron in your body. If this is low, iron therapy may well help reduce the weight of the period.

Migraine – see also *Headache* and *Cluster Headaches* Migraine affects 6 per cent of men and almost 20 per cent of women. Characterized by intense, localized pain, usually on one side of the head, migraine attacks can last from anywhere between two hours and several days. Some attacks may lead to severe symptoms such as intense, throbbing pain, nausea, vomiting and diarrhoea. About 75 per cent of migraine sufferers experience some loss of their ability to function normally during an attack, and almost a third of sufferers become totally incapacitated by at least some of their headaches.

There is good evidence that a major cause of migraine is food sensitivity (*refs* 1, 2, 3, 4). Certain foods are well known to trigger migraine. Sometimes referred to as 'the five Cs', these are: chocolate, cheese, claret (and other red wines), coffee (and other sources of caffeine) and citrus fruits. While these foods are commonly held to be the main culprits in migraine, research has suggested that the most common food trigger is actually wheat (*ref* 5). This research also found milk and egg to be other common precipitating foodstuffs. Identification and elimination of offending foods is often very effective in controlling migraine attacks. More information about this can be found in chapter 3, pages 34–43.

Migraine can sometimes be triggered if the level of sugar in the bloodstream gets too low (hypoglycaemia). This may explain why some individuals can wake up with a headache or be prone to an attack if a meal is skipped. To ensure a stable level of blood sugar, regular meals and snacks should be eaten, and the diet should be based around fresh fruits and vegetables, meat, fish, and wholegrain starches like wholemeal bread, wholewheat pasta, and brown rice. More details about stabilizing blood sugar, including supplements which may help with this, can be found on pages 69–84.

Nutritional deficiency can sometimes be a factor. One of the most important nutrients in this respect is magnesium. During a migraine attack the blood vessels around the brain tend to constrict (narrow) and then dilate (open out). The phase of dilation is believed to cause the pain characteristic of migraine. Magnesium deficiency increases the risk of spasm in the lining of the arteries, and the likelihood of subsequent dilation and pain. Indeed, migraine sufferers have been found to have lower levels of magnesium in their bloodstreams compared to non-sufferers. One report found that 80 per cent of women treated with magnesium (typical dose 200 mg per day) experienced an improvement in their headaches (*ref* 6). Magnesium deficiency is relatively common in our society, so I generally recommend that migraine sufferers take 200 to 250 mg of magnesium, once or twice a day.

A natural remedy that is often effective in the prevention and treatment of migraine is the herb feverfew (*Tanacetum parthenium*). The main active constituent is believed to be a substance called 'parthenolide'; this appears to inhibit the release of inflammatory substances that play a part in changing the blood vessels typical in migraine. Feverfew has been found to reduce the frequency, severity and duration of migraine attacks (*refs* 7, 8, 9), although it may take several weeks for benefits to become apparent. The recommended dose of parthenolide is 250 mg a day.

Mitral Valve Prolapse The heart is essentially divided into two. The right side of your heart pumps blood to the lungs, while the left side pumps blood to the rest of the body. Each side has an upper and lower chamber. The mitral valve sits between the upper and lower chambers on the left side of the heart. Its function is to ensure that when the heart beats blood is only pumped out of the heart towards the body's tissues, and not in the other direction.

In mitral valve prolapse (MVP), the mitral valve is slightly deformed, and this may eventually lead to some leakiness of the valve. If the condition is severe enough it may give rise to symptoms such as chest pain, palpitations, fatigue and breathlessness. MVP affects about 5 per cent of the adult population, and is most common in young to middle-aged women. Certain nutrients may help slow the progression of MVP and reduce the risk of symptoms.

Studies have shown that the majority of MVP sufferers are deficient in magnesium, and that magnesium supplementation can benefit MVP sufferers (*ref* 1). A reasonable dose is 250 to 350 mg of magnesium twice a day. Another nutrient which may help the symptoms of MVP is Coenzyme Q10. This helps energy production in the body, and seems to have particular benefits for the heart. In one study, children with MVP showed a marked benefit from this nutrient (*ref* 2); 30–50 mg should be taken three times a day.

Molluscum Contagiosum Molluscum contagiosum is actually a viral infection which gives rise to the presence of shiny, white, wart-like lumps on the skin. It can affect any part of the skin, but the face, genitals and inside of the thighs are commonly affected. More common in children than in adults, it usually clears up of its own accord within a year or so. In a small percentage of sufferers, however, problems can persist for longer.

One nutrient which seems to help clear molluscum contagiosum infection is the mineral selenium. Doses of 100 to 200 mcg of selenium per day in children and 300 to 400 mcg per day in adults may help to control the infection by inhibiting the reproduction of the molluscum virus. In addition, it may pay to apply something topically to the warts. Extracts of myrrh (*Commiphora molmol*) have potent anti-viral action and have been used historically to treat a wide range of infections. Ten drops of essential oil of myrrh should be dissolved in 100 mls of almond oil. This mixture should be rubbed into the affected area two or three times a day.

Morning Sickness Morning sickness is a common problem that usually starts before the sixth week of pregnancy and disappears by the twelfth week. Although morning sickness is almost always harmless, any woman who is experiencing severe or prolonged problems should consult her doctor. While nausea and vomiting in early pregnancy invariably cause discomfort and distress for sufferers, simple natural remedies can often be very effective in bringing symptoms under control.

It is often helpful to cut down on fatty foods such as red meat, dairy products and fried foods. These tend to make the feelings of sickness worse. Another good idea is to eat small meals (including breakfast) quite often during the day. This helps to keep the level of sugar in the bloodstream stable, which often alleviates symptoms.

One natural and effective remedy for morning sickness is ginger. Chewing a piece of root ginger throughout the day or drinking ginger tea made from grated or sliced root ginger may help relieve symptoms quite quickly. An alternative to fresh root ginger is ginger capsules or tablets. The equivalent of 250 mg of ginger should be taken up to four times a day. Another natural substance known to help women suffering from nausea in pregnancy is vitamin B6 (*refs* 1, 2); 25 mg should be taken, two or three times a day.

Mouth Ulcers (canker sores) Mouth ulcers can have a variety of causes. One common, and often overlooked, factor is an ingredient in toothpaste known as sodium lauryl sulphate (SLS). SLS is a foaming agent, but is also thought to cause erosion of a substance called 'mucin' which lines and protects the mouth. One study showed that individuals suffering from recurrent mouth ulcers found significant relief by avoiding SLS in toothpaste (*ref* 1). Natural, SLS-free toothpastes are often available in health food stores.

Mouth ulcers may also be related to nutritional deficiencies, especially of iron and B vitamins (*refs* 2, 3, 4). Taking a good quality multivitamin and mineral supplement in combination with a B-complex supplement may help clear mouth ulcers in time. Iron should not be supplemented unless there is a proven deficiency. The best blood test for iron levels measures the level of a compound called 'ferritin'.

A natural supplement that often works well for mouth ulcers is deglycyrrhizinated licorice (DGL). This has natural soothing properties and can reduce the healing time for mouth ulcers. DGL is thought to work by increasing mucin production in the mouth. A DGL tablet should be chewed twenty minutes before each meal. For topical relief, the contents from a soft gelatine vitamin E capsule can be applied directly on to the ulcers as often as necessary.

Multiple Sclerosis Multiple sclerosis (MS) is characterized by degeneration in the fatty, protective covering of nerve cells (myelin sheaths) in the brain and spinal cord. The disease is thought to be auto-immune in nature, which essentially means the body's immune system is responsible for the degeneration. It generally causes progressive paralysis and often leads to symptoms such as numbness, loss of vision, bladder problems, and loss of balance.

Auto-immune conditions often seem to have food sensitivity as a provoking factor, and this appears to be the case in some cases of MS (*ref* 1). While this may only be relevant to a minority of sufferers, it may be worthwhile considering this possibility. More details about how to identify individual sensitivities can be found on pages 34–43. Some doctors believe that infection with Candida albicans can be an important factor in some cases of MS. See pages 53–62 for more details about this.

One dietary approach that seems to have considerable merit in the treatment of MS is the Swank diet. Dr Roy Swank studied the effect of a low-fat diet in a hundred and fifty patients between 1949 and 1984. The diet restricted saturated fat to 20 g per day, and 'partially hydrogenated' fats such as margarine and many processed fats were eliminated. Healthy fats in the form of cod liver oil (5 g per day) and vegetable oils (10–40 g per day) were given. Compared with untreated individuals, those who adhered strictly to this regime had less deterioration in their condition. The treated group also enjoyed much better overall survival (about 70 per cent over the study period compared to about 20 per cent in the untreated group) (*ref* 2). There is some evidence that the sooner the Swank diet is started, the less risk there is of significant disability. Taking additional quantities of essential fatty acids (EFAs) has been shown to be of some benefit in MS. Three double-blind studies have shown that taking 17–23 g of linoleic acid (found in sunflower oil) each day reduced disability caused by the condition (*ref* 3).

One herbal remedy assessed as a treatment for MS is Padma 28 (see Useful Information at the back of the book under Cedar Health/Padma UK). This blend of twenty-eight herbs based on a Tibetan formula was given to about half of a group of a hundred people with MS. After a year, 44 per cent of those treated with Padma 28 were found to have an improved condition, increased strength or fewer neurological complications. In the untreated group, not a single person improved, and about 40 per cent experienced a deterioration in their condition (*ref* 4).

Nails – weak Weak nails are almost exclusively a female phenomenon, and are very often related to low levels of stomach acid (hypochlorhydria). The strength of the nails is dependent on the supply of certain nutrients, especially minerals, and the absorption of these nutrients is quite dependent on adequate levels of acid in the stomach. For more details about the diagnosis and treatment of hypochlorhydria, see pages 44–8.

Taking a good multivitamin and mineral formulation may help strengthen the nails in time. Some companies have produced formulations specifically for this purpose and these are almost certainly worth a try. One nutrient that seems to be of particular value in strengthening nails is biotin. In one study, thirty-five individuals were treated with 2,500 mcg per day of biotin. An improvement in the condition of their nails was reported by 63 per cent. The average length of time before improvement was seen was two months (*ref* 1).

Obesity Problems with overweight and obesity can have many underlying factors, more than one of which can coincide in the same individual. Identification and correction of individual imbalances is the key to successful, long-term weight loss. The most common underlying issues seen are emotional issues, blood sugar imbalance, low thyroid function, food sensitivity, yeast overgrowth, toxicity, unhealthy fat consumption, inefficient breathing, and insufficient exercise. These factors are discussed in depth in my book *BodyWise: 10 Steps to Permanent Weight Loss and Well-being*.

Oedema Oedema is the medical term for swelling. Many individuals, particularly women, complain of fluid retention, which often manifests as swollen ankles and feet, puffy hands and weight fluctuation from day to day of a few pounds or more. In practice, I find that food sensitivity is a common cause of fluid retention, with wheat seemingly being the most common culprit. See pages 34–43 for more details about the identification of individual food sensitivities. Low thyroid function often causes oedema too, and advice about how this problem can be identified and treated can be found in chapter 5.

Quite often, swollen ankles and feet may be caused by a condition known as chronic venous insufficiency (CVI). Blood is pumped from the heart to the tissues in the arteries and returns in the veins. Veins contain valves designed to ensure that blood travels towards the heart, but not in the other direction. However, in CVI the veins do not work as efficiently as they should, and this can cause blood to pool and stagnate in the lower legs. As a result, there is a risk that fluid will escape from inside the veins into the surrounding tissues. The tissues can therefore become 'waterlogged', causing swelling and puffiness in the feet, ankles and calves. This problem also often gives rise to a dull ache in the lower legs that comes on after prolonged standing.

One of the most useful natural remedies for the treatment of CVI is the herb horse chestnut (*Aeculus hippocastanum*). Horse chestnut contains a group of substances given the collective name 'aescin'. Aescin appears to help CVI through two distinct mechanisms. Once it makes its way into the circulation aescin helps to draw fluid out of the tissues back into the vessel. It also seems to help strengthen the lining of the vein walls, thereby reducing the risk that fluid will leak out. Horse chestnut is usually available in tablet and tincture form. Enough needs to be taken to give at least 50–75 mg of aescin, twice a day. Some benefit is likely to be seen within a few weeks, after which a lower dose is often enough to control the condition. The benefits of horse chestnut in the treatment of vein-related problems has been confirmed in double-blind research (*ref* 1).

Oesophageal Spasm The oesophagus takes food from the mouth to the stomach through a rhythmical contraction of muscle in the lining of the oesophagus which 'milks' food down into the stomach. However, in some individuals the muscle in the oesophagus may go into spasm (cramp). Oesophageal spasm is often felt as a central chest pain, which is not burning in nature, and often comes on after eating.

Probably the simplest approach to dealing with this problem is to take a supplement of the mineral magnesium. Magnesium is essential for normal muscle function, and a deficiency of this nutrient can lead to problems with spasm or 'cramp'. Because of its role in normalizing muscle function magnesium is usually effective in controlling oesophageal spasm. A dose of 250 to 500 mg should be taken each day.

Osgood-Schlatter disease The thigh muscles attach to the shinbone (tibia) via a tendon which runs underneath the kneecap (patella). This tendon inserts into the shin at a point called the tibial tuberosity. Osgood-Schlatter disease is a disease which is characterized by the painful enlargement of the tibial tuberosity. The pain is generally worse during exercise and the area below the knee is usually tender to the touch. The condition normally affects boys aged ten to fourteen. It usually clears up on its own over about six months or a year, though it is usually advised that the sufferer avoids running-based exercise during this time.

Dr Jonathan Wright, one of America's most renowned nutritional doctors, has found that a combination of vitamin E and selenium can be very effective in treating Osgood-Schlatter disease. A dose of 400 IU of vitamin E each day along with 100 mcg of selenium twice a day is likely to give relief within six weeks. After this, half the dose should be given for a further six weeks to reduce the risk of a recurrence. As a long-term preventive it can help a child to take a good quality multivitamin and mineral supplement containing selenium and vitamin E.

Osteoarthritis Of the hundred or so medically recognized joint conditions, osteoarthritis is the most common. It affects about one third of the population aged between forty-five and sixty-five. After this age, approximately three-quarters of individuals are affected to some degree. Traditionally, osteoarthritis is treated with painkillers known as non-steroidal anti-inflammatory drugs (NSAIDs) such as ibuprofen. However, there is good evidence that while these drugs may help dull the pain associated with the condition, they also speed up the rate at which the osteoarthritis progresses (*refs* 1, 2, 3).

Osteoarthritis is characterized by the degeneration of joint cartilage, and predominantly affects the major weight-bearing joints (hips, knees and spine). It is also common in the hands, particularly the last joints in the fingers and the base of the thumb. In the affected joint(s) problems may occur with pain and/or stiffness. It often progresses to cause major disability, with a significant number of sufferers eventually requiring surgical joint replacement.

There are a number of different dietary approaches which may prove effective in controlling osteoarthritis. Seemingly, the most successful approach is the elimination of foods from the nightshade (*solanaceae*) family, which include tomato, potato, pepper (capsicum) and aubergine. These foods contain a substance called 'solanine' which some scientists believe may be involved in the processes which cause osteoarthritis. The elimination of nightshade foods seems to work for about half of sufferers, but often takes about six months before real benefit is experienced.

Ginger is a natural substance which can have pain-relieving properties in the body. It does this through its ability to stimulate the production of natural anti-inflammatory substances. Ginger tea makes a very good alternative to regular tea and coffee. Freshly grated, chopped or sliced root ginger can be steeped in hot water for five or ten minutes. Ginger supplements may also be of benefit for pain control.

Many natural agents offer relief from osteoarthritis, and may even help to reverse the condition. One of the most widely researched natural remedies is glucosamine sulphate. This compound is an essential building block in the manufacture of cartilage tissue. Several double-blind clinical studies exist which show glucosamine to be an effective agent in the treatment of osteoarthritis (*refs* 4, 5 6). It has also been shown to control the symptoms of osteoarthritis as well as ibuprofen (400 mg, three times a day) after four weeks of continuous treatment (*ref* 7). The normal recommended dose of glucosamine sulphate is 500 mg three times a day. Once therapeutic benefit is achieved, it is usually possible to taper down to a once or twice a day dose.

Another agent often used in conjunction with glucosamine sulphate is chondroitin sulphate. This seems to work by attracting fluid into the joint cartilage tissue, which may improve the spongy, shock-absorbing qualities of the cartilage, and may also help bring essential nutrients to the area. A study which examined the effect of chondroitin sulphate on osteoarthritis found it to be significantly better than a placebo (inactive medication) at controlling symptoms such as pain and stiffness (*ref* 8). The normal recommended dose of chondroitin sulphate is 400 mg, three times a day. Again, this dose may often be reduced once symptoms have been controlled. Glucosamine and chondroitin are very often combined together in nutritional supplements designed to enhance joint health. Interestingly, an animal study showed that glucosamine and chondroitin appear to work best when used together (*ref* 9).

Green-lipped mussel extract has developed a reputation as a useful agent in the treatment of osteoarthritis. Research has identified a compound known as eicosatetraenoic acid (ETA) which has been found to have anti-inflammatory actions more potent than that of commonly prescribed painkillers. One study found that treatment with green-lipped mussel extract (1,050 mg per day of dried powder or 210 mg per day of a special extract) brought statistically significant improvements in the symptoms of osteoarthritis within three months (*ref* 10).

Another natural remedy for osteoarthritis is niacinamide – a form of vitamin B3. Studies have shown that niacinamide therapy can increase joint mobility, improve muscle strength and enhance energy in individuals with osteoarthritis (*refs* 11, 12, 13). A typical dose would be 250 mg, four to six times a day, though larger doses may be necessary for individuals with advanced osteoarthritis. Results can take twelve weeks or more to become apparent.

Osteoporosis Bone is living tissue and is constantly being renewed and replaced in the body. Osteoporosis (thinning bones) comes about when bone tissue is broken down faster than it is formed. When this happens the bones can become weakened and the chances of fracture increase, especially in the hips and spine. Osteoporosis is more common in women than men, and is usually related to hormonal changes after the time of menopause. While osteoporosis is generally regarded as a natural part of the ageing process, there is a lot that can be done to combat it using simple diet- and lifestyle-related changes.

Weight-bearing, and in particular, exercises that require weight bearing, can help keep bones strong. Studies have shown that gentle weight-bearing exercise reduces bone loss (*ref* 1), and may even increase bone density. Brisk walking or aerobics for twenty to thirty minutes each day is quite likely to help strengthen bones.

One of the main factors which have a bearing on bone strength is hormonal balance. Oestrogen, one of the principal female hormones, is thought to have a bone protective effect. This explains why osteoporosis is most common after the time of menopause, when oestrogen levels are low. Consuming foods rich in a class of substances called 'phytoestrogens' may help. These naturally occurring plant constituents, which are found in beans, lentils, chickpeas and soya products such as soya milk and tofu, mimic the effect of the hormone oestrogen in the body. There is increasing evidence to suggest that consuming a diet rich in phytoestrogens can help prevent osteoporosis in the long term. In one study, post-menopausal women were treated with calcium (1,000 mg per day) combined with ipriflavone (a synthetic phytoestrogen). After two years, individuals treated with both ipriflavone and calcium maintained their bone density, while those treated with calcium alone lost about 5 per cent of the bone density in their spine (*ref* 2). The dose of ipriflavone used in this study was 200 mg, three times a day. Other studies of women with osteoporosis showed that ipriflavone therapy actually increased bone density and reduced symptoms such as bone pain (*refs* 3, 4, 5).

Perhaps the best-known nutrient for bone health is calcium, and studies suggest that a good intake of this mineral can reduce the risk of osteoporosis (*ref* 6). Calcium supplementation also seems to enhance the bone-preserving action of hormone replacement therapy (*ref* 7). However, the effects of calcium on bone density are relatively small, and other nutrients are important for bone building.

Perhaps even more important than calcium appears to be the mineral magnesium. The more magnesium there is in the diet, the higher bone density tends to be. In addition, supplementing with magnesium appears to actually increase bone density. In one study, giving 250 to 750 mg of magnesium in supplement form stopped bone loss or increased bone density in twenty-seven out of thirty-one people over a two-year period (*ref* 8). Bearing in mind the relative importance of calcium and magnesium, anyone wanting to keep their bones strong would do well to eat a diet rich in foods which contain plenty of these. Green leafy vegetables, sardines, mackerel, seafood, and sesame seeds all fit the bill in this respect. Additional supplementation with magnesium (about 500 to 750 mg per day) and calcium (500 to 1,000 mg per day) is likely to be of benefit.

Other nutrients which appear to have a role in bone formation include zinc, copper, vitamin B6, folic acid, boron, manganese, strontium, vitamin K, vitamin C, vitamin D and silicon. Many nutritional supplements designed to enhance bone health now exist, the best ones generally being those that include a wide selection of these nutrients. A comprehensive approach to osteoporosis does seem to work best. In one study, women on hormone replacement therapy were advised to limit animal protein, salt, sugar, alcohol, tea, coffee, chocolate and tobacco. The women were also given 600 mg of magnesium and 500 mg of calcium per day along with other nutrients including zinc, copper, boron, manganese, vitamin C and vitamin D. In just eight to nine months, bone density in these women had increased by a massive 11 per cent (*ref* 9).

Essential fatty acids also have a role to play in bone formation. In one study, women who took 6 g per day of a combination of evening primrose oil (rich in omega-6 fatty acids) and fish oil (rich in omega-3 fatty acids) in addition to

600 mg of calcium per day enjoyed a rise in bone density of about 3 per cent over three years (*ref* 10).

p

Painful Periods (dysmenorrhoea) – see also *Menorrhagia* The body of the womb is made up of muscular tissue. During a period this muscle contracts to help expel the womb's bloody lining. Sometimes, the contractions can be very strong, and this can lead to severe pain and cramping. Painful periods – referred to as 'dysmenorrhoea' by the medical profession – affect about half of menstruating women. In a small but significant proportion of these, the symptoms can be very severe and incapacitating, and may necessitate rest and the use of painkillers for the first day or two of the period.

Niacin (a form of vitamin B3) may relieve menstrual cramps. A dose of 200 mg of niacin should be taken each day, increasing up to 100 mg every two or three hours on the days when cramps are experienced. Calcium and magnesium are essential to muscle function, and can be very effective in reducing menstrual cramps. A dose of 1,000 mg of calcium and 500 mg of magnesium should be taken each day. During the period itself, taking about 250 mg of calcium and 100 mg of magnesium every four hours can often help to relieve symptoms. When the symptoms are at their worst, it might also help to use a preparation of the herb cramp bark (*Viburnum opulus*). The normal dose is 1 teaspoon of tincture, three times a day during symptoms.

Pancreatitis The pancreas is an organ that lies in the upper abdomen behind the stomach. It secretes digestive enzymes into the small intestine, in addition to manufacturing hormones (including insulin), which play an important part in the regulation of blood sugar levels. The pancreas can be prone to bouts of inflammation (pancreatitis). Where attacks tend to be recurrent the condition is usually termed 'chronic pancreatitis'. Chronic pancreatitis may damage the pancreas over time and lead to potential complications such as diabetes. The condition may be associated with specific trigger factors such as gallstones (see pages 235–6) and alcohol. Often, however, there is no obvious underlying cause.

The cause of pancreatitis seems to be associated with damaging, destructive molecules called 'free radicals'. Supplementing the diet with antioxidants, which quench the action of free radicals, may reduce the risk of further pancreatitis attacks. Antox is a natural remedy which contains the antioxidant nutrients selenium, methionine (an amino acid), beta-carotene, and vitamins C and E. Work carried out at the Manchester Royal Infirmary has shown that Antox can reduce the frequency of pancreatitis attacks, and the need for surgery (*ref* 1). Although Antox contains only natural ingredients, it requires a prescription in the UK. More details about this product can be obtained from Pharma Nord (see Useful Information at the back of the book).

Parkinson's Disease Parkinson's disease is a nervous system disorder characterized by shaking (tremor), stiffness and weakness in the muscles. Sufferers usually have a rigid posture, expressionless faces, and move slowly using a shuffling, unbalanced walk. Parkinson's disease is related to a deficiency of the brain chemical dopamine, which has an important effect in the regulation of muscle movement. The mainstay of conventional treatment for Parkinson's is a drug called L-dopa. L-dopa is converted in the brain into dopamine, and can therefore help with symptoms and slow the progression of the illness. However, the effects of L-dopa tend to wear off in time, and its use is associated with certain side-effects including loss of appetite, insomnia and feelings of agitation.

One natural substance that seems to be of benefit is niacinamide adenine dinucleotide (NADH). NADH is believed to increase dopamine production in the brain's cells, thereby helping to control the symptoms of Parkinson's disease. Not only does NADH seem to help control the symptoms of Parkinson's, it also may help reduce depression and improve mood and brain function. The normal recommended dose of NADH is 5 mg, once or twice a day. Results generally take a few days to a few weeks to become apparent.

More information about natural approaches to Parkinson's disease can be found in *Parkinson's Disease – the Way Forward!*

Peptic Ulcer The lining of the gut is shielded from potentially damaging digestive secretions by a coating of protective mucus. Sometimes, this protective mechanism breaks down leading to the development of a raw area or ulcer in the wall of the intestine. The majority of ulcers develop in the part of the gut just after the stomach called the duodenum, though some develop in the stomach itself. Dietary changes and certain nutritional supplements may promote ulcer healing and help prevent a recurrence of the problem. Avoiding sugar, alcohol, coffee and tea, all of which seem to increase the risk of developing an ulcer or slow down its healing, can often help.

Vitamin A at a dose of 10,000 IU per day for women and a dose of 25,000 IU a day for men and zinc at a dose of 30 mg per day may both be beneficial because they enhance tissue healing. Another effective natural remedy for ulcers is deglycyrrhizinated licorice (DGL). DGL is thought to work by increasing secretion of protective mucin in the gut wall, and has been shown to be about as effective as conventional drugs in healing ulcers (*ref* 1). It is important that it is taken as a chewable tablet (*ref* 2). One or two 250 mg tablets should be chewed fifteen minutes before each meal and one to two hours before bedtime.

Many peptic ulcers are caused by infection with an organism known as Helicobacter pylori. Mastic gum – prepared from the resin of a tree which grows on an island in the Aegean Sea – has been shown to be effective in treating this infection. Experimentally, mastic gum has been shown to reduce symptoms in 80 per cent of sufferers, and heal 70 per cent of duodenal ulcers (*ref* 3). A supplement of 1 g of mastic gum should be taken each day for two weeks.

Polycystic Ovarian Syndrome (PCOS) As its name suggests, polycystic ovarian syndrome (PCOS) is characterized by multiple cysts in one or both ovaries. The condition is associated with hormonal disruption; principally, higher than normal levels of the hormone testosterone. In a man the testes start producing testosterone at around the time of puberty. Testosterone is the principal hormone involved in male sexual development, giving rise to body and facial hair growth, muscle development, and a deepening of the voice. In women testosterone is produced in the ovaries, but usually in very small amounts compared with men. In PCOS, larger than normal amounts of testosterone may lead to an increase in hair growth on the body and face (hirsutism). Other common symptoms of PCOS include acne, breast pain, weight gain and mood disturbance.

Precisely what causes PCOS is not known for sure, but there is emerging evidence that the higher than normal levels of testosterone are worsened by increased levels of another hormone – insulin. Insulin is released in response to carbohydrate foods (sugars and starches), and it makes sense to limit those foodstuffs which give rise to the highest insulin levels. Details about how to balance blood sugar levels and the nutrients which may help with this can be found in chapter 4.

The symptoms of excess testosterone can sometimes be helped by the herb saw palmetto. This herb slows down the conversion of testosterone into an even more active form of the hormone known as dihydrotestosterone. In this way, saw palmetto may reduce the impact of testosterone on the body, and help to reduce excess hair growth and other symptoms such as acne. The normal recommended dose is 250 to 350 mg per day. More information about PCOS can be obtained from the self-help organization Verity (see Useful Information at the back of the book).

Pre-eclampsia Pre-eclampsia (sometimes referred to as 'toxaemia of pregnancy') is a condition which may occur in the second half of pregnancy. It is characterized by raised blood pressure, oedema (fluid retention in the tissues) and the presence of protein in the urine. Pre-eclampsia is more common in first pregnancies and in women aged under twenty-five or over thirty-five. Untreated, it can eventually cause seizures (eclampsia), which may pose a risk to both mother and baby. Pre-eclampsia seems to be more common in women having their first baby, and in those who are obese, diabetic, or are suffering from high blood pressure related to the pregnancy. The conventional medical approach to pre-eclampsia is based on bed rest and the use of drugs to lower the blood pressure. However, by using a natural approach it might be possible to prevent or delay the progression of this condition.

It is wise for sufferers of pre-eclampsia to eat a diet moderately high in protein, to make up for the protein being lost in the urine. Calcium deficiency is associated with pre-eclampsia (*ref* 1), and several studies show that taking calcium supplements may protect against pre-eclampsia (*refs* 2, 3, 4, 5, 6). A review of several studies showed that calcium did not protect women at low risk (who tend to need little protection) of developing pre-eclampsia, but is a real benefit for women at high risk (*ref* 7). A good dose is 1,000 mg of calcium per day. Magnesium may also help protect against the condition (*ref* 8). A safe dose is 350 to 500 mg per day and may prove effective. Vitamin B6 has also been shown to help reduce the risk of pre-eclampsia (*ref* 9), even at quite a modest dose (5 mg, twice a day). It is probably a good idea for women wanting to give themselves maximum protection to take 25–50 mg of vitamin B6 per day.

Pre-menstrual Syndrome (PMS) Pre-menstrual syndrome (PMS) is a term used to describe a combination of various physical and mental symptoms that may occur in the week or two prior to menstruation. Typical features of PMS include irritability, depression, tearfulness, fatigue, food cravings, abdominal bloating, breast tenderness, fluid retention and weight gain. The condition is highly individual, with the exact blend of symptoms and their duration varying enormously between women.

PMS is due to hormonal fluctuations in the second half of the menstrual cycle and is thought to affect 80 per cent of women to some degree. The conventional medical approach is centred around symptom relief, such as diuretics for fluid retention, or the use of the oral contraceptive pill. However, many studies have documented that PMS can be very successfully treated with certain lifestyle changes and nutritional supplements.

In practice, sugar and caffeine both seem to increase the risk of PMS. The link between sugar and PMS has not been studied, but caffeine has been clearly implicated (*ref* 1). Another lifestyle factor that is well known to affect PMS in the long term is exercise (*ref* 2). Getting about half an hour's exercise such as jogging, aerobics, cycling or swimming on most days is quite likely to help control the symptoms of PMS.

Several nutrients may be of value in treating PMS. There is good evidence that vitamin B6 can help to control a variety of pre-menstrual symptoms including depression, bloating, and headaches (*refs* 3, 4). For most women 50 to 100 mg per day seems to be the effective dose. Magnesium deficiency also seems to be a factor (*ref* 5). In one study magnesium supplements helped to correct mood problems common in PMS (*ref* 6).

One herb that I find almost universally effective in PMS is agnus castus, which seems to increase progesterone production. This is important because many cases of PMS seem to be related to a condition commonly referred to as 'oestrogen dominance', essentially an excess of the hormone oestrogen in the body. Progesterone balances the effects of oestrogen, and this is perhaps why agnus castus is often effective in treating PMS. Forty drops of concentrated agnus castus liquid (either fluid extract or tincture) should be taken each morning.

Poor Circulation A common cause of poor circulation is Raynaud's disease (see *Raynaud's disease*). Another common but under-recognized factor in poor circulation is low thyroid function. This is quite likely to be an underlying feature if the sufferer also has other symptoms of low thyroid function such as general sensitivity to cold, fatigue, weight gain or dry skin. For more information on diagnosing and treating thyroid disease, see chapter 5.

Prostatitis Prostatitis is a condition in which the prostate gland is either infected or inflamed, giving rise to chronic pain in the groin and/or a painful, burning sensation on urination. It is not clear what really causes prostatitis; however, in a significant proportion of sufferers it seems that an initial infection can set off an inflammatory reaction that can persist for several months.

The prostate contains a high concentration of substances called prostaglandins which have an inflammatory or anti-inflammatory effect depending on their precise nature. Sufferers of prostatitis may do well to increase their consumption of essential fats, as these tend to encourage the production of anti-inflammatory prostaglandins in the body. At the same time, it is wise to avoid all foods and drinks that encourage inflammation such as red meat, sugar, caffeine and alcohol. Rye pollen is thought to have anti-inflammatory and anti-hormonal properties and has been found to be effective in relieving the symptoms of prostatitis in a significant proportion of sufferers (*ref* 1). The normal recommended dose is 500 mg, two or three times a day.

Psoriasis Psoriasis is a chronic skin condition which normally gives rise to raised, red, and scaly patches of skin, often on the knees, elbows, scalp and behind the ears. The condition seems to be linked to a rapid growth in the outer layers of the skin. A percentage of psoriasis sufferers develop a form of arthritis known as psoriatic arthritis.

Although the precise cause of psoriasis is unknown, it does seem to be linked to certain factors. Psoriasis can tend to run in families, suggesting that a predisposition to the condition may be inherited. The development of psoriasis may also be linked to our emotional state, with a significant number of sufferers reporting that the condition started after a time of particular stress. Other theories regarding the cause of psoriasis include the consumption of too much animal fat in the diet, a malfunctioning immune system and a build-up of toxins in the colon.

Some foods do seem to aggravate psoriasis including citrus fruits, fried foods, refined foods and sugar. Meat and dairy products should be particularly avoided because they contain the substance arachidonic acid, which can make the psoriatic lesions turn red and swell. Another thing to avoid is alcohol. Alcohol can put stress on the liver, reducing its ability to filter the blood efficiently. There is good evidence that alcohol consumption can considerably worsen psoriasis. Two underlying factors that tend to crop up in some (though not all) cases of psoriasis are food sensitivity and candida overgrowth. More information about how to diagnose and treat these problems can be found in chapter 3.

Two natural agents that often help to relieve psoriasis are essential fatty acids (EFAs) and the herb Oregon grape (*Mahonia aquifolium*). Psoriasis sufferers may do well to take 1 tablespoon each day of flaxseed oil, in addition to 1 teaspoon of Oregon grape tincture, three times a day. Oregon grape is often available as topical preparations (e.g. creams or lotions), and these are certainly worth a try.

Raynaud's Disease In Raynaud's (pronounced ray-nodes) disease circulation is poor in the extremities. Constriction in the vessels which supply blood to the fingers and/or toes leads to problems. Typically, when first exposed to the cold, the affected digits turn white, then blue, and then finally red once they warm up again. As they warm, it is not uncommon for the digits to become painful for some minutes. Although there really is no conventional medical treatment for Raynaud's disease, certain natural approaches may help.

Magnesium may reduce spasm in the vessels of the fingers and toes and can often reduce the frequency and severity of attacks. A dose of 300 to 500 mg should be taken every day. Another useful agent in the treatment of Raynaud's disease and general circulatory problems is the herb ginkgo biloba. There is a wealth of anecdotal evidence supporting the use of ginkgo in cases of Raynaud's disease. Sufferers often find tremendous relief from this herb during the winter when symptoms are usually at their worst.

Ginger has a warming effect on the body, and can help to keep circulatory symptoms at bay. Ginger tea, made by simmering about one inch cubed of grated or finely chopped root ginger in two pints of water for about ten minutes, can often help to stimulate the circulation if taken regularly as a drink.

Vitamin B3 is well known to enhance circulation. This nutrient comes in more than one form, one of which (niacin) induces flushing in the skin in doses as low as 50–100 mg per day. However, some people find this flushing effect quite unpleasant, and high doses of niacin can be associated with other symptoms including headache and nausea. An alternative to niacin is inositol hexaniacinate. Actually a molecule of inositol (loosely classified as a B vitamin) complexed with six molecules of niacin, this compound appears to help enhance the circulation without the side-effects common with niacin. Taking 500 mg of inositol hexaniacinate two to four times a day may help control the symptoms of poor circulation although it can take two months before improvement is seen.

Restless Legs Restless legs is a syndrome characterized by uncomfortable tickling, burning, prickling or aching sensations in the muscles of the legs. Sufferers usually find that symptoms develop at night while they are in bed. The condition is quite common, and is thought to affect as many as 15 per cent of the population. While conventional treatment options for restless legs are limited, natural approaches usually work very well to control or eliminate symptoms.

Caffeine seems to worsen or trigger the symptoms of restless legs (*ref* 1), so coffee, tea, caffeinated soft drinks and chocolate should be avoided. Restless legs is also associated with blood sugar fluctuation (*ref* 2), and taking steps to improve blood sugar control may be effective in controlling symptoms.

In practice, certain nutrients can be very effective in controlling restless legs. Magnesium can often be useful, and this may be related to the fact that it has a relaxant effect on muscle tissues. I generally advise 350 to 500 mg of magnesium each day in the first instance, though this dose can usually be reduced as symptoms improve. Taking a magnesium supplement seems to work particularly well in combination with vitamin E, which itself has been shown to improve the symptoms of restless legs (*ref* 3). A dose of 400 to 800 IU of vitamin E should be taken each day.

In some individuals, there seems to be a relationship between restless legs and iron deficiency (*refs* 4, 5), and iron supplementation often helps (*ref* 4). However, iron supplements should only really be used in people with proven iron deficiency. See pages 201–2 for more details about this.

Rheumatoid Arthritis Rheumatoid arthritis (RA) is an inflammatory condition characterized by inflammation in the joints of the fingers, toes, wrists or other joints of the
body. The affected joints are swollen and stiff and may become deformed in the
long term. The disease usually comes in waves, with painful periods being interspersed with times that are relatively symptom-free. The disease usually starts in
early adulthood or middle age but can sometimes start in childhood. RA affects 2
to 3 per cent of the population and about 75 per cent of sufferers are women.

RA is what is known as an 'auto-immune' disease – the immune system
mounts an immune response against the body's own tissues causing inflammation. In the case of rheumatoid arthritis, the part of the body that is affected
is the tissue that lines the joint known as the 'synovium'. While the cause of
rheumatoid arthritis is not known for sure, there is some evidence that it can be
triggered by food. In one study of twenty-two RA sufferers, twenty improved on
elimination of foods from the diet (*ref* 1). The worst offending foods in this study
were grains, milk, nuts, beef and egg. More information about the identification
of individual food sensitivities can be found on pages 34–43.

Those with RA may benefit from eating plenty of foods rich in healthy essential
fatty acids (EFAs). These are contained in oily fish such as mackerel, salmon
and trout, extra virgin olive oil and pumpkin, sunflower and sesame seeds. There
is some evidence that both omega-6 fatty acids in the form of borage oil (*refs*
2, 3), blackcurrant seed oil (*ref* 4) and evening primrose oil (*refs* 5, 6) and
omega-3 fatty acids in the form of fish oil (*refs* 7, 8, 9, 10, 11, 12) can be
effective in controlling the symptoms of RA. About 1.5 g of gamma-linolenic acid
and 10 g of fish oil supplements per day appear to be the effective doses.

Copper has an anti-inflammatory effect in the body and can often help
individuals with RA. In a double-blind study, wearing a copper bracelet helped to
relieve the symptoms of RA (*ref* 13). Copper can also be taken as a supplement,
at a dose of 2–4 mg per day.

Green-lipped mussel extract has developed a reputation as a useful agent
in the treatment of arthritis. Research has identified a compound known as
eicosatetaenoic acid (ETA) which was found to have anti-inflammatory actions
more potent than that of commonly prescribed painkillers. One study found that
treatment with green-lipped mussel extract (1,050 mg per day of dried powder
or 210 mg per day of a special extract) brought significant improvements in 68
per cent of RA sufferers (*ref* 14).

Rosacea Rosacea is a chronic skin disorder often with a red rash around the nose
and cheeks. Initially, the condition can start with flushing of the face, often after
drinking a hot beverage or alcohol, or eating spicy food. In time, rosacea may
develop into a chronic reddening of the face with acne-like lesions in the affected
area. The conventional medical treatment for this condition is usually long-term

antibiotics. While these may help suppress the condition to start with, they rarely provide a lasting solution to the problem, and may lead to problems with yeast overgrowth (see pages 53–62).

There is some evidence that sufferers of rosacea tend to suffer from low stomach acid secretion (hypochlorhydria) (*refs* 1, 2). More details about how to diagnose and treat this condition can be found on pages 44–8. Rosacea is also associated with certain nutrient deficiencies, particularly the B vitamins (*ref* 3). For this reason, it is wise for sufferers to take a B-complex supplement that contains about 25 mg of the vitamins B1, B2, B3, B5 and B6 each day.

S

Sarcoidosis Sarcoidosis is a chronic (long-term) progressive disease in which solid nodules form in various tissues and organs of the body. The areas that are commonly affected include the lungs, lymph nodes (glands), liver and skin. It is not known what causes the condition. Fortunately, most cases of sarcoidosis do not require treatment, and the condition often disappears of its own accord within a couple of years. However, about 10 per cent of people with sarcoidosis have persistent problems, and go on to develop severe lung disease. Steroid drugs may be used to treat this form of sarcoidosis, but they are often ineffective.

There is no widely recognized natural treatment for sarcoidosis. However, a few years ago there was a report in medical literature describing the treatment of sarcoidosis with melatonin (*ref* 1). Melatonin is a hormone that is produced by the pea-sized pineal gland in the brain. Although melatonin is best known as a sleep-inducing hormone, it can also regulate the immune system and appears to have the ability to slow down the accumulation of abnormal cells in the body. For these reasons, melatonin was tried in two patients with long-standing sarcoidosis who had failed to respond to steroids.

Each patient was treated with 20 mg of melatonin a day, and both experienced a gradual disappearance of the sarcoid nodules in their lungs. One patient also had skin lesions, and these resolved too, but came back when the melatonin was stopped. Once the melatonin was resumed, the skin cleared again. These reports suggest that melatonin might be an effective natural treatment for sarcoidosis. Despite being a natural substance, melatonin is only available by prescription in the UK.

Scalp – itchy Itching in the scalp is almost always related to yeast infection there. Underlying this is usually an overgrowth of candida in the gut, and correcting this problem usually leads to lasting relief from the scalp symptoms. See pages 53–62 for details on the diagnosis and treatment of candida in the body. Shampoos and scalp treatments based on tea tree oil (a natural anti-fungal) may help provide relief when used topically.

Scalp – painful Some children will experience quite severe pain when their hair is combed, brushed or pulled. Occasionally, the scalp may be tender to the touch too. This problem is usually related to a deficiency in vitamin D. In its severe form, vitamin D deficiency can give rise to a condition called rickets, which is characterized by bone abnormalities such as bow legs and curvature of the spine. It is possible that even mild vitamin D deficiency may interfere with normal growth and development.

Foods rich in vitamin D such as salmon, herring and mackerel should be emphasized in the diet. In addition, exposure to sunlight is important, as vitamin D is formed in the skin in response to sunlight. Vitamin D may be added in supplement form, but the dose should not exceed 200 IU per day.

Scarring Scarring in the skin, either from injury, surgery or a skin condition such as acne, can be unsightly and is notoriously difficult to treat. However, a natural remedy for scarring does exist in the form of Rosa Mosqueta oil. Rosa Mosqueta is oil extracted from rose hips, and contains beneficial fats which are essential for the development of new cells in the body, including the skin. Applied regularly for some months, Rosa Mosqueta can often be quite effective in reducing all forms of scarring. Rosa Mosqueta oil is available from Rio Trading (see Useful Information at the back of the book).

Schizophrenia Schizophrenia is a form of mental illness. There may be severe symptoms such as hallucinations (for example, the hearing of voices), delusions (abnormal, irrational beliefs), and abnormal speech and behaviour. The condition affects about 1 per cent of the population and usually leads to long-term mental and behavioural problems. The conventional medical approach to schizophrenia is based around the use of medications designed to correct chemical imbalance in the brain. However, there is growing evidence that schizophrenia can be helped through natural, nutritional approaches.

About half of schizophrenics have low levels of the chemical histamine in their blood. Such people are often helped by nutrients which can help increase histamine levels such as vitamin B3, folic acid, vitamin B12, zinc and manganese. Paradoxically, about 20 per cent of schizophrenics seem to have high, rather than low, levels of histamine in their bodies. Nutrients which may help these people include vitamin C, calcium and the amino acid methionine. Another group of schizophrenics has high levels of substances called 'kryptopyroles' in their bodies and may respond to supplementation with vitamin B6, zinc and manganese. Schizophrenia can also be associated with sensitivities to certain foods and chemicals, especially wheat, milk and tobacco.

Schizophrenia generally needs careful management, and I suggest this is done in conjunction with a practitioner experienced in the sorts of imbalances that appear to be common in the condition.

Scleroderma Scleroderma is most commonly characterized by thickening and tightening of the skin affecting the face and hands. Internal tissues can also be affected, including the lungs, kidneys, heart and digestive tract. The condition is what is known as an 'auto-immune disorder' – one in which the body's immune system attacks its own tissues – and is most common in middle-aged women. There really is no conventional treatment for scleroderma; steroids are sometimes used, but these are generally ineffective.

There are two nutrients which seem to be quite effective in controlling and relieving scleroderma. PABA (paraaminobenzoic acid) is a nutrient often considered to be a member of the B vitamin family. Large doses of PABA appear to reverse the accumulation of fibrous tissue (*refs* 1, 2, 3). The recommended dose of PABA is 3 g, four times a day. At this level, PABA may cause liver problems along with rash and fever. For this reason, PABA should really only be used under the supervision of a doctor experienced in its use.

Vitamin E may also help. Again, the doses needed are large – between 800 to 1,200 IU per day – though even at these levels vitamin E is considered to be safe.

Seasonal Affective Disorder (SAD) Seasonal affective disorder (SAD) is depression probably caused by reduced exposure to sunlight. Generally, the depression will start in the autumn or winter, and disappear in the spring. It is a common phenomenon, with estimates of 5 per cent of people being affected to some degree. In countries where daylight is very much reduced during the winter, such as the Scandinavian countries, SAD seems to be a particular problem, and rates of depression and suicide tend to rise significantly in the winter months.

The conventional treatment for SAD is anti-depressant drugs. However, natural approaches are often an effective alternative, and are less likely to give rise to unwanted side-effects. Because SAD is essentially caused by lack of sunlight, it makes sense to get as much natural daylight as possible. Even on a dull day, the amount of natural light available outside is far higher than levels found in most indoor settings. Brisk walking, jogging and cycling are ideal pastimes, because exercise is well known to help lift mood. It is also worthwhile considering purchasing a 'light box' for use at home or work. These devices, which give off light with the specific characteristics of the sun's rays, can often help to combat the symptoms of SAD.

Depression may be affected by certain dietary factors. For instance, caffeine, alcohol and sugar are commonly associated with depression, and eliminating them from the diet can help improve mood. It can be useful to eat plenty of oily fish such as salmon, trout, tuna, herring and mackerel, as the consumption of the healthy fats present in these fish seems to help ward off depression.

Many SAD sufferers find that taking a preparation based on the herb hypericum (St John's Wort) helps relieve their symptoms. This finding has also been supported scientifically (*refs* 1, 2). The usual dose of hypericum is 300 mg of standardized extract, three times a day.

Seborrhoeic Dermatitis Seborrhoeic dermatitis is characterized by a red, greasy, scaly rash that is usually found on the face, especially around the nose, forehead, chin and in the eyebrows. Other common sites include the armpit, groin and the skin over the breast bone (sternum) in the middle of the chest.

While the precise cause of seborrhoeic dermatitis is not known for sure, it often seems to be related to overgrowth of the yeast organism Candida albicans in the system. If the rash is itchy, then this is a bit of a clue that candida may be an underlying factor. More information about the diagnosis and treatment of candida can be found on pages 53–62.

Taking a daily B-complex supplement can sometimes benefit seborrhoeic dermatitis. Another useful natural approach is vitamin B6 cream (10 mg of B6 per gram of cream). One study showed that B6 cream could be quite effective in controlling seborrhoeic dermatitis (*ref* 1).

Shingles Shingles is caused by a reactivation of the chicken pox (herpes zoster) virus in the body, and usually gives rise to a red, painful, belt-like rash around one side of the torso. The pain that comes with the rash can last for many years after the attack and is often referred to by doctors as 'post-herpetic neuralgia'. High doses of vitamin E can often relieve long-term pain associated with shingles (*refs* 1, 2). However, it can take six months or more before real benefit is seen. The recommended dose is 1,200 to 1,600 IU of vitamin E each day.

Another natural approach is to apply capsaicin cream to the affected area(s). Capsaicin is the substance that gives cayenne pepper its 'heat'. Capsaicin creams of 0.025 and 0.075 per cent have been found to significantly reduce the pain of post-herpetic neuralgia when applied three or four times a day (*refs* 3, 4).

Sickle Cell Disease Oxygen is transported around the body in haemoglobin, a substance found in the red blood cells. In individuals with sickle cell disease, the haemoglobin is abnormal, causing the red blood cells to become distorted into a sickle-like shape. Cells affected in this way can become stuck in the body's smallest vessels, which in turn may lead to painful 'crises' requiring hospitalization and treatment with painkillers and intravenous fluids.

Certain nutrients seem to be able to help control the symptoms of sickle cell disease. Vitamin B6 appears to inhibit sickling of red blood cells and has been shown to improve well-being and significantly reduce the number of painful crises in sickle cell disease (*ref* 1). A dose of 50 mg of B6 should be taken twice a day. Vitamin E (450 IU per day) has been shown to reduce the number of diseased cells (*ref* 2).

Sinusitis Inflammation of the sinuses – sinusitis – can have many underlying causes. One factor that seems to come up a lot in practice is food sensitivity. Some foods seem to induce mucus formation in the sinuses, causing congestion there. Congested sinuses are also more likely to become infected. Mucus-forming foods include dairy products (especially milk and cheese), and foods based on white flour. However, because food sensitivities are an individual issue, it is often worthwhile assessing this problem on an individual basis. More details about how to go about doing this can be found on pages 34–43.

A natural remedy that is often helpful in clearing an attack of sinusitis is bromelain (*ref* 1). This extract of pineapple has the ability to break down protein in the body, and may therefore help to loosen up and help clear the congestion characteristic of the condition. A dose of 500 mg of bromelain should be taken three or four times a day between meals.

Smell – Loss of Sense of Loss of smell (also referred to as anosmia) can sometimes be related to smoking, or conditions such as nasal inflammation (rhinitis), or head injury. Usually, though, there is no discernible underlying cause, and treatment options tend to be limited as a result. In practice, natural agents may sometimes help improve the sense of smell. Zinc is often used for this purpose; 30–45 mg should be taken each day. As zinc supplements may cause copper deficiency in time, it is good practice to take 2–3 mg of copper at the same time. Magnesium may also help to improve the sense of smell. In one study, the majority of people who had failed to respond to other treatments found their sense of smell improved with taking magnesium (*ref* 1). A dose of 250 mg of magnesium should be taken each day.

Strep Throat Streptococcal bacteria can give rise to a number of different infections including tonsillitis, sore throat (sometimes referred to as 'strep throat'), and ear infections. Streptococcal infections are also responsible for scarlet fever, and may give rise to rheumatic fever, which can have potentially serious consequences. Conventionally, streptococcal infections are treated with antibiotics (usually penicillin), although there is evidence that strains of this type of bacteria are becoming resistant to treatment.

In practice, recurrent streptococcal infections appear to be related to the ingestion of dairy products. It has been noticed that if children exclude cow products from their diets, then the streptococcal infection is very unlikely to return. The reason is not known for sure, but it is possible that an immune sensitivity to dairy products (this is quite common in children) diverts the immune system, making it more likely for infections to take hold in the body. Another theory is that the mucus dairy products tend to induce in the throat and ears makes an ideal medium for the growth of organisms like streptococcus.

In the light of this observation, it makes sense for sufferers of recurrent strep throat to eliminate cow's milk, cheese, ice cream and yoghurt from the diet. Soya milk and cheese, as well as almond, oat and rice milk make good alternatives. If antibiotics have been taken, it is also wise for a supplement of healthy gut bacteria (also known as a 'probiotic') to be taken for two or three months. This helps to restore beneficial bacteria to the gut that may be depleted after several courses of antibiotics, and may help to prevent gut-related problems in future.

Stretch Marks Stretch marks, often referred to as 'striae' by the medical profession, are caused by thinning and a loss of elasticity in the deeper layers of the skin. They often start as raised red lines, flattening out and becoming shiny, purplish streaks in time. Stretch marks commonly develop on the hips and thighs of adolescent girls during their growth spurt. They are also a feature in about three-quarters of pregnant women, often developing on the breasts, lower abdomen and thighs. Occasionally, stretch marks are the result of an excess of steroid hormones in the body. This can happen as a result of long-term steroid use (Cushing's disease), or if excessive amounts of steroid hormones are being made by the body (Cushing's syndrome).

One nutrient that appears to help stop the development of stretch marks is zinc. This mineral plays an essential role in the healthy development and repair of skin tissues. Zinc deficiency is common in women, and the risk of this will increase as the body's requirements for nutrients rise during puberty. A dose of 30–45 mg of zinc should be taken each day, and because zinc supplements can cause copper deficiency, this should be balanced with 2–3 mg of copper each day too.

Topically, I have found the application of Rosa Mosqueta oil (see *Scarring*) to be quite effective in reducing the appearance of stretch marks if used consistently for several months. Rosa Mosqueta oil can be obtained from Rio Trading (see Useful Information at the back of the book).

Stroke Prevention (see also *Atherosclerosis*) The brain receives its blood supply via a network of vessels. An interruption in the blood supply to the brain can cause part of the brain to die, and this is what is commonly referred to as a 'stroke'. Common symptoms include weakness or paralysis down one side of the body, speech problems, unconsciousness and even death. The great majority of strokes are caused by the formation of a tiny blood clot in a blood vessel which is usually partially blocked with fatty deposits. A small proportion of strokes are due to the rupture of a blood vessel in or around the brain. Strokes are quite rare before the age of sixty, but become increasingly more common thereafter. The major risk factor for stroke is high blood pressure. See *Hypertension* for details of natural approaches to this problem.

Aspirin is frequently used to help reduce the risk of stroke because it has 'blood-thinning' effects. However, vitamin E may also offer protection for the same reason. Interestingly, there is a study that attempted to determine the stroke-protective qualities of aspirin and vitamin E. One group of people took aspirin (325 mg) each day, while another took aspirin combined with 400 IU of vitamin E (*ref* 1). The results showed that while aspirin was helpful, better protection was achieved when it was combined with vitamin E. As yet, no studies have looked at the effect of vitamin E alone on risk of stroke, but from what we know about its effects in the body, there is a good chance that it offers significant benefit in this area. A dose of 400 to 800 IU should be taken each day.

Surgery – Recovery From For speedy healing, it is always a good idea to give the body an adequate supply of the most important nutrients. Generally, supplementation should be started about a month before surgery, finishing about six weeks later.

One of the most important healing nutrients is vitamin C. This promotes the healing of the supporting tissues. A dose of 1 g of vitamin C should be taken, twice a day. Other important nutrients for healing include zinc, vitamin B12 and folic acid. The main function of these is to stimulate new cell formation. Doses of 30 mg of zinc and 500 to 1,000 mcg of vitamins B12 and folic acid should be taken each day. To this regime it often helps to add a supplement of the herb gotu kola (*Centella asiatica*). This natural agent has been found to reduce healing time and improve the strength of healing tissue (*refs* 1, 2); 500 mg should be taken, twice a day.

For two days before and ten days after surgery, it seems to help to take a supplement of the pineapple extract bromelain. Bromelain lessens swelling and inflammation and reduces healing time by helping in the clearing of tissue debris. Three capsules should be taken, three times a day on an empty stomach.

Sweating – Excessive The herb sage has a long history of use in herbal medicine in the treatment of excessive sweating and hot flushes. Sage tea can be made by steeping sage leaves in hot water for five or ten minutes. Drink several cups a day. Alternatively, sage can be taken in tincture (alcoholic extract) form. The normal dose is fifteen to twenty drops of tincture in water, three times a day.

Systemic Lupus Erythematosis (SLE) Systemic lupus erythematosis (SLE) is what is known as an 'auto-immune' disease – one in which the immune system attacks the body's own tissues. In SLE any tissue may be affected, and this can give rise to a wide variety of symptoms including arthritis, kidney disease, heart damage, skin sensitivity to light, fever, weight loss, neurological problems and a rash around the nose and cheeks. Potentially the condition can be very serious, and may actually prove fatal. Conventionally, the mainstay of treatment for SLE is steroids. These have a range of possible side-effects, and may not adequately contain the illness anyway.

There is some thought that, like other auto-immune disorders, SLE may be related to food sensitivity. Not a lot of research has been done into this, but I have to say, in my experience, food sensitivity is indeed an important provocative factor in many cases of SLE. Identification and elimination of individual food sensitivities is often very effective in controlling the symptoms. I have even seen patients revert from positive blood tests for SLE to negative using this approach. More information about food sensitivity can be found on pages 34–43.

In some patients I have seen, the yeast organism Candida albicans seems to be an important underlying factor, and successful treatment of this problem is often effective in controlling symptoms. More information about this can be found in pages 53–62.

Taste – Loss of Sense of Loss of the sense of taste quite often responds to an increase in zinc consumption. The diet should include plenty of foods rich in zinc such as sunflower and pumpkin seeds, seafood and fish. In addition, it usually helps to take a zinc supplement. Enough zinc ascorbate or zinc citrate should be taken to provide 30 mg of zinc each day for three or four months. Because zinc supplementation can induce copper deficiency, 1 mg of copper should be taken for each 15 mg of zinc taken. After this, the risk of zinc and other nutrient deficiencies may be reduced by taking a good quality combined multivitamin and mineral supplement containing zinc each day.

Tinnitus Tinnitus is a condition characterized by ringing or humming in the ears. It affects about one in ten adults in the UK, and can vary in severity. While some individuals suffer occasional, mild attacks of tinnitus which do not cause much distress, others may experience constant symptoms which can impact signifi-cantly on the quality of their life. Tinnitus is the result of malfunction in the inner ear – the part of the body responsible for both hearing and balance. While the precise cause of tinnitus is not known, it is thought that it can be related to a reduced blood supply to the inner ear. The natural approach to tinnitus is the same for that of a related condition – Ménière's disease (see *Ménière's disease*).

Thrombophlebitis Thrombophlebitis is characterized by inflammation in a vein near the surface of the skin, usually in the leg. Another feature of this condition is the formation of small blood clots (thrombi) around the site of inflammation. Typical symptoms of thrombophlebitis include swelling, redness and tenderness in and around the affected area. Conventional treatment is normally centred around the use of support stockings, bandaging and the administration of non-steroidal anti-inflammatory drugs (painkillers).

A major component of the tiny blood clots that occur in thrombophlebitis is a blood protein called fibrin. The body breaks down fibrin naturally in time, but certain foods such as garlic, onions, cayenne pepper and ginger accelerate this process. These foods can therefore help to relieve the symptoms of thrombophlebitis and plenty of them should be included in the diets of those prone to this condition.

There are two natural agents which may be of real benefit in thrombophlebitis. One of these, bromelain, is an extract of pineapple that has been shown to break down fibrin and therefore acts as a natural clot dissolver and blood thinner. Bromelain also has a strong anti-inflammatory effect and can help to reduce pain and swelling in and around the vein. A dose of 500 mg should be taken, three times a day. In this instance, bromelain should be taken on an empty stomach to ensure maximum effect. The other natural substance which can be very useful in combating thrombophlebitis is vitamin E. This nutrient also has blood-thinning properties and may therefore help to prevent the development of thrombi. About 800 IU of vitamin E should be taken each day.

Thrush (vaginal yeast infection) Thrush is caused by a yeast organism known as Candida albicans. Although it is normal to have some yeast in the body, too much can create problems. Thrush is characterized by vaginal itching with or without a white discharge and is a sign of candida overgrowth in this part of the body. The reservoir of candida in the body is actually the digestive tract, which is why treating only the vaginal source of the infection with pessaries and creams often fails to bring lasting relief. To really get to the bottom of this problem it is usually necessary to combat the overgrowth of candida in the intestinal tract. More information about this can be found in pages 53–62.

For topical relief I generally recommend the use of probiotic (healthy bacteria) supplements inserted vaginally (as a pessary). Increasing the number of healthy bacteria in and around the vagina does seem to help keep candida at bay. Acidophilus pessaries are available under the name YeastGuard from VitaTech (see Useful Information at the back of the book). One pessary should be inserted each week.

Tongue – Fissured Fissuring (cracking) of the tongue is very often related to a deficiency in B vitamins such as B2, B6, B12 and folic acid. Sometimes, iron is deficient too, though this should not be taken as a supplement unless there is a proven deficiency. The best test for this is the 'ferritin' blood test. The other nutrients are very safe to take in reasonable doses. I generally recommend that a good quality B-complex supplement that supplies 25–50 mg of the B vitamins B1, B2, B3, B5 and B6, along with B12 and folic acid be taken every day.

Tongue – Sore Certain vitamin deficiencies can lead to problems with soreness and discomfort on the tongue and inside the mouth. Perhaps the most important nutrients in terms of oral health are the B vitamins. Individuals lacking in folic acid tend to develop sore mouths and throats. Too little vitamin B3 (niacinamide) can cause soreness of the gums, mouth and tongue. If the discomfort in the mouth is like a 'burning' sensation, then B6 deficiency is likely. If cracks at the corners of the mouth are sore, this generally indicates a lack of vitamin B2 (riboflavin). Sore lips have also been noted to be related to deficiencies of folic acid, vitamin B5 (pantothenic acid) and vitamin B6.

As with a fissured tongue, I generally recommend that a good quality B-complex supplement that supplies 25–50 mg of the B vitamins B1, B2, B3, B5 and B6, along with B12 and folic acid be taken every day.

Tongue – Geographical Geographical tongue is characterized by the presence of irregular, discoloured patches on the tongue. These patches give the surface of the tongue an appearance similar to a map of the world, hence the term 'geo-graphical tongue'. The condition is rare, but there is no recognized conventional medical treatment.

In practice, geographical tongue usually responds to supplementation with certain nutrients. Folic acid, essential for the healthy division of cells, can be effective in returning health to the tongue; 1,000 to 2,000 mcg of folic acid should be taken each day until the condition starts to improve, reducing the dose to 400 mcg per day once this happens. Zinc can help in cases of geographical tongue; this also has an important part to play in cell replication. A daily dose of 30–45 mg of zinc should be taken for two to four months. Because taking zinc supplements can induce copper deficiency, 2–3 mg of copper should also be taken each day.

Tonsillitis Infections of the tonsils (tonsillitis) can essentially be caused by two different types of organisms: bacteria and viruses. Viral infections are more common and tend to produce red, inflamed tonsils, but no white spots. Viral tonsillitis will not tend to respond to antibiotics. In bacterial tonsillitis, the tonsils will often develop white spots and tend to respond to antibiotics.

Like streptococcal infections of the throat, tonsillitis does often seem to be related to sensitivity to dairy products, especially milk and cheese. When these are eliminated from the diet, attacks tend to become much less frequent or disappear altogether. More information about food sensitivity can be found on pages 34–43.

A useful nutrient for combating tonsillitis is zinc. Sucking a zinc lozenge every two waking hours does seem to help reduce the symptoms of tonsillitis, which may be related to the nutrient's immune-stimulating and virus-killing activity. The precise form of the zinc in the lozenge is important – it should be zinc *gluconate*. Other forms of zinc may not actually liberate sufficient quantities of zinc to exert a significant effect. The lozenge should not contain citric acid, tartaric acid, mannitol or sorbitol either, as these can inactivate the zinc.

The herb echinacea has gained quite a reputation over the last few years as a potent infection fighter. Echinacea is proven to stimulate the immune system, and may help to clear a tonsil infection. There are two main species of echinacea used therapeutically – purpurea and angustifolia. As each has some distinct properties, I generally recommend that they be taken in combination.

Travel Sickness Balance in the body is governed by delicate organs in the inner ear. Travel sickness is thought to be related to the effect of movement and vibration here, but it is not known why some individuals seem to be more sensitive to this than others.

Certain natural remedies may help reduce or even prevent the nausea and sickness that is characteristic of travel sickness. One substance often very effective in this respect is ginger. The ancient Chinese mariners would ward off sea sickness by keeping a slice of fresh root ginger between their cheek and gum. These days, ginger is available in capsule and tablet form. A dose of 500 mg should be taken, three times a day. Ginger at this dose is perfectly safe to be taken regularly for extended periods.

Tremor Tremor or shaking can be related to a number of underlying factors including the use of certain prescription medications (e.g. antidepressants) and some conditions (e.g. Parkinson's disease or an overactive thyroid). When a tremor does not seem to be related to any specific underlying cause it is often referred to as an 'essential tremor'. Essential tremors may run in families, in which case they are sometimes referred to as 'familial tremors'. Essential and familial tremors tend to get worse during movement, and can make even simple everyday tasks such as writing quite difficult.

On a dietary level, it is a good idea to eliminate all forms of caffeine from the diet. Coffee, tea, chocolate and some over-the-counter remedies are the main sources. Caffeine can increase levels of arousal and even anxiety, and this is very likely to worsen any existing tremor. Certain supplements may help to control tremor. I have found magnesium very helpful. Magnesium helps to normalize muscle function, and it is quite possible that it is through this mechanism that it helps to reduce shaking. A dose of 150 to 250 mg of magnesium should be taken, twice a day. Another nutrient that appears to help reduce shaking is vitamin B6. Taking a B-complex supplement which contains at least 25 mg of vitamin B6 each day can often help. Finally, there is some thought that taking healthy fats known as essential fatty acids (EFAs) can help reduce familial tremor (*ref* 1). These fats may possibly work by contributing to the health of the insulating sheaths which surround the nerves. A dose of 2 g of safflower oil should be taken, twice a day.

Trigeminal Neuralgia The trigeminal nerve carries sensation from the face to the brain as well as participating in the processes of taste, chewing, salivation and the production of tears. Sufferers of trigeminal neuralgia experience episodes of intense pain in one side of the face which usually last from a few seconds to a few minutes. Attacks tend to come in batches which last several weeks at a time. The condition is uncommon before the age of fifty. Sometimes, anti-epileptic drugs can help relieve the condition, though these are often ineffective or may be associated with significant side-effects.

Trigeminal neuralgia is not an easy condition to treat, either with conventional or complementary medicine. However, there is a case study in the scientific literature of a woman who had complete relief from her symptoms by adopting a caffeine-free diet (*ref* 1). It is not known how caffeine may trigger trigeminal neuralgia, though it is likely to be connected with its nerve-stimulating action. However, it is certainly worthwhile trying the elimination of caffeine from the diet.

Trigger Finger Trigger finger is when one or more fingers are stuck in a bent position, often requiring extra force than normal to straighten. In practice, this problem seems to respond to vitamin B6 – 100 mg should be taken three times a day. This approach is often successful, sparing the sufferer the need for surgery, but it can take several months before the condition resolves.

Ulcer – Mouth (see *Mouth Ulcers*)

Ulcer – Peptic (see *Peptic Ulcer*)

Ulcer – Skin Skin ulcers are more common in individuals with reduced blood supply to the leg (peripheral vascular disease), varicose veins and diabetes. Whatever the underlying cause of an ulcer, its healing can often be helped by supplementing with certain nutrients. In particular, vitamin C (*ref* 1) and zinc (*refs* 2, 3) have both been shown to speed up the healing of ulcers, sometimes cutting down the healing time by half. In addition to their effect on tissue healing, these nutrients also stimulate the immune system. This is important because this can reduce the risk of infection – a common complication of leg ulcers. A reasonable dose is 1 g of vitamin C taken two or three times a day along with 90 to 150 mg of zinc each day. Zinc can induce copper deficiency so this should be balanced with 6–10 mg of copper. As the ulcer heals, it is usually possible to reduce the zinc dose. A maintenance dose of 15–30 mg per day may help to prevent ulcers from recurring.

Certain herbs may also help ulcers to heal. Ginkgo biloba can be useful because it helps stimulate the circulation, improving the transport of healing elements to the ulcer. Another useful herb is horse chestnut (*aesculus*). This strengthens blood vessels (including veins), and also helps prevent tissues becoming waterlogged and prone to breakdown and infection. Gotu kola (*Centella asiatica*) contains substances called saponins which seem to have a beneficial effect on collagen, a protein-based material essential for skin health and healing. One review found that gotu kola can help heal wounds (*ref* 4). A dose of 10–20 mls of tincture should be taken each day; alternatively, 60 mg of standardized extract should be taken, once or twice a day.

Ulcerative Colitis Ulcerative colitis is characterized by inflammation in the lining of the large bowel. Typical symptoms include pain, bloating, and diarrhoea that can be bloody. The symptoms tend to come and go, with attacks being interspersed with relatively symptom-free periods. The condition is most common in young and middle-aged adults.

Although the cause of ulcerative colitis is not known for sure, there is some evidence that it may be triggered by food in some cases (*refs* 1, 2). More information about the identification of potential trigger foods can be found on pages 34–43.

Some people with ulcerative colitis have difficulty digesting starches and sugars, which can lead to the fermentation of carbohydrate in the gut by bacteria and/or yeast. This in turn leads to irritation and ulceration of the bowel wall. Reducing or excluding fermentable carbohydrates such as grains, potatoes and sugar has helped a significant proportion of people with the condition. For more details about this specific approach, read *Breaking the Vicious Cycle* by Elaine Gottschall.

Urinary Frequency Frequent urination, particularly when only small volumes are passed, may be related to a condition known as 'detrusor instability'. The detrusor is a muscle in the pelvis, a proportion of which makes up the outer muscular coat of the bladder. In detrusor instability, it is thought that this muscle does not function normally, giving rise to certain symptoms which may include frequent urination, the need to pass water at night and incontinence.

Caffeine has been shown to worsen the symptoms of detrusor instability and should be avoided (*ref* 1). In any condition in which muscle seems to contract abnormally such as cramping or twitching, magnesium is always worth a try because it helps relax muscle tissue naturally. In one study, magnesium was found to help symptoms of detrusor instability in a good proportion of women (*ref* 2). A dose of 250 mg of magnesium should be taken, one to three times a day.

Urinary Tract Infection Urinary tract infection is the medical term for what is commonly referred to as 'cystitis' or 'urine infection'. Cystitis is the most common bacterial infection in women. Women tend to become more prone to cystitis as they age: while the condition affects about 10 per cent of younger women, the incidence after menopause is roughly double this. Overall, one in four women will suffer from cystitis at some point in their lives. For some women, cystitis tends to recur, and gives rise to troublesome and persistent symptoms such as pain on urination, frequent urination, and even incontinence. Conventional treatment for cystitis is based on antibiotics.

The most common cause of UTI is a bacterium known as E. coli. This organism is often to be found on the skin in the genital area. From here, E. coli organisms can make their way up the pipe that takes urine from the bladder to the outside (the urethra). Here, they may set up camp by attaching to the inner surface of the bladder. E. coli germs generally originate in the bowel, and a few basic approaches can often be effective in reducing the risk of this organism getting the opportunity to become established in the bladder.

Drinking plenty of water throughout the day helps to flush out organisms in and around the urethra and bladder before they get a foothold. For most women 1.5 to 2 litres of water is about right. Urinating as soon as possible after sexual intercourse is of particular importance, because sex increases the risk of E. coli being introduced into the urethra and bladder. Personal hygiene is obviously important, and washing should be done on at least a daily basis using a mild, unscented soap. Again, this is especially important around the time of sex. When using the lavatory, wiping from the front to the back reduces the risk of organisms being brought into the vicinity of the urethra.

In addition to these basic measures, natural substances may prove effective in controlling UTIs. Over the last decade there has been a lot of interest in the role of cranberry in this respect. Cranberry contains substances called 'proanthocyanidins', which help to prevent E. coli sticking to the bladder wall. In one study, women taking 400 mg per day of cranberry solids had a reduced risk of UTI compared to women taking inactive medication (placebo) over a three-month period (*ref* 1). Cranberry supplements are available from health food stores.

While cranberry reduces the risk of E. coli sticking to the bladder wall, taking calcium supplements actually increases the risk of this happening. This is relevant because women are most likely to take calcium supplements after the time of menopause to protect against osteoporosis (thinning bones), and these women are also those that tend to be at the highest risk of UTI. For most women, this factor is unlikely to be of any relevance. However, women experiencing recurrent UTIs who are also taking calcium in supplement form might benefit from either reducing their dose of calcium or possibly taking a cranberry supplement to counterbalance the effects of the calcium.

A common folk remedy for the prevention of UTIs is 'live' yoghurt. Yoghurt contains organisms known as lactobacilli which may help to 'crowd out' unhealthy organisms such as E. coli in and around the vagina, thereby helping to prevent infections. Lactobacilli also make the vagina more acidic, which helps to inhibit E. coli. Acidophilus pessaries are available under the name YeastGuard from VitaTech (see Useful Information at the back of the book). One pessary should be inserted each week.

The reason why post-menopausal women could be at increased risk of UTIs may be related to low levels of the hormone oestrogen. Oestrogen helps to maintain the vaginal tissue, and increase its content of glycogen – a carbohydrate that lactobacilli use as fuel. One study compared a twice weekly oestrogen cream application with an inactive cream. Over the eight months that the study ran for, the women using the oestrogen cream had significantly fewer infections than the women taking a placebo (*ref* 2).

There is some evidence that oestrogen therapy can increase the risk of certain conditions including cancers of the womb and breast. There are three principal types of oestrogen which occur naturally in the body. The one used in this study quoted above – oestriol – is believed to be safe for use by women who still have a womb. However, to be on the safe side, oestriol cream should be avoided by women who have a history of breast cancer, liver disease or the formation of blood clots (e.g. deep vein thrombosis). In the UK, oestriol cream is available by prescription under the name 'Ovestin'.

Urticaria – see *Hives*

V

Varicose Veins Blood is pumped by the heart around the body along the arteries, and returns to the heart along the veins. The veins contain valves that ensure the blood flows towards the heart, but not in the opposite direction. However, sometimes the valves in the veins in the legs can fail, causing blood to collect there. When this happens, the vein may enlarge and distort, giving rise to what are commonly referred to as varicose veins. Varicose veins can be uncomfortable, and can bleed if injured. In addition, they can be associated with other conditions including discoloration of the skin, eczema and ulcers in the lower leg.

Activity stimulates the circulation, which can help reduce the risk of varicose veins getting any worse. It is advisable for varicose vein sufferers to walk briskly, jog or cycle for about half an hour a day. When sitting for long periods, the feet should be put up on a chair or stool as this will help blood-flow in the veins. Crossing of the legs should be avoided as this tends to hinder circulation, increasing the risk of further varicose vein development.

A commonly used and often effective natural treatment is the herb horse chestnut (*Aesculus hippocastanum*). Horse chestnut contains a substance called 'aescin' which is believed to strengthen the vein walls, reducing the risk of further damage. Horse chestnut can be applied directly to the veins (via a gel or cream) or taken internally. The normal recommended dose is 300 mg of standardized extract, three times a day.

Warts Warts are a common, contagious skin condition that may affect many different parts of the body including the hands, feet and genital region. Warts are caused by a virus known as the human papillomavirus (HPV) of which there are several different types. Many warts disappear of their own accord within a few months, but treatment is often necessary in more persistent cases. Conventional treatments include cryosurgery (burning with liquid nitrogen), and the topical application of agents such as podophyllin and salicylic acid.

In natural medicine, extracts of the plant greater celandine (*Chelidonium majus*) are often used to treat warts topically. Greater celandine contains substances which appear to inhibit the wart virus. This treatment seems to work best if the top of the wart (or verruca) is abraded with a pumice stone or emery board before application.

Wound Healing – see *Surgery – Recovery From*

References

2. Give Your Body Water

1. Borghi L., et al., 'Urinary Volume, Water and Recurrences of Idiopathic Calcium Nephrolithiasis: a 5-year Randomised Prospective Study', *Urology* 1996; 155: 839–43
2. Curhan G. C., et al., 'Dietary Factors and Kidney Stone Formation', *Comprehensive Therapy* 1994; 20: 485–9
3. Goldfarb S. 'The Role of Diet in the Pathogenesis and Therapy of Nephrolithiasis', *Endocrinology and Metabolism Clinics of North America* 1990; 19: 805–20
4. Hughes J., et al., 'Diet and Calcium Stones', *Canadian Medical Association Journal* 1992; 146: 137–43
5. Iguchi M., et al., 'Clinical Effects of Prophylactic Dietary Treatment on Renal Stones', *Urology* 1990; 144: 229–32
6. Pin N. T., et al., 'Dehydration from Outdoor Work and Urinary Stones in a Tropical Environment', *Occupational Medicine* 1992; 42: 30–2
7. Embon O. M., et al., 'Chronic Dehydration Stone Disease', *British Journal of Urology* 1990; 66: 357–62
8. Hiatt R. A., et al., 'Randomized Controlled Trial of a Low Animal Protein, High Fiber Diet in the Prevention of Recurrent Calcium Oxalate Kidney Stones', *American Journal of Epidemiology* 1996; 144: 25–33
9. Ackermann D., 'Prophylaxis in Idiopathic Calcium Urolithiasis', *Urological Research* 1990; 18 (suppl 1): S37–S40
10. Bitterman W. A., et al., 'Environmental and Nutritional Factors Significantly Associated with Cancer of the Urinary Tract Among Different Ethnic Groups', *Urologic Clinics of North America* 1991; 18: 501–8
11. Wilkens, L. R., et al., 'Risk Factors for Lower Urinary Tract Cancer: the Role of Total Fluid Consumption, Nitrites and Nitrosamines, and Selected Foods', *Cancer Epidemiology, Biomarkers and Prevention* 1996; 5: 116–66
12. Shannon J., et al., 'Relationship of Food Groups and Water Intake to Colon Cancer Risk', *Cancer Epidemiology, Biomarkers and Prevention* 1996; 5: 495–502

13. Stookey, J. D., et al., Correspondence re: Shannon J., et al., 'Relationship of Food Groups and Water Intake to Colon Cancer Risk', *Cancer Epidemiology, Biomarkers and Prevention* 1997; 6: 657–8

14. Sansevero A. C., 'Dehydration in the Elderly: Strategies for Prevention and Management', *Nurse Practitioner* 1997; 22: 41–2, 51–7, 63–72

15. Sagawa S., et al., 'Effect of Dehydration on Thirst and Drinking During Immersion in Men', *Journal of Applied Physiology* 1992; 72: 128–34

16. Armstrong L. E., et al., 'Urinary Indices of Hydration Status', *International Journal of Sports Nutrition* 1994; 4: 265–79

17. Ludwig D. S., et al., 'Relation Between Consumption of Sugar-Sweetened Drinks and Childhood Obesity: a Prospective, Observational Analysis', *Lancet* 2001; 357: 505–8

18. Robert D., et al., 'Chlorination, Chlorination By-products, and Cancer: a Meta-analysis', *American Journal of Public Health*, July 1992; 82(7): 955–63

19. Cantor K. P., et al., 'Drinking Water Source and Chlorination By-products in Iowa', III. Risk of Brain Cancer. *American Journal of Epidemiology*, 1999; 150(6): 552–60

20. McDonagh M., et al., 'Systematic Review of Water Fluoridation', *British Medical Journal* 2000; 321: 855–9

21. Rubenowitz E., et al., 'Magnesium and Calcium in Drinking Water and Death from Acute Myocardial Infarction', *Epidemiology* 1999; 10(1): 31–6

22. Gurwitz D., et al., 'Magnesium in Mineral Bottled Waters and Cerebrovascular Stroke', *American Journal of Medicine* 1999; 107: 189–90

23. Yang C-Y., 'Calcium and Magnesium in Drinking Water and Risk of Death from Cerebrovascular Disease', *Stroke* 1998; 29: 411–14

24. Yang C-Y., et al., 'Magnesium in Drinking Water and Risk of Death Due to Diabetes Mellitus', *Magnesium Research* 1999; 12(2): 131–7

25. Yang C-Y., et al., 'Calcium and Magnesium in Drinking Water and Risk of Death Due to Prostate Cancer', *Journal of Toxicology and Environmental Health* 2000; 60 (part A): 17–26

3. Detoxify the System

1. Faulstich J., et al., 'Silibinin Inhibition of Amatoxin Uptake in the Perfused Rat Liver', *Arzneimittel-Forschung Drug Research* 1980; 30: 452–4

2. Tuchweber B., et al., 'Prevention by Silibinin of Phalloidin Induced Toxicity', *Toxicology and Applied Pharmacology* 1979; 51: 265–75

3. Feher J., et al., 'Free Radicals in Tissue Damage in Liver Disease and Therapeutic Approach', *Tokai Journal of Experimental and Clinical Medicine* 1986; 11: 121–34

4. Sonnenbichler J., et al., 'Stimulating Influence of a Flavonolignan Derivative on Proliferation, RNA Synthesis and Protein Synthesis in Liver Cells', Assessment and Management of Hepatobiliary Disease. Berlin: Springer-Verlag 1987

5. Plummer N., 'The Lactic Acid Bacteria – their Role in Human Health', BioMed Publications 1992

4. *Balance Your Blood Sugar*

1. Chalew S. A., et al., 'Diagnosis of Reactive Hypoglycaemia: Pitfalls in the Use of the Oral Glucose Tolerance Test', *Southern Medical Journal* 1986; 79: 285–7

2. Kraft J., 'Detection of Diabetes Mellitus In Situ (occult diabetes)', *Laboratory Medicine* 1975 (Feb): 10

3. Wurtman R. J., 'Neurochemical Changes Following High Dose Aspartame with Dietary Carbohydrates', *New England Journal of Medicine* 1983: 429–30

4. Blundell J. E., et al., 'Paradoxical Effects of an Intense Sweetener (Aspartame) on Appetite', *Lancet* 1986; 1: 1092–3

5. Rogers P. J., et al., 'Separating the Actions of Sweetness and Calories: Effects of Sacharin and Carbohydrates on Hunger and Food Intake in Human Subjects', *Physiology and Behaviour* 1989; 45: 1093–9

6. Jorgensen H., 'The Influence of Saccharin on Blood Sugar', *Acta Physiologica Scandinavica* 1950; 20: 33–7

7. Anderson R. A., et al., 'Effects of Supplemental Chromium on Patients with Symptoms of Reactive Hypoglycaemia', *Metabolism* 1987; 36(4): 351–5

8. Anderson R. A., et al., 'Chromium Supplementation in Humans with Hypoglycaemia', *Federation Proceedings* 1984; 43: 471

9. Wimhurst J. M., et al., 'Comparison of the Ability of Magnesium and Manganese to Activate the Key Enzymes of Glycolysis', *FEBS Letters* 1972; 27: 321–6

10. Paolisso G., et al., 'Daily Magnesium Supplements Improve Glucose Handling in Elderly Subjects', *American Journal of Clinical Nutrition* 1992; 55: 1161–7

11. Bou-Holaigh, I., et al., 'Is Neurally Mediated Hypotension an Unrecognised Cause of Chronic Fatigue?' Rowe, P. C., et al., *Lancet* 1995; 345: 624 'The Relationship Between Neurally Mediated Hypotension and Chronic Fatigue Syndrome', *Journal of the American Medical Association* 1995; 274(12): 961–7

12. Scott, L. V., et al., 'Small Adrenal Glands in Chronic Fatigue Syndrome:

a Preliminary Computer Tomography Study', *Psychoneuroendocrinology* 1999; 24(7): 759–68
13. Cleare A. J., et al., 'Low-Dose Hydrocortisone in Chronic Fatigue Syndrome: a Randomised Crossover Trial', *Lancet* 1999; 353: 455–8

5. *Maintain Thyroid Function*

1. Barnes, B. and Galton, L., *Hypothyroidism: the Unsuspected Illness*, Harper & Row 1976

References for Ultimate Health A–Z

Acne Vulgaris
1. Snider B., et al., 'Pyridoxine Therapy for Premenstrual Acne Flare', *Archives of Dermatology* 1974; 110: 130–1
2. Amann W., 'Improvement of Acne Vulgaris with Agnus Castus (Agnolyt™)', *Ther Gegenw* 1967; 106: 124–6 (in German)
3. Slayden S. M., et al., 'Hyperandrogenemia in Patients Presenting with Acne', *Fertility and Sterility* 75 (2001): 5; 889–92
4. Hillstom L., et al., 'Comparison of Oral Treatment with Zinc Sulphate and Placebo in Acne Vulgaris', *British Journal of Dermatology* 1977; 97: 679–84
5. Michaelsson G., et al., 'A Double-Blind Study of the Effect of Zinc and Oxytetracycline in Acne Vulgaris', *British Journal of Dermatology* 1977; 97: 561–6

Alcoholism
1. Pekkanen L., 'Effects of Thiamine Deprivation and Antagonism on Voluntary Ethanol Intake in Rats', *Journal of Nutrition* 1980; 110: 937–44
2. Brown R. V., 'Vitamin Deficiency and Voluntary Alcohol Consumption in Mice', *Quarterly Journal of Studies on Alcohol* 1969; 30: 592–7
3. Williams R. J., et al., 'Dietary Deficiencies in Animals in Relation to Voluntary Alcohol and Sugar Consumption', *Quarterly Journal of Studies on Alcohol* 1955; 16: 234–44
4. Smith J. A., et al., 'The Treatment of Alcoholism by Nutritional Supplements', *Quarterly Journal of Studies on Alcohol* 1951; 12: 381–5
5. Trulson M. F., et al., 'Vitamin Medication in Alcoholism', *Journal of the American Medical Association* 1954; 155: 114–19
6. Horrobin D. F., 'A Biochemical Basis for Alcoholism and Alcohol-induced Liver Damage Including the Fetal Alcohol Syndrome and Cirrhosis: interference with essential fatty acid and prostaglandin metabolism', *Medical Hypotheses* 1980; 6: 929–42
7. Horrobin D. F., 'Essential Fatty Acids, Prostaglandins, and Alcoholism: an overview', *Clinical and Experimental Research* 1987; 11: 2–9
8. Rogers L. L., et al., 'Glutamine in the Treatment of Alcoholism', *Quarterly Journal of Studies on Alcohol* 1957; 18: 581–7

Alzheimer's Disease

1. Candy J. M., et al., 'Aluminosilicates and Senile Plaque Formation in Alzheimer's Disease', *Lancet* 1986 Feb 15: 354–7

2. Good P. F., et al., 'Selective Accumulation of Aluminum and Iron in the Neurofibrillary Tangles of Alzheimer's Disease: a laser microprobe (LAMMA) study', *Annals of Neurology* 1992; 31(3): 286–92

3. Graves A. B., et al., 'The Association Between Aluminum-Containing Products and Alzheimer's Disease', *Journal of Clinical Epidemiology* 1990; 43(1): 35–44

4. Landsberg J. P., et al., 'Absence of Aluminum in Neuritic Plaque Cores in Alzheimer's Disease', *Nature* 1992; 360: 65–8

5. Grant W. B., 'Dietary Links to Alzheimer's Disease', *Journal of Alzheimer's Disease* (1999 update) 1999; 1: 197–201

6. Grundman M., 'Vitamin E and Alzheimer Disease: the Basis for Additional Clinical Trials', *American Journal of Clinical Nutrition* 2000; 71: 630S–636S

7. Glueck C. J., et al., 'Evidence that Homocysteine is an Independent Risk Factor for Atherosclerosis in Hyperlipidemic Patients', *American Journal of Cardiology* 1995; 75: 132–6

8. Ubbink J. B., et al., 'Vitamin B12, Vitamin B6, and Folate Nutritional Status in Men with Hyperhomocysteinemia', *American Journal of Clinical Nutrition* 1993; 57: 47–53

9. Ubbink J. B., et al., 'Vitamin Requirements of Hyperhomocysteinemia in Humans', *Journal of Nutrition* 1994; 124: 1928–33

10. Calvani M., et al., 'Action of Acetyl-L-Carnitine in Neurodegeneration and Alzheimer's Disease', *Annals of the New York Academy of Science* 1992; 663: 483–6

11. Le Bars P. L., et al., 'A Placebo-Controlled, Double-Blind, Randomized Trial of an Extract of Ginkgo Biloba for Dementia', North American EGb Study Group. *Journal of the American Medical Association* 1997; 278: 1327–32

12. Hofferberth B., 'The Efficacy of EGb 761 in Patients with Senile Dementia of the Alzheimer Type: a Double-Blind, Placebo-Controlled Study on Different Levels of Investigation', *Human Psychopharmacology* 1994; 9: 215–22

13. Kanowski S., et al., 'Proof of Efficacy of the Ginkgo Biloba Special Extract EGb 761 in Outpatients Suffering from Mild to Moderate Primary Degenerative Dementia of the Alzheimer Type or Multi-Infarct Dementia', *Pharmacopsychiatry* 1996; 29: 47–56

14. Maurer K., et al., 'Clinical Efficacy of Ginkgo Biloba Special Extract

EGb 761 in Dementia of the Alzheimer's Type', *Journal of Psychiatric Research* 1997; 31: 645–55

Anaemia – Iron Deficiency

1. Salonen J. T., et al., 'High Stored Iron Levels Associated with Excess Risk of Myocardial Infarction in Western Finnish Men', *Circulation* 1992; 86: 803–11

Anaemia – Pernicious

1. Kondo H., 'Haematological Effects of Oral Cobalamin Preparations on Patients with Megaloblastic Anaemia', *Acta Haematologica* 1998; 99(4): 200–5
2. Berlin R., et al., 'Vitamin B12 Body Stores During Oral and Parenteral Treatment of Pernicious Anaemia', *Acta Medica Scandinavia* 1978; 204(1–2): 81–4

Aneurysm

1. Tilson M. D., et al., 'Deficiencies of Copper and a Compound with Ion-Exchange Characteristics of Pyridinoline in Skin from Patients with Abdominal Aortic Aneurysms', *Surgery* 1983; 94: 134–41
2. Tilson M. D., 'Decreased Hepatic Copper Levels: a Possible Chemical Marker for the Pathogenesis of Aortic Aneurysms in Men', *Archives of Surgery* 1982; 117: 1212–13

Angina

1. Cohen L., et al., 'Magnesium Sulphate in the Treatment of Variant Angina', *Magnesium* 1984; 3: 46–9
2. Cohen L., et al., 'Prompt Termination and/or Prevention of Cold-Pressor Stimulus-Induced Vasoconstriction of Different Vascular Beds by Magnesium Sulphate in Patients with Prinzmetal's Angina', *Magnesium* 1986; 5: 144–9
3. Kamikawa T., et al., 'Effects of Coenzyme Q10 on Exercise Tolerance in Chronic Stable Angina Pectoris', *American Journal of Cardiology* 1985; 56: 247–51
4. Kamikawa T., et al., 'Effects of L-Carnitine on Exercise Tolerance in Patients with Stable Angina Pectoris', *Japanese Heart Journal* 1984; 25: 587–97
5. Cherchi A., et al., 'Effects of L-Carnitine on Exercise Tolerance in Chronic Stable Angina: a Multicentre, Double-Blind, Randomized, Placebo Controlled, Crossover Study', *International Journal of Clinical Pharmacology, Therapeutics and Toxicology* 1985; 23: 569–72

6. Chappell, L. T., et al., 'The Correlation Between EDTA Chelation Therapy and Improvement in Cardiovascular Function: a Meta-analysis', *Journal of Advancement in Medicine* 1993; 6: 139–60

Anorexia

1. Safi-Kutti S., 'Oral Zinc Supplementation in Anorexia Nervosa', *Acta Psychiatrica Scandinavia Supplementum* 1990; 361: 14–17
2. Birmingham C. L., et al., 'Controlled Trial of Zinc Supplementation in Anorexia Nervosa', *International Journal of Eating Disorders* 1994; 15: 251–5

Anxiety

1. Boulenger J-P., et al., 'Increased Sensitivity to Caffeine in Patients with Panic Disorders: Preliminary Evidence', *Archives of General Psychiatry* 1984; 41: 1067–71
2. Minzler E., et al., 'Effect of a Special Kava Extract in Patients with Anxiety-, Tension- and Excitation-States of Non-Psychotic Genesis' – double blind study with placebos over four weeks. *Arzneimittel-Forschung* 1991; 41: 584–8

Asthma

1. Ogle K. A., et al., 'Children with Allergic Rhinitis and/or Bronchial Asthma Treated with Elimination Diet', *Annals of Allergy* 1977; 39: 8–11
2. Hodge L., et al., 'Increased Consumption of Polyunsaturated Oils May Be a Cause of Increased Prevalence of Childhood Asthma', *Australian and New Zealand Journal of Medicine* 1994; 24: 727
3. Hodge L., et al., 'Consumption of Oily Fish and Childhood Asthma Risk', *Medical Journal of Australia* 1996; 164: 137–40
4. Burney P. G., et al., 'The Effect of Changing Dietary Sodium on the Bronchial Response to Histamine', *Thorax* 1981; 44(1): 36–41
5. Durlach J., 'Magnesium and Allergy: Experimental and Clinical Relationships Between Magnesium and Hypersensitivity', *Rev Franc Allergol* 1975; 15: 133–46
6. Collipp P. J., et al., 'Pyridoxine Treatment of Childhood Bronchial Asthma', *Annals of Allergy* 1975; 35: 153–8
7. Reynolds R. D., et al., 'Depressed Plasma Pyridoxal Phosphate Concentrations in Adult Asthmatics', *American Journal of Clinical Nutrition* 1985; 41: 684–8
8. Li M., et al., 'Clinical Observations of the Therapeutic Effect of Ginkgo Leaf Concentrated Oral Liquor on Bronchial Asthma', *Chinese Journal of Integrative & Western Medicine* 1997; 3: 264–7

Atherosclerosis

1. Von Schacky C., et al., 'The Effect of Dietary Omega-3 Fatty Acids on Coronary Atherosclerosis' – a randomized, double-blind, placebo-controlled trial. *Annals of Internal Medicine* 1999; 130: 554–62
2. Kummerow F. A., et al., 'Swine as an Animal Model in Studies on Atherosclerosis', *Federation Proceedings* 1975; 33: 235
3. Willett W. C., et al., 'Intake of Trans Fatty Acids and Risk of Coronary Heart Disease Among Women', *Lancet* 1993; 341: 581–5
4. Oster K. A., et al., *The XO Factor*, Park City Press, New York, 1983, pp. 44–5
5. Gaby A. R., 'Nutritional Factors in Cardiovascular Disease', *Journal of Natural Medicine* 1983; 5(2): 107–20
6. Yudkin J., et al., 'Sugar Intake and Myocardial Infarction', *American Journal of Clinical Nutrition* 1967; 20: 503–6
7. Glueck C. J., et al., 'Evidence that Homocysteine is an Independent Risk Factor for Atherosclerosis in Hyperlipidemic Patients', *American Journal of Cardiology* 1995; 75: 132–6
8. Ubbink J. B., et al., 'Vitamin B12, Vitamin B6, and Folate Nutritional Status in Men with Hyperhomocysteinemia', *American Journal of Clinical Nutrition* 1993; 57: 47–53
9. Ubbink J. B., et al., 'Vitamin Requirements of Hyperhomocysteinemia in Humans', *Journal of Nutrition* 1994; 124: 1927–33
10. Stampfer M. J., et al., 'Vitamin E Consumption and the Risk of Coronary Heart Disease in Women', *New England Journal of Medicine* 1993; 328: 1444–9
11. Rimm E. B., et al., 'Vitamin E Consumption and the Risk of Coronary Heart Disease in Men', *New England Journal of Medicine* 1993; 328: 1450–6
12. Stephens N. G., et al., 'Randomised Controlled Trial of Vitamin E in Patients with Coronary Disease': Cambridge Heart Antioxidant Study (CHAOS), *Lancet* 1996; 347: 781–6
13. Mitchinson M. J., et al., 'Mortality in the CHAOS Trial', *Lancet* 1999; 353: 381–2

Atrial Fibrillation

1. Dobmeyer D. J., et al., 'The Arrhythmogenic Effects of Caffeine in Human Beings', *New England Journal of Medicine* 1983; 308: 814–16
2. Tsuji H., et al., 'The Associations of Levels of Serum Potassium and Magnesium with Ventricular Premature Complexes' – the Framingham Heart Study, *American Journal of Cardiology* 1994; 74: 232–5
3. Al Makdessi S., et al., 'Protective Effect of Crataegus Oxycantha Against

Reperfusion Arrhythmias After Global No-flow Ischaemia of the Rat Heart', *Basic Research in Cardiology* 1999; 94: 71.77

Back Pain
1. Greenwood J., Jr., 'Optimum Vitamin C Intake as a Factor in the Preservation of Disc Integrity', *Medical Annals of DC* 1966; 33: 274–6

Benign Prostatic Hypertrophy
1. Terry P., et al., 'Fatty Fish Consumption and Risk of Prostatic Cancer', *Lancet* 2001; 357: 1764
2. Hart J. P., et al., 'Vitamin F in the Treatment of Prostatic Hypertrophy', Report Number 1, Lee Foundation for Nutritional Research, Milwaukee, Wisconsin, 1941
3. Wilt T. J., Ishani A., Stark G., et al., 'Saw Palmetto Extracts for the Treatment of Benign Prostatic Hyperplasia: a Systematic Review', *Journal of the American Medical Association* 1998; 280: 1604–9
4. Andro M. C., Riffaud J. P., 'Pygeum Africanum Extract for the Treatment of Patients with Benign Prostatic Hyperplasia: a Review of 25 Years of Published Experience', *Current Therapeutic Research* 1995; 56: 796–817

Breath-Holding Attacks
1. Daoud A. S., et al., 'Effectiveness of Iron Therapy on Breath-holding Spells', *Journal of Pediatry* 1997; 130: 547–50

Bronchitis
1. Grassi C., et al., 'A Controlled Trial of Intermittent Oral Acetylcysteine in the Long-term Treatment of Chronic Bronchitis', *European Journal of Clinical Pharmacology* 1976; 9: 393–6

Bulimia Nervosa
1. Dalvit-McPhillips S., 'A Dietary Approach to Bulimia', *Physiological Behaviour* 1984; 33: 769–75
2. Mira M., et al., 'L-Tryptophan as an Adjunct to Treatment of Bulimia Nervosa', *Lancet* 1989; 2: 1162–3

Bursitis
1. Klemes I. S., 'Vitamin B12 in Acute Subdeltoid Bursitis', *Industrial Medicine and Surgery* 1957; 26: 290–2

Carpal Tunnel Syndrome
1. Ellis J. M., 'Vitamin B6 Deficiency in Patients with a Clinical Syndrome

Including the Carpal Tunnel Defect – Biochemical and Clinical Response to Therapy with Pyridoxine', *Research Communications in Chemical Pathology and Pharmacology* 1976; 13(4): 743–57

2. Ellis J. M., et al., 'Survey and New Data on Treatment with Pyridoxine of Patients Having a Clinical Syndrome Including the Carpal Tunnel and Other Defects', *Research Communications in Chemical Pathology and Pharmacology* 1977; 17(1): 165–77

Cataract

1. Christen W. G., et al., 'Smoking Cessation and Risk of Age-Related Cataract in Men', *Journal of the American Medical Association* 2000; 284(6): 713–16
2. Mares-Perlman J. A., et al., 'Vitamin Supplement Use and Incident Cataracts in a Population-Based Study', *Archives of Ophthalmology* 2000; 118: 1556–63
3. Seddon J., et al., 'The Use of Vitamin Supplements and the Risk of Cataracts Among U.S. Male Physicians', *Journal of Public Health* 1994; 84(5): 788–92
4. Jacques P. F., et al., 'Long-term Vitamin C Supplement Use and Prevalence of Early Age-Related Lens Opacities', *American Journal of Clinical Nutrition* 1997; 66: 911–16
5. Hankinson S. E., et al., 'Nutrient Intake and Cataract Extraction in Women: a Prospective Study', *British Medical Journal* 1992; 305: 335–9
6. Chasan-Taber L., et al., 'A Prospective Study of Carotenoid and Vitamin A Intakes and Risk of Cataract Extraction in US Women', *American Journal of Clinical Nutrition* 1999; 70: 509–16

Cervical Dysplasia

1. Palan P. R., et al., 'Plasma Levels of Antioxidant Beta-carotene and Alpha-tocopherol in Uterine Cervix Dysplasia and Cancer. *Nutrition and Cancer* 1991; 15: 13–20
2. Ho G. Y., et al., 'Viral Characteristics of Human Papillomavirus Infection and Antioxidant Levels as Risk Factors for Cervical Dysplasia', *International Journal of Cancer* 1998; 78: 594–9
3. Dawson, E. B., et al., 'Serum Vitamin and Selenium Changes in Cervical Dysplasia', *Federation Proceedings* 1984; 43: 612
4. Wassertheil-Smoller S., et al., 'Dietary Vitamin C and Uterine Cervical Dysplasia', *American Journal of Epidemiology* 1981; 114: 714–24
5. Romney S. L., et al., 'Retinoids and the Prevention of Cervical Dysplasias', *American Journal of Obstetrics and Gynecology* 1981; 114: 890–4
6. Kanetsky P. A., et al., 'Dietary Intake and Blood Levels of Lycopene:

Association with Cervical Dysplasia Among Non-Hispanic, Black Women', *Nutrition and Cancer* 1998; 31: 31–40

Cholecystitis

1. Breneman J. C., 'Allergy Elimination Diet as the Most Effective Gallbladder Diet', *Annals of Allergy* 1968; 26: 83–7
2. Capper W. L., et al., 'Gallstones, Gastric Secretion and Flatulent Dyspepsia', *Lancet* 1967; 1: 413–15

Cluster Headaches

1. Leone M., et al., 'Melatonin Versus Placebo in the Prophylaxis of Cluster Headache' – a double-blind pilot study with parallel groups. *Cephalalgia* 1996; 16: 494–6

Cold and Flu

1. Sanchez A., et al., 'Role of Sugars in Human Neutrophilic Phagacytosis', *American Journal of Clinical Nutrition* 1973; 26: 180
2. Bernstein J., et al., 'Depression of Lymphocyte Transformation Following Oral Glucose Ingestion', *American Journal of Clinical Nutrition* 1977; 30: 613 (abstract)
3. Anderson T. W., et al., 'Vitamin C and the Common Cold' – a double-blind trial, *Canadian Medical Association Journal* 1972; 107: 503–8
4. Eby G. A., et al., 'Reduction in Duration of Common Colds by Zinc Gluconate Lozenges in a Double-Blind Study', *Antimicrobial Agents and Chemotherapy* 1984; 25: 20–4
5. Barret B., et al., 'Echinacea for Upper Respiratory Infection', *Journal of Family Practice* 1999; 48: 628–35
6. Mumcuoglu M., et al., 'Inhibition of Several Strains of Influenza Virus and Beneficial Effect of Sambucol in the Treatment of Naturally Occurring Influenza B in a Double-Blind Preliminary Study', 6th International Congress for Infectious Diseases, Prague April 26–30, 1994, Abstract no. 1271, p. 392

Cold Sores

1. Flodin N. W., 'The Metabolic Roles, Pharmacology, and Toxicology of Lysine', *Journal of the American College of Nutrition* 1997; 16: 7–21
2. Terezhalmy G. T., et al., 'The Use of Water-Soluble Bioflavonoid-Ascorbic Acid Complex in the Treatment of Recurrent Herpes Labialis', *Oral Surgery* 1978; 45: 56–62
3. Nead D. E., 'Effective Vitamin E Treatment for Ulcerative Herpetic Lesions', *Dental Survey* 1976; 52(7): 50–1

4. Fink M., et al., 'Treatment of Herpes Simplex by Alpha-Tocopherol (Vitamin E)', *British Dental Journal* 1980; 148: 246 (letter)

Colic

1. Lothe L., et al., 'Cow's Milk Whey Protein Elicits Symptoms of Infantile Colic in Colicky Formula-Fed Infants' – a double-blind crossover study. *Pediatrics* 1989; 83(2): 262–6
2. Lothe L., et al., 'Cow's Milk as a Cause of Infantile Colic' – a double-blind study. *Pediatrics* 1982; 70(1): 7–10
3. Lust K. D., et al., 'Maternal Intake of Cruciferous Vegetables and Other Foods and Colic Symptoms in Exclusively Breast-Fed Infants', *Journal of the American Dietetic Association* 1996; 96: 47–8
4. Taubman B., 'Clinical Trial of the Treatment of Colic by Modification of Parent–Infant Interaction', *Pediatrics* 1984; 74: 998–1003

Cradle Cap

1. Nisenson A., 'Seborrhoeic Dermatitis of Infants and Leiner's Disease: a Biotin Deficiency', *Journal of Pediatrics* 1957; 51: 537

Cramp

1. Dahle L. O., et al., 'The Effect of Oral Magnesium Substitution on Pregnancy-Induced Leg Cramps', *American Journal of Obstetrics and Gynecology* 1995; 173: 175–80

Crohn's Disease

1. Heaton K. W., et al., 'Treatment of Crohn's Disease with an Unrefined Carbohydrate, Fibre Rich Diet', *British Medical Journal* 1979; 2: 764–6
2. Riordan A. M., et al., 'Treatment of Active Crohn's Disease by Exclusion Diet', East Anglian Multicentre Controlled Trial, *Lancet* 1993; 342: 1131–4
3. Mate J., et al., 'Does Dietary Fish Oil Maintain the Remission of Crohn's Disease: a Case Control Study', *Gastroenterology* 1991; 100: A228 (abstract)

Depression

1. Schmidt U., et al., 'St John's Wort Extract in the Ambulatory Therapy of Depression. Attention and Reaction Ability are Preserved', *Fortschritte der Medizin* 1993; 111(19): 339–42
2. Muller W. E., et al., 'Effects of Hypericum Extract (LI 160) in Biochemical Models of Antidepressant Activity', *Pharmacopsychiatry* 1997; 30: 102–7

Diabetes

1. Karjalainen J., et al., 'A Bovine Albumin Peptide as a Possible Trigger of

Insulin-Dependent Diabetes Mellitus', *New England Journal of Medicine* 1992; 327: 302–7

2. Kostraba J. N., et al., 'Early Exposure to Cow's Milk and Solid Foods in Infancy, Genetic Predisposition, and Risk of IDDM', *Diabetes* 1993; 42: 288–95

3. Fava D., et al., 'Relationship Between Dairy Product Consumption and Incidence of IDDM in Childhood in Italy', *Diabetes Care*, 1994; 17: 1488–90

Ear Infections

1. Nsouli T. M., et al., 'Role of Food Allergy in Serous Otitis Media', *Annals of Allergy* 1994; 73: 215–19

Eczema

1. Atherton D. J., et al., 'A Double Blind Controlled Crossover Trial of an Antigen Avoidance Diet in Atopic Eczema', *Lancet* 1978; 1: 401–3

2. Sampson H. A., et al., 'Food Hypersensitivity and Atopic Dermatitis: Evaluation of 113 Patients', *Journal of Pediatrics* 1985; 107: 669–75

3. Manku M. S., et al., 'Essential Fatty Acids in the Plasma Phospholipids of Patients with Atopic Eczema', *British Journal of Dermatology* 1984; 110: 643–8

4. Schalin-Karrila M., et al., 'Evening Primrose Oil in the Treatment of Atopic Eczema', *British Journal of Dermatology* 1987; 117: 11–19

5. Wright S., et al., 'Oral Evening Primrose Oil Improves Atopic Eczema', *Lancet* 1982; ii: 1120–2

Emphysema

1. Fujimoto S., et al., 'Effects of Coenzyme Q10 Administration on Pulmonary Function and Exercise Performance in Patients with Chronic Lung Disease', *Clinical Investigation* 1993; 71: S162–6

2. Dal Negro R., et al., 'L-Carnitine and Physiokinesiotherapy in Chronic Respiratory Insufficiency', *Clinical Trials Journal* 1985; 22: 353–60

Endometriosis

1. Rier S. E., et al., 'Endometriosis in Rhesus Monkeys Following Chronic Exposure to 2,3,7,8 Tetrachlorodibenzo-p-dioxin', *Fundamental and Applied Toxicology* 1993; 21: 433–41

2. Damewood M. D., 'Pathophysiology and Management of Endometriosis', *Journal of Family Practice* 1993; 37(1): 68–75

3. Cust M. P., 'A Risk-Benefit Assessment of Estrogen Therapy in Postmenopausal Women', *Drug Safety* 1990; 5(5): 345–58

Epilepsy

1. Egger J., et al., 'Oligoantigenic Diet Treatment of Children with Epilepsy and Migraine', *Journal of Pediatrics* 1989; 114: 51–8
2. Hagberg B., et al., 'Tryptophan Load Tests and Pyridoxal-5-Phosphate Levels in Epileptic Children', *Acta Paediatrica Scandinavica* 1966; 55: 371–84
3. Ogunmekan A. O., et al., 'A Randomized, Double-Blind, Placebo-Controlled Clinical Trial of D-Alpha-Tocopheryl Acetate (vitamin E), as Add-on Therapy, for Epilepsy in Children', *Epilepsia* 1989; 30: 84–9

Fatigue

1. D'Angelo L., et al., 'A Double-Blind Placebo-Controlled Clinical Study on the Effect of Standardized Ginseng Extract on Psychomotor Performance in Healthy Volunteers', *Journal of Ethnopharmacology* 1986; 16: 15–22
2. Hallstrom C., Fulder S., Carruthers M., 'Effect of Ginseng on the Performance of Nurses on Night Duty', *Comparative Medicine East and West* 1982; 6: 277–82
3. Wagner H., et al., 'Plant Adaptogens', *Phytomed* 1994; 1: 63–76
4. Farnsworth N. R., et al., 'Siberian Ginseng: Current Status as an Adaptogen', In *Economic and Medicinal Plant Research*. Vol 1. Academic Press, London, 155–215 (1985)
5. Asano K., et al., 'Effect of Eleutherococcus Senticosus Extract on Human Physical Working Capacity', *Planta Medica* 1986; 53: 175–7

Fibrocystic Breast Disease

1. Minton J. P., et al., 'Caffeine, Cyclic Nucleotides, and Breast Disease', *Surgery* 1979; 86: 105–8
2. Minton J. P., et al., 'Clinical and Biochemical Studies on Methylxanthine-Related Fibrocystic Breast Disease', *Surgery* 1981; 90: 299–304
3. Rose D. P., et al., 'Low Fat Diet in Fibrocystic Disease of the Breast with Cyclic Mastalgia: a Feasibility Study', *American Journal of Clinical Nutrition* 1985; 41(4): 856
4. Boyd N. F., et al., 'Effect of a Low-Fat High-Carbohydrate Diet on the Symptoms of Cyclical Mastopathy', *Lancet* 1988; ii: 128–32
5. Abrams A. A., 'Use of Vitamin E in Chronic Cystic Mastitis', *New England Journal of Medicine* 1965; 272(20): 1080–1
6. London R. S., et al., 'Endocrine Parameters and Alpha-Tocopherol Therapy of Patients with Mammary Dysplasia', *Cancer Research* 1981; 41: 3811–13
7. Mansel, R. E., et al., *Effects of Essential Fatty Acids on Cyclic Mastalgia and Noncyclical Breast Disorders*, 'Omega-6 essential fatty acids: Pathophysiology and roles in clinical medicine', Alan R. Liss, New York, 1990, 557–66

8. Preece P. E., et al., 'Evening Primrose Oil (EFAMOL) for Mastalgia', in *Clinical Uses of Essential Fatty Acids*, ed. D. F. Horrobin, Montreal: Eden Press, 1982, 147–54

Fibromyalgia

1. Romano T., et al., 'Magnesium Deficiency and Fibromyalgia Syndrome', *Journal of Nutritional Medicine* 1994; 4: 165–7
2. Abraham G. E., et al., 'Management of Fibromyalgia: Rationale for the Use of Magnesium and Malic Acid', *Journal of Nutritional Medicine* 1992; 3: 49–59

Gingivitis

1. El-Ashiry G. M., et al., 'Local and Systemic Influences in Periodontal Disease II.' Effect of prophylaxis and natural and synthetic vitamin C upon gingivitis. *Journal of Periodontology* 1964; 35: 250–9
2. Wilkinson E. G., et al., 'Bioenergetics in Clinical Medicine VI.' Adjunctive treatment of periodontal disease with coenzyme Q10. *Research Communications in Chemical Pathology and Pharmacology* 1976; 14: 715–19

Glaucoma

1. Raymond L. F., 'Allergy and Chronic Simple Glaucoma', *Annals of Allergy* 1964; 22: 146
2. Berens C., et al., 'Allergy in Glaucoma. Manifestations of Allergy in Three Glaucoma Patients as Determined by the Pulse-Diet Method of Coca', *Annals of Allergy* 1947; 5: 526
3. McGuire R., 'Fish Oil Cuts Ocular Pressure', *Medical Tribune* 1991; 19: 25
4. Stocker F. W., 'Clinical Experiments with New Ways of Influencing the Intraocular Tension II.' Use of rutin to enhance the tension-reducing effect of miotics by reducing the permeability of the blood-aqueous barrier. *Archives Ophthalmology* 1949; 73: 429–35

Gout

1. Emmerson B. T., 'Effect of Oral Fructose on Urate Production', *Annals of the Rheumatic Diseases* 1974; 33: 276–80
2. Blau L. W., 'Cherry Diet Control for Gout and Arthritis', *Texas Reports on Biology and Medicine* 1950; 8: 309–11

Haemorrhoids

1. Nini G., et al., 'Controlled Clinical Evaluation of a New Anti-Haemorrhoid Drug, Using a Completely Randomized Experimental Plan', *Clinical Therapeutics* 1978; 86: 545–9 (in Italian)

Hay Fever

1. Holmes H. M., et al., 'Hay Fever and Vitamin C', *Science* 1942; 96: 497
2. Ruskin S. L., 'High Dose Vitamin C in Allergy', *American Journal of Digestive Diseases* 1945; 12: 281

Hearing Loss

1. Houston D. K., et al., 'Age-Related Hearing Loss, Vitamin B-12, and Folate in Elderly Women', *American Journal of Clinical Nutrition* 1999; 69: 564–71
2. Attias J., et al., 'Oral Magnesium Intake Reduces Permanent Hearing Loss Induced by Noise Exposure', *American Journal of Otolaryngology* 1994; 15: 26–32

Heart Failure

1. Bashir Y., et al., 'Effects of Long-Term Oral Magnesium Chloride Replacement in Congestive Heart Failure Secondary to Coronary Artery Disease', *American Journal of Cardiology* 1993; 72: 1156–62
2. Folkers K., et al., 'Therapy of Coenzyme Q10 of Patients in Heart Failure Who are Eligible or Ineligible for Transplant', *Biochemical and Biophysical Research Communications* 1992; 15: 247–53
3. Leuchtgens H., 'Crataegus Special Extract (WS 1442) in Cardiac Insufficiency', *Fortschritte der Medizin* 1993; 111: 352–4
4. Schmidt U., et al., 'Efficacy of the Hawthorn (Crataegus) Preparation LI 132 in 78 Patients with Chronic Congestive Heart Failure Defined as NYHA Functional Class II', *Phytomed* 1994; 1: 17–24

High Cholesterol

1. Reaven P. D., et al., 'Leisure Time Exercise and Lipid and Lipoprotein Levels in an Older Population', *Journal of the American Geriatric Society* 1990; 38: 847–54
2. Brown W. V., 'Niacin for Lipid Disorders', *Postgraduate Medicine* 1995; 98: 185–93
3. Press R. I., et al., 'The Effect of Chromium Picolinate on Serum Cholesterol and Apolipoprotein Fractions in Human Subjects', *Western Journal of Medicine* 1990; 152: 41–5
4. Hermann J., et al., 'Effects of Chromium of Copper Supplementation on Plasma Lipids, Plasma Glucose and Serum Insulin in Adults Over Age Fifty', *Journal of Nutrition for the Elderly* 1998; 27–45
5. Riales R., et al., 'Effect of Chromium Chloride Supplementation on Glucose Tolerance and Serum Lipids Including High Density Lipoprotein of Adult Men', *American Journal of Clinical Nutrition* 1981; 34: 2670–8

6. Roeback J. R., et al., 'Effects of Chromium Supplementation on Serum High-Density Lipoprotein Cholesterol Levels in Men Taking Beta-Blockers', *Annals of Internal Medicine* 1991; 115: 917–24

7. Uberg M., et al., 'Hypocholesterolemic Effects on Nicotinic Acid and Chromium Supplementation', *Journal of Family Practice* 1988; 27: 603–6

8. Davis W. H., et al., 'Monotherapy with Magnesium Increases Abnormally Low High Density Lipoprotein Cholesterol: a Clinical Assay', *Current Therapeutic Research* 1984; 36: 341–6

9. Niyanand S., et al., 'Clinical Trials with Guggulipid – a New Hypolipidemic Agent', *Journal of the Association of Physicians of India* 1989; 37: 323–8

High Triglycerides

1. Reiser S., 'Effect of Dietary Sugars on Metabolic Risk Factors Associated with Heart Disease', *Nutrition and Health* 1985; 3: 203–16

2. Szanto S., et al., 'The Effect of Dietary Sucrose on Blood Lipids, Serum Insulin, Platelet Adhesiveness and Body Weight in Human Volunteers', *Postgraduate Medicine* 1969; 45: 602–7

3. Steinberg D., et al., 'Alcohol and Atherosclerosis', *Annals of Internal Medicine* 1991; 114: 967–76

4. Silagy C., et al., 'Garlic as a Lipid-Lowering Agent: a Meta-Analysis', *Journal of the Royal College of Physicians, London* 1994; 28: 39–45

5. Holzgartner J., et al., 'Comparison of the Efficacy of a Garlic Preparation vs. Bezafibrate', *Arzneimittel-Forschung* 1992; 42: 1473–7

6. Niyanand S., et al., 'Clinical Trials with Guggulipid – a New Hypolipidemic Agent', *Journal of the Association of Physicians of India* 1989; 37: 323–8

7. Agarwal R. C., et al., 'Clinical Trial of Guggulipid New Hypolipidemic Agent of Plant Origin in Primary Hyperlipidemia', *Indian Journal of Medical Research* 1986; 84: 626–34

Hives (urticaria)

1. Henz B. M., et al., 'Most Chronic Urticaria is Food-Dependent, Not Idiopathic', *Experimental Dermatology* 1998; 7: 139–42

2. Lessof M. H., 'Reactions to Food Additives', *Clinical and Experimental Allergy* 1995; 25 (supplement 1): 27–8

3. Juhlin L., 'Additives and Chronic Urticaria', *Annals of Allergy* 1987; 59: 119–23

4. Kulczycki A. Jr., 'Aspartame-Induced Urticaria', *Annals of Internal Medicine* 1986; 104: 207–8

5. Rawls W. B., et al., 'Chronic Urticaria Associated with Hypochlorhydria or Achlorhydria', *Review of Gastroenterology* 1951; 18: 267–71

Hyperactivity (attention deficit hyperactivity disorder)

1. Mitchell E. A., et al., 'Clinical Characteristics and Serum Essential Fatty Acid Levels in Hyperactive Children', *Clinical Pediatrics* 1987; 26: 406–11
2. Stevens L. J., et al., 'Essential Fatty Acid Metabolism in Boys with Attention-Deficit Hyperactivity Disorder', *American Journal of Clinical Nutrition* 1995; 62: 761–8
3. Starobrat-Hermelin B., et al., 'The Effects of Magnesium Physiological Supplementation on Hyperactivity in Children with Attention Deficit Hyperactivity Disorder (ADHD). Positive Response to Magnesium Oral Loading Test', *Magnesium Research* 1997; 10: 149–56

Hypertension (high blood pressure)

1. Stamler J., et al., 'Findings of the International Cooperative INTERSALT Study', *Hypertension* 1991; 17(1): 9–15
2. Cappuccio F. P., MacGregor G. A., 'Does Potassium Supplementation Lower Blood Pressure? A Meta-Analysis of Published Trials', *Journal of Hypertension* 1991; 9: 465–73
3. Silagy C., Neil A. W., 'A Meta-Analysis of the Effect of Garlic on Blood Pressure', *Journal of Hypertension* 1994; 12: 463–8
4. Griffith L. E., et al., 'The Influence of Dietary and Non-Dietary Calcium Supplementation on Blood Pressure. An Updated Meta-Analysis of Randomized Controlled Trials', *American Journal of Hypertension* 1999; 12: 84–92
5. Resnick L. M., 'The Role of Dietary Calcium in Hypertension: a Hierarchical Review', *American Journal of Hypertension* 1999; 12: 99–112
6. Motoyama T., Sano H., Fukuzaki H., et al., 'Oral Magnesium Supplementation in Patients with Essential Hypertension', *Hypertension* 1989; 13: 227–32
7. Gigiesi V., Cantini F., Brodbeck B., 'Effect of Coenzyme Q10 in Essential Hypertension', *Current Therapeutic Research* 1990; 47: 841–5
8. Singh R. B., Niaz M. A., Rastogi S. S., et al., 'Effect of Hydrosoluble Coenzyme Q10 on Blood Pressures and Insulin Resistance in Hypertensive Patients with Coronary Artery Disease', *Journal of Human Hypertension* 1999; 13: 203–8

Impotence

1. Sohn M., et al., 'Ginkgo Biloba Extract in the Therapy of Erectile Dysfunction', *Journal of Sex Education and Therapy* 1991; 17: 53–61

Incontinence

1. Arya L. A., et al., 'Dietary Caffeine Intake and the Risk for Detrusor Instability: a Case-Control Study', *Obstetrics and Gynaecology* 2000; 96(1): 85–9

2. Gordon D., et al., 'Double-Blind, Placebo-Controlled Study of Magnesium Hydroxide for Treatment of Sensory Urgency and Detrusor Instability: Preliminary Results', *British Journal of Obstetrics and Gynaecology* 1998; 105: 667–9

Indigestion
1. Al-Habbal M. J., et al., 'A Double-Blind Controlled Clinical Trial of Mastic and Placebo in the Treatment of Duodenal Ulcer', *Journal of Clinical and Experimental Pharmacology and Physiology* 1984; 11: 541–4

Infertility – female
1. Howe G., et al., 'Effects of Age, Cigarette Smoking, and Other Factors on Fertility: Findings in a Large Prospective Study', *British Medical Journal* 1985; 290: 1697–9
2. Grodstein F., et al., 'Infertility in Women and Moderate Alcohol Use', *American Journal of Public Health* 1994; 84: 1429–32
3. Czeizel A. E., et al., 'The Effect of Preconceptional Multivitamin Supplementation on Fertility', *International Journal for Vitamin and Nutrition Research* 1996; 66: 55–8
4. Bayer R., 'Treatment of Infertility with Vitamin E', *International Journal of Fertility* 1960; 5: 70–8
5. Propping D., et al., 'Treatment of Corpus Luteum Deficiency', *Zeitschr Allgemeinmedizin* 1987; 63: 932–3

Infertility – male
1. Hurley D., 'Pollutants Blamed for Steady Decline in Sperm Counts, Ejaculate Volume', *Medical Tribune* 1992: 14
2. Comhaire F., et al., 'Declining Sperm Quality in European Men', *Andrologia* 1996; 28: 300–1
3. Anonymous, 'Sperm Swim Singly After Vitamin C Therapy', *Journal of the American Medical Association* 1983; 249: 2747–51
4. Marmar J. L., et al., 'Semen Zinc Levels in Infertile and Postvasectomy Patients and Patients with Prostatitis', *Fertility and Sterility* 1975; 26: 1057–63
5. Costa M., et al., 'L-Carnitine in the Idiopathic Asthenozoospermia: a Multicenter Study', *Andrologia* 1994; 26: 155–9

Insomnia
1. Hollingworth H. L., et al., 'The Influence of Caffeine on Mental and Motor Efficiency', *Archives of Psychology* 1912; 20: 1–66

Intermittent Claudication

1. Smulski H. S., et al., 'Placebo-Controlled, Double-Blind Trial to Determine the Efficacy of the Tibetan Plant Preparation Padma 28 for Intermittent Claudication', *Alternative Therapy* 1995; 1(2): 44–9

Kidney Stones

1. Robertson W. G., et al., 'The Cause of Idiopathic Calcium Stone Disease: Hypercalcuria or Hyperoxaluria?', *Nephron* 1980; 26: 105–10
2. Curhan G. C., et al., 'A Prospective Study of Dietary Calcium and Other Nutrients and the Risk of Symptomatic Kidney Stones', *New England Journal of Medicine* 1993; 328: 833–8
3. Curhan G. C., et al., 'Comparison of Dietary Calcium and Supplemental Calcium and Other Nutrients as Factors Affecting the Risk of Kidney Stones in Women', *Annals of Internal Medicine* 1997; 126: 497–504
4. Prien E. L., et al., 'Magnesium Oxide-Pyridoxine Therapy for Recurrent Calcium Oxalate Calculi', *Journal of Urology* 1974; 112: 509–12

Leukoplakia

1. Toma S., et al., 'Selenium Therapy in Patients with Precancerous and Malignant Oral Cavity Lesions: Preliminary Results', *Cancer Detection and Prevention* 1991; 15: 491–4

Macular Degeneration

1. Goldberg J., et al., 'Factors Associated with Age-Related Macular Degeneration', *American Journal of Epidemiology* 1988; 128: 700–10
2. Seddon J. M., et al., 'Dietary Carotenoids, Vitamin A, C and E and Advanced Age-Related Macular Degeneration', *Journal of the American Medical Association* 1994; 272: 1413–20
3. Lebuisson D. A., et al., 'Treatment of Senile Macular Degeneration with Ginkgo Biloba Extract: a Preliminary Double-Blind Study Versus Placebo'. In *Rokan (Ginkgo Biloba): Recent Advances in Pharmacology and Clinic*, Fünfgeld F. W. ed., Berlin: Springer-Verlag 1988, pp. 231–6

Memory and Concentration – poor

1. Perrig W. J., et al., 'The Relation Between Antioxidants and Memory Performance in the Old and Very Old', *Journal of the American Geriatric Society* 1997; 45(6): 718–24
2. Allain H., et al., 'Effects of Two Doses of Ginkgo Biloba Extract (EGb 761) on the Dual-Coding Test in Elderly Subjects', *Clinical Therapeutics* 1993; 15(3): 549–58
3. Rai G. S., et al., 'A Double-Blind, Placebo-Controlled Study of Ginkgo

Biloba Extract ("Tanakan") in Elderly Patients with Mild to Moderate Memory Impairment', *Current Medical Research and Opinion* 1991; 12(6): 350–5

4. Cipolli C., et al., 'Effects of L-Acetylcarnitine on Mental Deterioration in the Aged: Initial Results', *Clinical Therapeutics* 1990; 132(6): 479–510 (in Italian)

5. Salvioli G., et al., 'L-Acetylcarnitine Treatment of Mental Decline in the Elderly', *Drugs Under Experimental and Clinical Research* 1994; 20(4): 169–76

Ménière's Disease

1. Yanick P. Jr., 'Dietary and Lifestyle Influences on Cochlear Disorders and Biochemical Status: a 12-Month Study', *Journal of Applied Nutrition* 1988; 40(2): 75–84

2. Haguenauer J. P., et al., 'Treatment of Equilibrium Problems with Extract of Ginkgo Biloba. A Multicenter, Double-Blind, Placebo-Controlled Study', *Presse Med* 1986; 15: 1569–72 (in French)

Menopause

1. Hemminki E., et al., 'Impact of Postmenopausal Hormone Therapy on Cardiovascular Events and Cancer: Pooled Data from Clinical Trials', *British Medical Journal* 1997; 315: 149–53

2. Hulley S., et al., 'Randomized Trial of Estrogen Plus Progestin for Secondary Prevention of Coronary Heart Disease in Postmenopausal Women', *Journal of the American Medical Association* 1998; 280: 605–13

3. Collaborative Group on Hormonal Factors in Breast Cancer, 'Breast Cancer and Hormone Replacement Therapy: Collaborative Reanalysis of Data from 51 Epidemiological Studies of 52,705 Women with Breast Cancer and 108,411 Women Without Breast Cancer', *Lancet* 1997; 350: 1047–59

4. Perloff W. H., 'Treatment of the Menopause', *American Journal of Obstetrics and Gynecology* 1949; 58: 684–94

5. Gozan H. A., 'The Use of Vitamin E in the Treatment of the Menopause', *New York State Journal of Medicine* 1952; 52: 1289

6. Christy C. J., 'Vitamin E in Menopause: Preliminary Report of Experimental and Clinical Study', *American Journal of Obstetrics and Gynecology* 1945; 50: 84

7. Finkler R. S., 'The Effect of Vitamin E in the Menopause', *Journal of Clinical Endocrinology and Metabolism* 1949; 9: 89–94

8. Rubenstein B. B., 'Vitamin E Reduces the Vasomotor Symptoms of Menopause', *Federation Proceedings* 1948; 7: 106

9. Lieberman S., 'A Review of the Effectiveness of Cimicifuga Racemosa

(black cohosh) for the Symptoms of Menopause', *Journal of Women's Health* 1998; 7: 525–9

Menorrhagia
1. Lithgow D. M., et al., 'Vitamin A in the Treatment of Menorrhagia', *South African Medical Journal* 1977; 51: 191–3

Migraine
1. Monro J., et al., 'Food Allergy in Migraine', *Lancet* 1980; ii: 1–4
2. Egger J., et al., 'Is Migraine Food Allergy? A Double-Blind Trial of Oligoantigenic Diet Treatment', *Lancet* 1983; ii: 865–9
3. Hughs E. C., et al., 'Migraine: a Diagnostic Test for Etiology of Food Sensitivity by a Nutritionally Supported Fast and Confirmed by Long-Term Report', *Annals of Allergy* 1985; 55: 28–32
4. Egger J., et al., 'Oligogenic Diet Treatment of Children with Epilepsy and Migraine', *Journal of Pediatrics* 1989; 114: 51–8
5. Grant E. C., 'Food Allergies and Migraine', *Lancet* 1979; I: 966–9
6. Weaver K., 'Magnesium and Migraine', *Headache* 1990; 30: 169 (letter)
7. Murphy J. J., et al., 'Randomized Double-Blind Placebo Controlled Trial of Feverfew in Migraine Prevention', *Lancet* 1988; ii: 189–92
8. Johnson E. S., et al., 'Efficacy of Feverfew as Prophylactic Treatment of Migraine', *British Medical Journal* 1985; 291: 569–73
9. Palevitch D., et al., 'Feverfew (Tanacetum Parthenium) as a Prophylactic Treatment for Migraine: a Double-Blind Placebo-Controlled Study', *Phytotherapy Research* 1997; 11: 508–11

Mitral Valve Prolapse
1. Lichodziejewska B., et al., 'Clinical Symptoms of Mitral Valve Prolapse are Related to Hypomagnesemia and Attenuated by Magnesium Supplementation', *American Journal of Cardiology* 1997; 79: 768–72
2. Oda T., et al., 'Effect of Coenzyme Q10 on the Stress-Induced Decrease of Cardiac Performance in Pediatric Patients with Mitral Valve Prolapse', *Japanese Circulation Journal* 1984; 48: 1387

Morning Sickness
1. Sahakian V., et al., 'Vitamin B6 is Effective Therapy for Nausea and Vomiting of Pregnancy: a Randomized, Double-Blind, Placebo-Controlled Trial', *Obstetrics and Gynaecology* 1991; 78: 33–6
2. Vutyavanich T., et al., 'Pyridoxine for Nausea and Vomiting of Pregnancy: a Randomized, Double-Blind, Placebo-Controlled Trial', *American Journal of Obstetrics and Gynecology* 1995; 173: 881–4

Mouth Ulcers (canker sores)

1. Herlofson B. B., et al., 'The Effect of Two Toothpaste Detergents on the Frequency of Recurrent Aphthous Ulcers', *Acta Odontologica Scandinavia* 1996; 54: 150–3
2. Porter S. R., et al., 'Hematologic Status in Recurrent Aphthous Stomatitis Compared to Other Oral Disease', *Oral Surgery, Oral Medicine, Oral Pathology* 1988; 66: 41–4
3. Palopoli J., et al., 'Recurrent Aphthous Stomatitis and Vitamin B12 Deficiency', *Southern Medical Journal* 1990; 83: 475–7
4. Wray D., et al., 'Nutritional Deficiencies in Recurrent Aphthae', *Journal of Oral Pathology* 1978; 7: 418–23

Multiple Sclerosis

1. Ehrentheil O. F., et al., 'Role of Food Allergy in Multiple Sclerosis', *Neurology* 1952; 2: 412–26
2. Swank R. L., et al., 'Effect of a Low Saturated Fat Diet in Early and Late Cases of Multiple Sclerosis', *Lancet* 1990; 336: 37–9
3. Dworkin R. H., et al., 'Linoleic Acid and Multiple Sclerosis: a Reanalysis of Three Double-Blind Trials', *Neurology* 1984; 34: 1441–5
4. Korwin-Piotrowska T., et al., 'Experience of Padma 28 in Multiple Sclerosis', *Phytotherapy Research* 1992; 6: 133–6

Nails – weak

1. Hochman L. G., et al., 'Brittle Nails: Response to Daily Biotin Supplementation', *Cutis* 1993; 51: 303–5

Oedema

1. Diehm C., et al., 'Medical Oedema Protection – Clinical Benefits in Patients with Chronic Deep Vein Incompetence. A Placebo Controlled Double Blind Study', *Vasa* 1992; 21: 188–92

Osteoarthritis

1. Brandt K. D., 'Effects of Non-Steroidal Anti-Inflammatory Drugs on Chondrocyte Metabolism in Vitro and in Vivo', *American Journal of Medicine* 1987; 83: 29–34
2. Shield M. J., 'Anti-Inflammatory Drugs and Their Effects on Cartilage Synthesis and Renal Function', *European Journal of Rheumatology and Inflammation* 1993; 13: 7–16
3. Brooks P. M., et al., 'NSAID and Osteoarthritis – Help or Hindrance?', *Journal of Rheumatology* 1982; 9: 3–5

4. Pujalte J. M., et al., 'Double Blind Clinical Evaluation of Oral Glucosamine Sulphate in the Basic Treatment of Osteoarthrosis', *Current Medical Research and Opinion* 1980; 2: 110–14

5. Dovanti A., et al., 'Therapeutic Activity of Oral Glucosamine Sulphate in Osteoarthritis: a Placebo-Controlled Double-Blind Investigation', *Clinical Therapeutics* 1980; 3(4): 266–72

6. Noack W., et al., 'Glucosamine Sulphate in Osteoarthritis of the Knee', *Osteoarthritis and Cartilage* 1994; 2: 51–9

7. Muller-Fabbender H., et al., 'Glucosamine Sulphate Compared to Ibuprofen in Osteoarthritis of the Knee', *Osteoarthritis and Cartilage* 1994; 2: 61–9

8. Leeb B. F., et al., 'A Meta-Analysis of Chondroitin Sulfate in the Treatment of Osteoarthritis', *Journal of Rheumatology* 2000; 27: 205–11

9. Lippiello L., et al., 'Beneficial Effect of Cartilage Disease-Modifying Agents Tested in Chondrocyte Cultures and a Rabbit Instability Model of Osteoarthrosis', American College of Rheumatology 1999 Annual Meeting, Boston, MA

10. Gibson S. L. M., et al., 'The Treatment of Arthritis with a Lipid Extract of Perna Canaliculus: a Randomized Trial', *Complementary Therapy and Medicine* 1998; 6: 122–6

11. Kaufman W., 'The Use of Vitamin Therapy for Joint Mobility. Therapeutic Reversal of a Common Clinical Manifestation of the "Normal" Aging Process', *Connecticut State Medical Journal* 1953; 17(7): 584–9

12. Kaufman W., 'The Use of Vitamin Therapy to Reverse Certain Concomitants of Aging', *Journal of the American Geriatric Society* 1955; 11: 927

13. Hoffer A., 'Treatment of Arthritis by Nicotinic Acid and Nicotinamide', *Canadian Medical Association Journal* 1959; 81: 235–8

Osteoporosis

1. Chow R., et al., 'Effect of Two Randomised Exercise Programmes on Bone Mass of Healthy Postmenopausal Women', *British Medical Journal* 1987; 295: 1441–4

2. Gennari C., et al., 'Effect of Ipriflavone – a Synthetic Derivative of Natural Isoflavones – on Bone Mass Loss in the Early Years After the Menopause', *Menopause* 1998; 5(1): 9–15

3. Agnusdei D., et al., 'Efficacy of Ipriflavone in Established Osteoporosis and Long-Term Safety', *Calcified Tissue International* 1997; 61: 19–22

4. Passeri M., et al., 'Effects of 2-Year Therapy with Ipriflavone in Elderly Women with Established Osteoporosis', *Italian Journal of Mineral and Electrolyte Metabolism* 1995; 9: 137–44

5. Kovacs A. B., et al., 'Efficiency of Ipriflavone in the Prevention and Treatment of Postmenopausal Osteoporosis', *Agents and Actions* 1994; 41(1–2): 86–7

6. Reid I. R., et al., 'Long-Term Effects of Calcium Supplementation on Bone Loss and Fractures in Postmenopausal Women: a Randomized Trial', *American Journal of Clinical Nutrition* 1999; 70: 97–103

7. Nieves J. W., et al., 'Calcium Potentiates the Effect of Oestrogen and Calcitonin on Bone Mass: Review and Analysis', *American Journal of Clinical Nutrition* 1998; 67: 18–24

8. Stendig-Lindberg G., et al., 'Trabecular Bone Density in a Two Year Controlled Trial of Peroral Magnesium in Osteoporosis', *Magnesium Research* 1993; 6: 155–63

9. Abraham G. E., et al., 'A Total Dietary Programme Emphasizing Magnesium Instead of Calcium', *Journal of Reproductive Medicine* 1990; 35: 503–7

10. Kruger M. C., et al., 'Calcium, Gamma-Linolenic Acid and Eicosapentaenoic Acid Supplementation in Senile Osteoporosis', *Aging* 1998; 10: 385–94

Pancreatitis

1. McCloy, R., 'Chronic Pancreatitis at Manchester, UK', *Digestion* 1998; 59(4): 36–48

Peptic Ulcer

1. Brogden R. N., et al., 'Deglycyrrhizinated Licorice: a Report of its Pharmacological Properties and Therapeutic Efficacy', *Drugs* 1974; 8: 330–9

2. Gaby A. R., 'Deglycyrrhizinated Licorice Treatment of Peptic Ulcer', *Townsend Letter for Doctors* 1988; July: 306 (review)

3. Al-Habbal M. J., et al., 'A Double-Blind Controlled Clinical Trial of Mastic and Placebo in the Treatment of Duodenal Ulcer', *Journal of Clinical and Experimental Pharmacology and Physiology* 1984; 11: 541–4

Pre-eclampsia

1. Hojo M., et al., 'Calcium Metabolism in Normal and Hypertensive Pregnancy', *Seminars in Nephrology* 1995; 15: 504–11

2. Hojo M., et al., 'Calcium Metabolism in Preeclampsia: Supplementation May Help', *Medscape Women's Health* 1997; 2: 5

3. Moutquin J. M., et al., 'Report of the Canadian Hypertension Society Consensus Conference: 2. Nonpharmacologic Management and Prevention of Hypertensive Disorders in Pregnancy', *Canadian Medical Association Journal* 1997; 157: 907–19

4. Crowther C. A., et al., 'Calcium Supplementation in Nulliparous Women

for the Prevention of Pregnancy-Induced Hypertension, Preeclampsia and Preterm Birth: an Australian Randomized Trial', FRACOG and the ACT study group. *Australian and New Zealand Journal of Obstetrics and Gynaecology* 1999; 39: 12–18

5. Bucher H. C., et al., 'Effect of Calcium Supplementation on Pregnancy-Induced Hypertension and Preeclampsia: a Meta-Analysis of Randomized Controlled Trials', *Journal of the American Medical Association* 1996; 275: 1113–17

6. Belizan J. M., 'Calcium Supplementation to Prevent Hypertensive Disorders of Pregnancy', *New England Journal of Medicine* 1991; 325: 1399–1405

7. DerSimonian R., et al., 'Resolving Discrepancies Between Meta-Analysis and a Subsequent Large Controlled Trial', *Journal of the American Medical Association* 1999; 282: 664–70

8. Conradt A., et al., 'Magnesium Deficiency, a Possible Cause of Preeclampsia: Reduction of Frequency of Premature Rupture of Membranes and Premature or Small-for-Date Deliveries After Magnesium Supplementation', *Journal of the American College of Nutrition* 1985; 4: 321

9. Wachstein M., et al., 'Influence of Vitamin B6 on the Incidence of Preeclampsia', *Obstetrics and Gynaecology* 1956; 8: 177–80

Pre-Menstrual Syndrome (PMS)

1. Rossignol A. M., 'Caffeine-Containing Beverages and Premenstrual Syndrome in Young Women', *American Journal of Public Health* 1985; 75: 1337

2. Prior J. C., et al., 'Conditioning Exercise Decreases Premenstrual Symptoms: a Prospective, Controlled 6-Month Trial', *Fertility and Sterility* 1987; 47: 402–8

3. Abraham G. E., et al., 'Effect of Vitamin B6 on Premenstrual Symptomatology in Women with Premenstrual Tension Syndrome: a Double-Blind Crossover Study', *Infertility* 1980; 3: 155–65

4. Kerr G. D., 'The Management of Premenstrual Syndrome', *Current Medical Research and Opinion* 1977; 4: 29–34

5. Sherwood R. A., et al., 'Magnesium and the Premenstrual Syndrome', *Annals of Clinical Biochemistry* 1986; 23: 667–70

6. Facchinetti F., et al., 'Oral Magnesium Successfully Relieves Premenstrual Mood Changes', *Obstetrics and Gynaecology* 1991; 78: 177–81

Prostatitis

1. Rugendorff E. W., et al., 'Results of Treatment with Pollen Extract (Cermilton N) in Chronic Prostatitis and Prostatodynia', *British Journal of Urology* 1993; 71: 433–8

Restless Legs

1. Lutz E. G., 'Restless Legs, Anxiety and Caffeinism', *Journal of Clinical Psychiatry* 1978; 39: 693–8
2. Roberts H. J., 'Spontaneous Leg Cramps and "Restless Legs" Due to Diabetogenic (Functional) Hyperinsulinism: Observations of 131 Patients', *Journal of the American Geriatric Society* 1965; 13: 602–8
3. Ayres S. Jr., et al., '"Restless Legs" Syndrome: Response to Vitamin E', *Journal of Applied Nutrition* 1973; 25: 8–15
4. O'Keeffe S. T., et al., 'Iron Status and Restless Legs Syndrome in the Elderly', *Age and Ageing* 1994; 23: 200–3
5. Eckborn K. A., 'Restless Legs Syndrome', *Neurology* 1960; 1868–73

Rheumatoid Arthritis

1. Hicklin J. A., et al., 'The Effect of Diet in Rheumatoid Arthritis', *Clinical Allergy* 1980; 10: 463
2. Leventhal L. J., et al., 'Treatment of Rheumatoid Arthritis with Gamma-Linolenic Acid', *Annals of Internal Medicine* 1993; 119: 867–73
3. Zurier R. B., et al., 'Gamma-Linolenic Acid Treatment of Rheumatoid Arthritis: a Randomized, Placebo-Controlled Trial', *Arthritis and Rheumatism* 1996; 39: 1808–17
4. Leventhal L. J., et al., 'Treatment of Rheumatoid Arthritis with Black-currant Seed Oil', *British Journal of Rheumatology* 1994; 33: 847–52
5. Brzeski M., et al., 'Evening Primrose Oil in Patients with Rheumatoid Arthritis and Side Effects of Non-Steroidal Anti-Inflammatory Drugs', *British Journal of Rheumatology* 1991; 30: 370–2
6. Jantti J., et al., 'Evening Primrose Oil and Olive Oil in the Treatment of Rheumatoid Arthritis', *Clinical Rheumatology* 1989; 8: 238–44
7. Kremer J. M., et al., 'Fish Oil Fatty Acid Supplementation in Patients with Rheumatoid Arthritis', *Annals of Internal Medicine* 1987; 106(4): 497–503
8. Kremer J. M., et al., 'Dietary Fish Oil and Olive Oil Supplementation in Patients with Rheumatoid Arthritis', *Arthritis and Rheumatology* 1990; 33(6): 810–20
9. Geusens P., et al., 'Long-Term Effect of Omega-3 Fatty Acid Supplementation in Active Rheumatoid Arthritis', *Arthritis and Rheumatology* 1994; 37: 824–9
10. Van der Tempel H., et al., 'Effects of Fish Oil Supplementation in Rheumatoid Arthritis', *Annals of Rheumatic Disease* 1990; 49: 76–80
11. Cleland L. G., et al., 'Clinical and Biochemical Effects of Fish Oil Supplements in Rheumatoid Arthritis', *Journal of Rheumatology* 1988; 15: 471–5
12. Kremer, J. M., et al., 'Effects of High Dose Fish Oil on Rheumatoid

Arthritis After Stopping Nonsteroidal Anti-Inflammatory Drugs', *Arthritis and Rheumatology* 1995; 38: 1107–14
13. Walker W. R., et al., 'An Investigation of the Therapeutic Value of the "Copper Bracelet". Dermal Assimilation of Copper in Arthritic Rheumatoid Conditions', *Agents and Actions* 1976; 6: 454–9
14. Gibson R. G., et al., 'Perna Canaliculus in the Treatment of Arthritis', *Practitioner* 1980; 224: 955–60

Rosacea
1. Ryle J. A., et al., 'Gastric Analysis in Acne Rosacea', *Lancet* 1920; 2: 1195
2. Brown W. H., et al., 'Fractional Gastric Analysis in Disease of the Skin: Further Observation in 316 Cases, with Special Reference to Rosacea', *British Journal of Dermatology and Syphilology* 1935; 47: 181
3. Tulipan L., 'Acne Rosacea: a Vitamin B Complex Deficiency', *Archives of Dermatology and Syphilology* 1947; 56: 589

Sarcoidosis
1. Cagnoni M. L., et al., 'Melatonin for Treatment of Chronic Refractory Sarcoidosis', *Lancet* 1993; 346: 1230–1

Scleroderma
1. Zarafonetis C. J. D., 'The Treatment of Scleroderma: Results of Potassium Para-Amonobenzoate in 104 Cases'. In Mills L. C., Moyer J. H., eds., *Inflammation and Diseases of Connective Tissue*, W. B. Saunders: Philadelphia, 1961, 688–96
2. Zarafonetis C. J. D., et al., 'Retrospective Studies in Scleroderma: Effect of Potassium Para-Amonobenzoate on Survival', *Journal of Clinical Epidemiology* 1988; 41: 193–205
3. Zarafonetis C. J. D., et al., 'Retrospective Studies in Scleroderma: Pulmonary Findings and Effect of Potassium Para-Amonobenzoate on Vital Capacity', *Respiration* 1989; 56: 22–33

Seasonal Affective Disorder (SAD)
1. Kim H. L., et al., 'St John's Wort for Depression: a Meta-Analysis of Well-Defined Clinical Trials', *Journal of Nervous and Mental Disease* 1999; 187: 532–8
2. Wheatley D., 'Hypericum in Seasonal Affective Disorder (SAD)', *Current Medical Research and Opinion* 1999; 15: 33–7

Seborrhoeic Dermatitis
1. Shreiner A. W., et al., 'A Local Defect in the Metabolism of Pyridoxine

in the Skin of Persons with Seborrhoeic Dermatitis of the "Sicca" Type',
Journal of Investigative Dermatology 1952; 19: 95–6

Shingles

1. Ayres S. Jr., et al., 'Post-Herpes Zoster Neuralgia: Response to Vitamin
   E Therapy', *Archives of Dermatology* 1973; 108: 855–66
2. Ayres S. Jr., et al., 'Post-Herpes Zoster Neuralgia: Response to Vitamin
   E Therapy', *Archives of Dermatology* 1975; 111: 396
3. Bernstein J. E., et al., 'Treatment of Chronic Postherpetic Neuralgia with
   Topical Capsaicin', *Journal of the American Academy of Dermatology* 1987;
   17: 93–6
4. Bernstein J. E., et al., 'Topical Capsaicin Treatment of Chronic Postherpetic Neuralgia', *Journal of the American Academy of Dermatology* 1989; 21:
   265–70

Sickle Cell Disease

1. Natta C. L., et al., 'Antisickling Properties of Pyridoxine Derivatives',
   Annals of the New York Academy of Science 1990; 585: 505–9
2. Natta C. L., et al., 'A Decrease in Irreversibly Sickled Erythrocytes in
   Sickle Cell Anemia Patients Given Vitamin E', *American Journal of Clinical
   Nutrition* 1980; 33: 968–71

Sinusitis

1. Sletzer A. P., 'Adjunctive Use of Bromelain in Sinusitis: a Controlled
   Study', *EENT* Monthly 1967: 46(10): 1281–8

Smell – Loss of Sense of

1. Henkin R. I., 'Changes in Smell Function in Patients with Hyposmia
   After Magnesium Treatment', *Journal of the American College of Nutrition*
   1991; 10: 548

Stroke Prevention

1. Steiner N., 'Vitamin E May Enhance the Benefits of Aspirin in Preventing
   Stroke', *American Family Physician*, 1995; 51(8): 1977

Surgery – Recovery From

1. Morisset R., et al., 'Evaluation of the Healing Activity of Hydrocotyle
   Tincture in the Treatment of Wounds', *Phytotherapy Research* 1987;
   1: 117–21
2. Kartnig T., 'Clinical Applications of Centella Asiatica' (L) Urb. In *Herbs,
   Spices, and Medicinal Plants: Recent Advances in Botany, Horticulture, and*

Pharmacology, vol. 3, eds., L. E. Craker, J. E. Simon. Oryx Press: Phoenix AZ, 1986, 145–73

Tremor

1. Lieb J., 'Linoleic Acid in the Treatment of Lithium Toxicity and Familial Tremor', *Prostaglandins and Medicine* 1980; 4: 275–9

Trigeminal Neuralgia

1. Glore S., et al., 'Trigeminal Neuralgia: Case Study of Pain Cessation with a Low-Caffeine Diet', *Journal of the American Dietetic Association* 1991; 91: 1120–1

Ulcer – Skin

1. Taylor T. V., et al., 'Ascorbic Acid Supplementation in the Treatment of Pressure-Sores', *Lancet* 1974; ii: 544–6
2. Carruthers R., 'Oral Zinc Sulphate and Bedsores', *Lancet* 1969; 1: 1264
3. Cohen C., 'Zinc Sulphate and Bedsores', *British Medical Journal* 1968; 2: 561
4. Kartnig T., 'Clinical Applications of Centella Asiatica' (L) Urb, In: *Herbs, Spices and Medicinal Plants: Recent Advances in Botany, Horticulture and Pharmacology*, vol. 3, eds., L. E. Craker, J. E. Simon. Oryx Press: Phoenix AZ, 1986, 145–73

Ulcerative Colitis

1. Rowe A. H., 'Chronic Ulcerative Colitis – Allergy in its Etiology', *Annals of Internal Medicine* 1942; 17: 83–100
2. Andresen A. F. R., 'Ulcerative Colitis – an Allergic Phenomenon', *American Journal of Digestive Disease* 1942; 9: 91–8

Urinary Frequency

1. Creighton S. M., et al., 'Caffeine: Does It Affect Your Bladder?' *British Journal of Urology* 1990; 66: 613–14
2. Gordon D., et al., 'Double-Blind, Placebo-Controlled Study of Magnesium Hydroxide for Treatment of Sensory Urgency and Detrusor Instability: Preliminary Results', *British Journal of Obstetrics and Gynaecology* 1998; 105: 667–9

Urinary Tract Infection

1. Edward B., et al., 'Cranberry Concentrate: UTI Prophylaxis', *The Journal of Family Practice* 1997; 45(2): 167–8
2. Raz R., et al., 'A Controlled Trial of Intravaginal Estriol in Postmenopausal Women With Recurrent Urinary Tract Infections', *The New England Journal of Medicine* 1993; 329: 753–6

Bibliography

Atkins, Robert C., *Dr Atkins' New Diet Revolution*, Evans 1992/1999

Barnes MD, Broda, and Galton, Lawrence, *Hypothyroidism: The Unsuspected Illness*, Harper and Row 1976

Batmanghelidj, Dr F., *Your Body's Many Cries for Water*, Tagman Press 2000

Braly MD, James, *Dr Braly's Food Allergy and Nutrition Revolution*, Keats Publishing, 1992

Brand-Miller, Jennie and Wolever, Thomas, *The Glucose Revolution: the Authoritative Guide to the Glycemic Index*, Marlowe & Company, NY, USA 1999

Briffa, Dr John, *BodyWise: 10 Steps to Permanent Weight Loss and Well-being*, Cico Books 2000

Brostoff, Dr Jonathan, and Gamlin, Linda, *The Complete Guide to Food Allergy and Intolerance*, Bloomsbury 1989/1992

Cleghorn, Patricia, *The Secrets of Self-Esteem*, Element 1996

Day, Laura, *Practical Intuition*, Vermillion 1996

DesMaisons PhD., Kathleen, *Potatoes Not Prozac*, Simon & Schuster 1998

Gottschall, Elaine, *Breaking the Vicious Cycle*, Kirkton Press, Ontario, Canada 1996

Holden, Richard, *Happiness Now!*, Hodder & Stoughton 1998

Jacobs, Jill, *Candida Albicans – a user's guide to treatment and recovery*, Optima 1990/1994

Jefferies, Dr McK, *Safe Uses of Cortisol Acetate*, Charles C. Thomas Ltd, Springfield, Illinois 1996

Kavounas, Alice, *Water: Pure Therapy*, Kyle Cathie 2000

Krystal, Phyllis, *Cutting the Ties that Bind*, Weiser 1993

Langer MD, Stephen E., and Scheer, James F., *Solved: The Riddle of the Illness*, Keats Publishing 1984/1995

Leader, Geoffrey, Leader, Lucille, Rossi, Aroldo et al., *Parkinson's Disease – the Way Forward. An integrated approach including drugs, surgery, nutrition, bowel and muscle function, self-esteem, sexuality, stress control and carers*, Denor Press 2001

Marsden, Kathryn, *The Food Combining Diet*, Thorsons 1993

McWhirter, Jane, *The Practical Guide to Candida*, All Hallows House Foundation 1995

Murray, Michael, *Encyclopedia of Nutritional Supplements*, Prima 1996

Ornish, Dean, *Love and Survival*, HarperCollins 1997

Rama, Swami, Ballentine, Rudolph, and Hymes, Alan, *The Science of Breath*, Himalayan Institute Press 2000

Renshaw, Ben, *Together but Something Missing*, Vermillion 2001

Sears PhD., Barry, with Bill Lawren, *The Zone*, Reagan Books 1995

Shapiro, Debbie, *Your Body Speaks Your Mind*, Piatkus 1996

Weller, Stella, *The Breath Book*, Thorsons 1999

Useful Information

Supplement Suppliers

VitaTech
Lakeside
180 Lifford Lane
Kings Norton
Birmingham B32 2HR
Tel: 0121 433 8729

Suppliers of supplements of the
VitaTech range (including
Hepranol, Thyranol, Glucoguard,
Adrenol, Acidol and pepsin,
Enzyme Forte, Replant,
Acidophilus Forte, Permaguard,
Yeast Guard and Canditrol) by
mail order.

Cedar Health/Padma UK
Pepper Rd
Hazelgrove
Stockport SK7 5BW
Tel: 0161 483 4662

Nutri-Chem Pharmacies
Ottawa
Canada
Tel: 001 613 820 4200

Pharma Nord UK Ltd
Telford Court
Morpeth
Northumberland NE61 2DB
Tel: 0800 591 756

Rio Trading Company
2 Centenary Estate
Hughes Rd
Brighton
East Sussex BN2 4AW

Specialist Services

Allergycare Ltd
1 Church Square
Taunton
Somerset TA1 1SA
Tel: 01823 325022

Providers of allergy related products
including specialist foods.
Allergycare also has a countrywide
food sensitivity testing service
(electro-dermal testing) available
through health food stores. Contact
Allergycare for more details.

BioLab
9 Weymouth Street
London W1N 3FF
Tel: 020 7636 5959

Specialist laboratory providing a
range of tests including the gut
fermentation test and a test for
stomach acidity. Tests need to be
accessed via a practitioner. Contact
BioLab for details.

York Nutritional Laboratory
Murton Way
Osbalwick
York YO19 5US
Tel: 0800 0746184

Providers of IgG blood testing for
food sensitivity.

Department of Microbiology
Chapel Allerton Hospital
Chapeltown Road
Leeds LS7 4SA
Tel: 0113 292 4657

Specialist parasite testing laboratory.

Practitioner Bodies

General Council and Register of
   Naturopaths
Goswell House
2 Goswell Road
Street
Somerset BA16 0JG

Provides a list of registered
naturopathic practitioners.

The British Society for Allergy,
Environmental and Nutritional
Medicine
PO Box 28
Totton
Southampton SO40 2ZA

Holds a list of naturally orientated
medical practitioners.

Society for the Promotion of
Nutritional Therapy
PO Box 47
Heathfield
East Sussex TN21 8ZX

Holds a list of non-medically
qualified nutritionists.

Verity
52–54 Featherstone St
London EC1Y 8RT

Dr John Briffa can be contacted at:
Woolaston House
25 Southwood Lane
Highgate
London N6 5ED

For more information about all
aspects of health and to email
Dr Briffa visit his website at:
www.drbriffa.com

Index

Figures in italics refer to captions; those in bold refer to the A-Z of health issues.

diet
  anti-candida 58–62
  elimination 38–42
  fasting 29
  liver-supporting 26–7, 67
  stabilizing blood sugar levels 82–3,
    99
  Stone Age 42
digestion 21, 32–4, *33*, 44–8, 52, 68,
  69, 156
dihydroepiandrosterone (DHEA) 87,
  93, 97, 100
diverticular disease **228**
dong quai 258
doubt 151–2
Down's Syndrome **228–9**
dry eyes (Sicca syndrome) 12, **229**
duodenal ulcer 49
dysmenorrhoea *see* painful periods

ear infections 34, 35, 66, **230**
echinacea 214, 222, 286
  angustifolia 222
  purpurea 222
eczema 34, 36, 44, 51, **230–31**
eggs 39, 40, 42, 47, 59, 61, 62, 68, 78,
  82, 85, 99
elderberries, black (*Sambucus nigra* L.)
  222
emotions 155, 156, 162, 164, 166, 167,
  170, 178
emphysema 1, 7, **231**
endometriosis **231–2**
energy levels 60, 66, 67, 69, 72, 80,
  85, 86, 88, 98, 100, 103, 113,
  139
Enzyme Forte 49–50, 51
enzymes 11, 13, 31, 32, 33, 45, 46,
  49–50, 51, 68, 83
epilepsy **232**
evening primrose oil 231, 275
excitement 148–53
exercise xi, 28, 90, 99, 115–32
expiration 3
eyes, dry (Sicca syndrome) **229**

fainting 97, 98, 99
fast foods 26
fasting 29
fat, body 71–2
fatigue 12, 22, 23, 24, 27, 34, 41, 50,
  51, 52, 68, 70, 81, 84, 88, 90, 96,
  98, 99, 101, 103, 139, 140, 156,
  233
  mental 54, 102–3
fats 26, 31, 33, 49
fatty acids 33
fatty foods 67
fear 178–80, 183
feng shui 169
feverfew (*Tanacetum parthenium*) 259
fibre 28
fibrocytic breast disease **234**
fibromyalgia **234–5**
fish 29, 33, 39, 42, 47, 51, 59, 62, 68,
  77, 78, 82, 83, 85, 99
flatulence 53
flavourings 26
fluid retention 34, 35, 50–51, 72, 102
fluoride 16, 17, 18, 22
folic acid 44
food cravings 35, 39, 51, 52, 54, 60–61,
  64, 66–9, 71, 73, 79, 84, 85, 86
food sensitivity 140
  see also under detoxification
forgiveness 158, 159–61, 164
free radicals 31
fruit 26, 28, 29, 42, 47, 60, 61, 67, 69,
  77, 80, 82, 85, 99
  dried 47, 58, 60
fruit juices 15, 58, 69
fulfilment 154, 155, 161, 190
fungal infections **235**
future, projecting into 152–3

gallbladder 25, 33, 44
gallstones 25, **235–6**
garlic 65, 246
gas exchange 2, 3, 4
gastritis 49
Gilbert's disease **236**